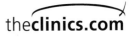

CLINICS IN OCCUPATIONAL AND ENVIRONMENTAL MEDICINE

Low Back Pain

GUEST EDITOR
Gerard A. Malanga, MD

Volume 5 • Number 3

SAUNDERS

An Imprint of Elsevier, Inc.
PHILADELPHIA   LONDON   TORONTO   MONTREAL   SYDNEY   TOKYO

W.B. SAUNDERS COMPANY
A Division of Elsevier Inc.

Elsevier Inc., 1600 John F. Kennedy Blvd., Suite 1800, Philadelphia, PA 19103-2899

http://www.occmed.theclinics.com

CLINICS IN OCCUPATIONAL AND	Volume 5, Number 3
ENVIRONMENTAL MEDICINE	ISSN 1526-0046
Editor: Catherine Bewick	ISBN 1-4160-3932-5

Clinics in Occupational and Environmental Medicine (ISSN 1526-0046) is published quarterly in February, May, August, and November by Elsevier Inc., 360 Park Avenue South, New York, NY, 10010. Business and editorial offices: 1600 John F. Kennedy Blvd., Suite 1800, Philadelphia, PA 19103-2899. Customer Service Office: 6277 Sea Harbor Drive, Orlando, FL 32887-4800. Subscription prices are $120.00 per year for US individuals, $166.00 per year for US institutions, $60.00 per year for US students and residents, $135.00 per year for Canadian individuals, $204.00 per year for Canadian institutions, $155.00 per year for international individuals, $204.00 per year for international institutions and $78.00 per year for Canadian and foreign students/residents. Foreign air speed delivery is included in all *Clinics* subscription prices. All prices are subject to change without notice. **Customer Service: 1-800-654-2452 (US). From outside of the US, call 1-407-345-4000. E-mail: hhspcs@wbsaunders.com. POSTMASTER:** Send address changes to *Clinics in Occupational and Environmental Medicine*, Elsevier Periodicals Customer Service, 6277 Sea Harbor Drive, Orlando, FL 32887-4800.

Clinics in Occupational and Environmental Medicine is indexed in *Index Medicus*

Printed in the United States of America.

GUEST EDITOR

GERARD A. MALANGA, MD, Director, Pain Management, Overlook Hospital, Summit, New Jersey; Director, Sports Medicine, Mountainside Hospital, Montclair, New Jersey; Associate Professor, Department of Physical Medicine and Rehabilitation, UMDNJ—New Jersey Medical School, Newark, New Jersey

CONTRIBUTORS

MICHAEL Y. CHANG, DO, University Rehabilitation Associates, Newark, New Jersey

STEPHEN J. COHEN, MD, University of Medicine and Dentistry of New Jersey, Newark, New Jersey

ROBIN L. DENNIS, MD, Physiatrist, Spine Center, Resurgens Orthopaedics, Atlanta, Georgia

SHEILA A. DUGAN, MD, Assistant Professor, Rush Medical College, Chicago, Illinois

FRANK J.E. FALCO, MD, Medical Director, Mid Atlantic Spine and Pain Specialists, P.A., Newark, Delaware; Clinical Assistant Professor and Director, Pain Medicine Fellowship, Physical Medicine and Rehabilitation Department, Temple University Medical School, Philadelphia, Pennsylvania

LEE IRWIN, MD, Pain Medicine Fellow, Mid Atlantic Spine and Pain Specialists, P.A., Newark, Delaware

KIM JANECK, PT, The Center for Physical Therapy and Sports Rehabilitation, Atlantic Health, Morristown, New Jersey

BRYAN D. KAPLANSKY, MD, Summit Spine and Sports Medicine P.C., Fort Wayne, Indiana

RICHARD T. KATZ, MD, Professor of Clinical Neurology (Physical Medicine and Rehabilitation), Washington University School of Medicine, St. Louis, Missouri

JOSHUA LEVY, DO, University Rehabilitation Associates, Newark, New Jersey

GERARD A. MALANGA, MD, Director, Pain Management, Overlook Hospital, Summit, New Jersey; Director, Sports Medicine, Mountainside Hospital, Montclair, New Jersey; Associate Professor, Department of Physical Medicine and Rehabilitation, UMDNJ-New Jersey Medical School, Newark, New Jersey

GREGORY J. MULFORD, MD, Atlantic Health, Morristown, New Jersey

SCOTT F. NADLER, DO, University Rehabilitation Associates, Newark, New Jersey

MARK V. REECER, MD, Fort Wayne Physical Medicine, Fort Wayne, Indiana

MITCHELL F. REITER, MD, Assistant Professor of Orthopaedic Surgery, UMDNJ—New Jersey Medical School, Newark, New Jersey

BARBARA REUVEN, PT, The Center for Physical Therapy and Sports Rehabilitation, Atlantic Health, Morristown, New Jersey

CHRISTOPHER T. ROMANO, MS, PT, The Kessler Institute for Rehabilitation, West Orange, New Jersey

RANDOLPH B. RUSSO, MD, Orthopaedic Associates of Grand Rapids, PC; Clinical Assistant Professor, Department of Physical Medicine and Rehabilitation, Michigan State University, Grand Rapids, Michigan

RANDY A. SHELERUD, MD, Assistant Professor, Spine Center, Department of Physical Medicine and Rehabilitation, Mayo Clinic, Rochester, Minnesota

TODD P. STITIK, MD, University Rehabilitation Associates, Newark, New Jersey

MICHAEL VIVES, MD, Associate Professor of Orthopaedic Surgery, UMDNJ—New Jersey Medical School, Newark, New Jersey

FRANK Y. WEI, MD, Southdale Office Center, Edina, Minnesota

JIE ZHU, MD, Pain Medicine Fellow, Mid Atlantic Spine and Pain Specialists, P.A., Newark, Delaware

CONTENTS

Preface   xi
Gerard A. Malanga

Epidemiology of Occupational Low Back Pain   501
Randy A. Shelerud

> There have been significant advances in our understanding of oc-
> cupational low back pain over the last decade largely because of
> a noteworthy improvement in the number and quality of prospec-
> tive trials. More recent work confirms that genetic factors may
> drive a large portion of the risk factors. The importance of physical
> fitness and spine support muscle fitness is believed to protect
> against future occurrences. Psychosocial factors can play a role in
> increasing the risk of future low back pain and acute pain becom-
> ing chronic. Some of the psychological influence may be through
> a muscular pain component. It is arguable that an emphasis should
> be placed on resources, education, and support to allow workers to
> be productive whether suffering from back pain or not.

Prevention Strategies for Occupational Low Back Pain   529
Bryan D. Kaplansky, Frank Y. Wei, and Mark V. Reecer

> The authors investigate the effects of worker education and train-
> ing, exercise, and ergonomics on the incidence of low back pain
> in occupational settings. Prevention strategies that involve risk fac-
> tor modification, worker selection, and lumbar orthotics also are
> examined.

Occupational Low Back Pain   545
Todd P. Stitik, Michael Y. Chang, Joshua Levy, and
Scott F. Nadler

> Low back injury is one of the most common conditions in the
> workplace. The causes are multifactorial and must be sought during
> the physician's examination. Failure to perform a comprehensive

history and physical examination ultimately can lead to treatment failure and injury recurrence. A comprehensive history and physical may help clinicians to differentiate organic and nonorganic causes of low back pain. Different diagnoses need specific rather than generalized treatment programs. Teaching clinicians the nuances of the history and physical examination in a setting with an injured worker is the goal of this article.

Diagnosis of Low Back Pain: Role of Imaging Studies 571
Randolph B. Russo

Approximately 70% of North Americans experience low back pain during their lifetime, with most of them demonstrating improvement within 2 to 4 weeks. The use of early radiographic evaluation is often unnecessary for uncomplicated acute low back injuries. Select patient populations have been identified for early evaluation. If the following red flags are associated with the pain, spinal imaging is indicated: possible fracture, neoplasm, infection, and cauda equina syndrome. High suspicion for the presence of one of these entities should prompt more formal evaluation of the spine. This article provides an overview of the commonly used diagnostic procedures in the evaluation of lumbar spine disorders.

The Role of Electrodiagnosis in the Evaluation of Low Back Pain 591
Gregory J. Mulford and Stephen J. Cohen

Establishing a specific diagnosis is important in the effective management of individuals who present with a complaint of low back pain. Electrodiagnostic studies are an integral part of the diagnostic evaluation when the history or physical examination suggests that neural structures may contribute as symptom generators. Lumbosacral radiculopathies, plexopathies, and peripheral nerve injuries are of primary concern when evaluating individuals with low back pain, and electrodiagnostic studies assist in identifying and quantifying neurophysiologic injuries and abnormalities using techniques. A thorough, thoughtful, and individualized electrodiagnostic study performed by qualified physicians as an extension of a detailed history and physical examination can be an important and useful component in the proper evaluation of individuals with low back pain.

The Role of Exercise in the Prevention and Management of Acute Low Back Pain 615
Sheila A. Dugan

The transition from acute pain to chronic pain and onward to disability is burdensome emotionally and financially to individual sufferers, loved ones, employers, and the health care system. Up to 40% of acute low back pain cases can become chronic and lead to disability in some cases. Treatments that reduce the risk of chronic pain by successful management of acute low back pain are highly desirable. Prevention of acute low back pain is even more desirable. Exercise has been part of the armamentarium of treating and preventing acute low back pain, especially as a means of avoiding disability. This article critically reviews studies of the role of exercise in the management and prevention of low back pain.

Spinal Stabilization Exercises for the Injured Worker   633
Kim Janeck, Barbara Reuven, and Christopher T. Romano

Returning the injured worker to his previous occupation can be a difficult and complex rehabilitation process. The goal of standard stabilization exercises (SSE) is to facilitate the active system for improved dynamic spinal stability. Improving dynamic spinal stability can decrease the forces placed on the intervertebral joints, which minimizes the chance of reinjury. When used in conjunction with industrial rehabilitation, SSEs offer the optimal environment for an injured worker to practice his occupational demands while using appropriate spinal stabilization.

Use of Medications in the Treatment of Acute Low Back Pain   643
Gerard A. Malanga and Robin L. Dennis

The prescription of medications continues to be one of the mainstays of treatment for acute low back pain episodes. The goals of pharmacologic treatment for acute low back are reduction of pain and return of normal function. Often, nociception is a result of secondary inflammation and muscle spasm after the acute injury of a structure of the spine, which may include muscle, tendon, ligament, disc, or bone. An understanding of the appropriate use of medications to address the underlying pain generator and the current evidence for using these medications is essential for any physician who sees and treats patients with acute low back pain.

Lumbar Spine Injection and Interventional Procedures in the Management of Low Back Pain   655
Frank J.E. Falco, Lee Irwin, and Jie Zhu

Lumbar spine injections play a role in the evaluation and treatment of low back pain and lumbar radiculopathy. These injection procedures have been demonstrated to be effective in determining the pain generator for low back pain. There is still debate as to the long-term pain relief from epidural and intra-articular facet joint injections, and no controlled studies have examined the long-term effects of SI joint injections. Additional investigation is certainly warranted to evaluate further the long-term benefits and determine which patients would benefit the most from these injections. Current evidence validates that these injections provide temporary relief of low back and radicular leg pain up to several months, if not longer. This duration of pain relief creates an opportunity to maximize rehabilitation efforts while symptoms are minimal.

Surgical Issues in the Injured Worker with Lower Back Pain
Mitchell F. Reiter and Michael Vives

703

Although most workers who sustain lower back injuries can be managed without surgery, a carefully selected subset of patients benefit from operative intervention. When evaluating these patients, care must be taken to identify surgical emergencies, including patients with cauda equina syndrome and progressive neurologic deficits and patients with certain historical red flags that should prompt further evaluation. Conditions that may benefit from surgery include lumbar disc herniations, discogenic back pain, spinal stenosis, and spondylolisthesis. This article reviews the indications for surgery in injured workers and expected postoperative outcomes.

Impairment and Disability Rating in Low Back Pain
Richard T. Katz

719

Many publications emphasize the theoretical relationship between impairment, disability, and the workplace. This article is intended to provide the reader with some framework in this regard, but its main intent is to create a practical how-to guide in the evaluation of impairment and disability that result from low back pain.

Index

741

FORTHCOMING ISSUES

Volume 5:4

Exposure to Airbone Particles
Mark W. Frampton, MD, and
Mark J. Utell, MD, *Guest Editors*

RECENT ISSUES

Volume 5:2 (published May 2006)

**Occupational Injuries and Disorders
of the Upper Extremity**
Jane Derebery, MD, Morton Kasdan, MD,
and Roberto Gonzalez, MD, *Guest Editors*

Volume 5:1 (published February 2006)

Tobacco's Impact on Industry
Virginia Cullen Reichert, NP,
Arunabh Talwar, MD, and
Alan M. Fein, MD, *Guest Editors*

Volume 4:4

Industrial Solvents and Human Health, Part II
Scott D. Phillips, MD, and
Gary R. Krieger, MD, MPH, *Guest Editors*

Volume 4:3

Industrial Solvents and Human Health, Part I
Scott D. Phillips, MD, and
Gary R. Krieger, MD, MPH, *Guest Editors*

ELSEVIER
SAUNDERS

Clin Occup Environ Med
5 (3) xi–xii

CLINICS IN
OCCUPATIONAL AND
ENVIRONMENTAL
MEDICINE

Preface

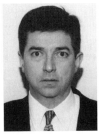

Gerard A. Malanga, MD
Guest Editor

I am pleased to serve as Editor to another issue devoted to low back pain. Since the time of the previous issue, which published in *Occupational Medicine: State of the Art Reviews* in 1998, there have been advances in the treatment of acute low back pain, particularly in the areas interventional and surgical procedures for low back pain. Unfortunately, the outcomes from these seemingly curative procedures have, over time, failed to produce long-term outcomes that were initially promised. Procedures such as intradiscal electrothermoplasty initially reported incredible outcomes only to have randomized controlled studies demonstrate no significant benefit. Surgically, disc arthroplasty has generated great excitement; however, short- and long-term outcomes are yet to be truly tested in the injured worker environment. Despite prior and more recent "advances," lost time from work and disability from low back pain continues to increase. It seems that addressing solely the structural component of low back pain is missing a large, more important aspect of this problem. In this issue, simple measures are reviewed that can facilitate reactivation and return to work of injured workers after a low back pain episode.

Disability from low back pain is in many cases iatrogenic. The path toward disabling patients begins with the fact that many primary care and spine physicians believe that low back pain can (and often will) result in a disabling condition. This belief system is transferred to patients by the recommendations often given to patients, such as resting, staying out of work, or restricting lifting and exercise. The language used when we speak to our patients and how diagnoses are presented to patients plant the seed for acute

1526-0046/06/$ - see front matter © 2006 Elsevier Inc. All rights reserved.
doi:10.1016/j.coem.2006.05.006   *occmed.theclinics.com*

low back pain to develop into disabling pain. This includes statements such as "you have a degenerative spine" or "I see a huge disc on your MRI."

Pain itself can be addressed in various ways, such as appropriate medications, judicious use of injections, and active physical therapy techniques. Pain, in and of itself, does not cause long-term disability from low back pain; rather it is pain from superimposed psychological influences, such as fear, anxiety, anger, or dissatisfaction with life or work, that ultimately evolves into the chronic low back pain state. Clearly, treating these issues in a mechanical fashion with a procedure does not (and historically has not) result in a successful outcome (ie, return to work). A cognitive behavioral approach that fully addresses these psychosocial issues has been validated in providing the best approach to this problem.

Ultimately, disability from low back pain returns back to the treating physician. Education of healthcare providers who have first contact with patients with acute low back pain is paramount. A clear understanding of the best ways to enhance the best outcome in our patients hopefully will lead to a reversal of the trend of increasing disability from this relatively benign condition. Understanding that low back pain is a condition that requires reactivation as soon as possible, that findings on imaging studies should not be overemphasized, or that nearly all episodes of pain can be treated successfully should guide the daily clinical practice of primary care physicians. Hopefully this issue of *Clinics in Occupational and Environmental Medicine* will provide material that is beneficial to occupational medicine physicians and primary care physicians in general.

I would like to thank all the contributors of this issue for their diligent work and thoughtful approach to their articles. I would like to thank Catherine Bewick for her assistance in putting this issue together. As always, I would like to thank my wife, Carrie, and our family for their love and support in this and all of my projects.

Gerard A. Malanga, MD
Department of Pain Management
Overlook Hospital
99 Beauvoir Avenue
Summit, NJ 07902, USA

Department of Physical Medicine and Rehabilitation
UMDNJ—New Jersey Medical School
30 Bergen Street
Newark, NJ 07101, USA

E-mail address: gmalanga@pol.net

ELSEVIER
SAUNDERS

Clin Occup Environ Med
5 (3) 501–528

CLINICS IN
OCCUPATIONAL AND
ENVIRONMENTAL
MEDICINE

Epidemiology of Occupational Low Back Pain

Randy A. Shelerud, MD

*Spine Center, Department of Physical Medicine and Rehabilitation, Mayo Clinic,
200 First Street, SW, Rochester, MN 55905, USA*

Back problems are the single most expensive of all musculoskeletal problems in industrial countries. In fact, the direct cost of occupational low back pain (LBP) may threaten to exhaust resources that provide workers' compensation benefits in some of these countries. Our understanding of the various aspects of this costly and disabling problem has come as a result of extensive study in the epidemiology of LPB. Any discussion concerning occupational LBP must use epidemiologic methods to discuss the extent of the impact of LBP on industry, discuss the etiology and natural history of the disease, and explore possible associations between personal and work-related factors and the presence or absence of LBP. Within this framework, this article focuses on the most recent and pertinent literature while acknowledging the wealth of past writings.

Since the last writing of this article, significant advances in the understanding of occupational LBP have continued to evolve [1]. The natural history of acute LBP is better understood as a symptom with often incomplete recovery and predictable recurrence. Prospective studies looking at psychosocial factors have clarified the risk of future LBP and chronicity of symptoms in the setting of certain psychological factors. There is also a much better understanding of the true prevalence of LBP thanks to work by Leboeuf-Yde and Kyvik, showing that LBP is an issue in adolescents and approaches adult prevalence rates by age 18 to 20.

The understanding of work-specific risk factors for LBP also have improved, calling into question some of the long agreed upon philosophies, such as lifting with the legs compared with back lifting. Also in question is the apparent "myth" of the risk of static sitting at work and its risk for future LBP. Worker fitness continues to be an important tool toward minimizing disability, particularly of spine support muscles, in which

E-mail address: shelerud.randy@mayo.edu

minimizing anterior shear, segmental buckling, and minimizing fatigue are better understood as important goals of fitness.

Probably the most notable and exciting research in the area of LBP has been the study of the role of genetic factors. Several studies of twins suggest that genetic and early life shared environmental factors may account for the lion's share of the risk of developing spinal degenerative changes and LBP in otherwise young, healthy workers. This work also suggests that most other traditionally agreed upon risk factors for LBP, such as obesity, smoking, and whole-body vibration, only play a minor role. Finally, a significant portion of the variance in risk may still be from unknown factors.

Back pain in the workplace: the extent of the problem

The US Bureau of Labor Statistics estimates that more than 6.7 million work-related illnesses and injuries occurred in the United States in 1990 and account for a sizable amount of morbidity and disability [2]. LBP traditionally has been among the most common of these work-related problems. In Rowe's investigation that followed plant workers for a decade, LBP ranked second only to upper respiratory tract infections in the amount of secondary absenteeism [3]. True prevalence rates are difficult to assess, however. Occupational LBP statistics must be distinguished from LBP statistics in general. The lifetime prevalence drops further to 13.8% if people are asked about LBP lasting at least 2 weeks versus at any time [4]. Based on this study and others, Frymoyer [5] concludes that the manner in which the question is asked and what populations are questioned markedly influence the assessment of the magnitude of the problem. Nevertheless, 85% of older adults report having back problems that interfere with work and recreational activity [6–8]. In fact, a year without an episode of backache is thought to be abnormal [9]. Making sense of an enormous amount of prevalence data is further confounded by variations in definitions of back pain, the nongeneralizability of individual industry studies, and underreporting of injury. Biering-Sorensen [10] noted that 23% of workers had LBP resulting in absenteeism but that 70% of workers had LBP at some time during the study. Others agree that not all workers with LBP file workers' compensation claims, and if they do file, not all miss work [11,12].

Back problems are an enormous expense in industrialized countries. Nachemson [13] reported that in Sweden, permanent disability caused by LBP has increased 6000% from 1952 to 1987. Most of this rise occurred in the 1980s and is thought to be related to newer workers' compensation laws. The resource drain that results could threaten Sweden's social welfare system. Similar trends have been noted by Fordyce [14] in the United States, where filed workers' compensation claims increased 2700% from 1956 to 1976. It comes as no surprise that back problems have become the most common cause of disability in persons younger than age 45 [15,16]. Approximately 10% of workers with chronic LBP consume 75% to 79% of medical costs and compensation payments [11,17]. Abenhaim and Suissa [17] estimated compensation costs at $45,000 per case per worker or a yearly cost for occupational LBP in Quebec of more than $125 million.

Vitally important to the occupational medicine physician are data concerning LBP prevalence measured by a common tool in various industries. Behrens and colleagues [18] studied data from interviews with 30,074 adults who had worked any time during the previous 12 months. Prevalence data were gathered for back pain caused by an injury and for back pain caused by repeated activities. The overall 12-month prevalence rate was 2.5% for work-related back injury and 4.5% for work-related back pain from repeated activities. The breakdown by occupation is shown in Table 1, with each occupation reflecting 1.1 to 11 million people. Truck drivers had the highest prevalence of back pain (6.7%), whereas mechanics had the highest prevalence of repetitive activity–related pain (10.5%). The scope of LBP in the workforce was further broadened by Klein and colleagues [19], who analyzed workers' compensation claims from 26 states for 1979 (Table 2).

Table 1
12 month prevalence of back pain in selected US, working populations

Occupation	Back pain from injury at work % (Standard Error)	Back pain from repeated activities at work % (Standard Error)	Occupation
Truck drivers	6.7 (1.1)	10.5 (1.3)	Mechanics, heavy machine repair
Operators of extractive, mining, material moving equipment	5.6 (1.4)	10.4 (2.1)	Operators of extractive, mining, material moving equipment
Construction trades	5.3 (0.8)	10.1 (1.0)	Construction trades
Cleaning and building service	4.9 (0.8)	9.2 (1.9)	Operators of machines processing stone, glass, metal, plastic
Firefighters, police	4.8 (1.1)	9.0 (2.8)	Mechanics, electrical equipment
Mechanics, heavy machine repair	4.6 (0.9)	8.3 (1.9)	Personal service occupations
Mechanics, electrical equipment	4.4 (1.4)	7.5 (1.3)	Truck drivers
Healthcare therapists, technicians	4.4 (0.9)	7.5 (1.2)	Agriculture, forestry, fishing
Physicians, dentists, nurses, and related	4.2 (1.1)	7.3 (1.0)	Health care therapists, technicians
Agriculture, forestry, fishing	4.1 (0.8)	7.0 (1.1)	Production laborers, handlers, cleaners

Adapted from Behrens V, Seligman P, Cameron L, et al. The prevalence of back pain, hand discomfort, and dermatitis in the United States working population. Am J Public Health 1994; 84:1780–1785.

Table 2
Ratios of compensation claims in 26 states because of back strains/sprains by occupation

Occupation	Claims per 100 workers
Miscellaneous laborers	12.3
Garbage collectors	11.1
Warehouse workers	9.3
Miscellaneous mechanics	5.6
Nursing aides	3.6
Nonspecific laborers	3.4
Material handlers	3.4
Lumber workers	3.3
Practical nurses	3.3
Construction laborers	2.8

Adapted from Klein BP, Jenson RC, Sandstrom LM. Assessment of workers' compensation claims for back strains/sprains. J Occup Med 1984;26:443–8.

Compensation claims peaked in the 20- to 24-year-old age group for men and the 30- to 34-year-old age group for women (Fig. 1). Incidence ratios were calculated (claims per 100 workers) by occupation (Table 3). Laborers and garbage collectors had the highest compensation ratios (12.3 and 11.1 claims per 100 workers, respectively). Their results also were in agreement with earlier studies on several points, including the fact that most claims

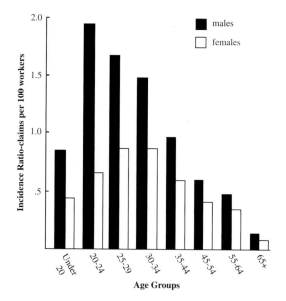

Fig. 1. Incidence ratio (claims per 100 workers) of compensation claims in 26 US states caused by strains/sprains of the back. (*Adapted from* Klein BP, Jenson RC, Sandstrom LM. Assessment of workers' compensation claims for back strains/sprains. J Occup Med 1984;26:443–8; with permission.)

Table 3
Prevalence and lifetime incidence of low back pain as determined by several studies

Study	Lifetime incidence (%)	Prevalence (%) Point	Period	N	Age (y)	Sex
Biering-Sorensen (1982)	62.6	12.0	—	449	30–60	M
	61.4	15.2	—	479	30–60	F
Hirsch et al (1969)	48.8	—	—	692	15–72	F
Hult (1954)	60.0	—	—	1193	25–59	M
Frymoyer et al (1983)	69.9	—	—	1221	28–55	M
Magora & Taustein (1969)	—	12.9	—	3316		MF
Nagi et al (1973)	—	18.0	—	1135	18–64	MF
Svensson & Andersson (1983)	61	—	31	716	40–47	M
(1988)	67	—	35	1640	38–64	F
Valkenburg & Haanen (1982)	51.4	22.2	—	3091	20+	M
	57.8	30.2	—	3493	20+	F

Adapted from Andersson GBJ. Epidemiology of spinal disorders. In: Frymoyer JW, editor. The adult spine: principles and practice. 3rd edition. Philadelphia: Lippincott-Raven; 1997.

are submitted by men, back injury claims make up approximately 20% to 25% of all claims and represent the single largest category of claims, and lifting objects is the most frequently cited form of overexertion [20–23]. These findings are similar to later work by Spitzer and colleagues [24], who studied Canadian data as part of the Quebec Task Force on Spinal Disorders. Klein pointed out that the data from this extensive study should not become synonymous with true incidence data, because many workers did not have access to or qualify for workers' compensation (most notably, railroad workers, federal employees, farmers, and harbor workers). Many workers also were reassigned to different duties within the same company while recuperating from their injuries, which skewed the data further.

The epidemiology of herniated lumbar intervertebral disc has been clarified in a prospective study by Heliövaara and colleagues [25] that involved 57,000 adults. During 11 years of study, the incidence data were collected only on patients who were admitted to the hospital. Approximately 30% of admissions for back disease were diagnosed as herniated lumbar intervertebral disc and 24% were diagnosed as sciatica (1537 patients). Men had a 1.6-fold risk of herniated nucleus pulposus (HNP) and a 1.3-fold risk of sciatica compared with women. Sciatica prevalence was 5.3% for men and 3.7% for women. Prevalences for true herniated disc were 1.9% for men and 1.3% for women. Risk factors for HNP or sciatica were sex, occupation, workload, and body height. In a related study, Heliövaara [26] compared relative risk of HNP or sciatica in different occupations. The results reflect the highest risk of HNP in occupations that involve motor vehicle driving and metal or machine work compared with white-collar work (Fig. 2). The next highest risk occupations included construction, forestry, and service work. In contrast, Kelsey found that sedentary jobs, chronic cough, and lack of physical exercise increased the risk of HNP [27–30]. Later

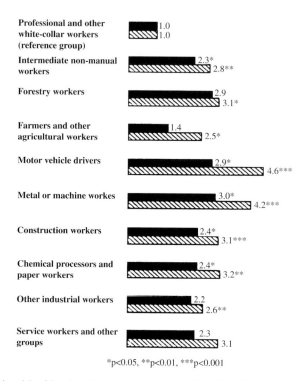

Professional and other
white-collar workers
(reference group)   1.0 / 1.0

Intermediate non-manual
workers   2.3* / 2.8**

Forestry workers   2.9 / 3.1*

Farmers and other
agricultural workers   1.4 / 2.5*

Motor vehicle drivers   2.9* / 4.6***

Metal or machine workes   3.0* / 4.2***

Construction workers   2.4* / 3.1***

Chemical processors and
paper workers   2.4* / 3.2**

Other industrial workers   2.2 / 2.6**

Service workers and other
groups   2.3 / 3.1

*p<0.05, **p<0.01, ***p<0.001

Fig. 2. Relative risk of herniated lumbar intervertebral disc (*black bars*) and herniated disc or sciatica combined (*lined bars*) in men. (*Adapted from* Heliovaara M. Occupation and risk of herniated lumbar intervertebral disk or sciatica leading to hospitalization. J Chronic Dis 1987;40: 259–64; with permission.)

work also showed a correlation with lifting and twisting work activities [31,32]. Disability because of back illness in Heliövaara's study was approximated at 3.5% for men and 4.5% for women [26].

Causative aspects of back pain

Patients with what is considered idiopathic LBP represent the vast majority of all back-related disorders in workers [24,33]. This LBP is clearly described as being aggravated by mechanical factors such as activity; it worsens over the day and is relieved by rest. A thorough history and physical examination only define pathogenesis in 20% of cases, however [34]. Traditionally, degenerative disc disease is believed to be the cause of nonspecific LBP [8,33,35]. Kuslich and colleagues [36] directly stimulated spinal elements during lumbar surgery and found that the most pain was produced when the anulus fibrosus was stimulated (with the exception of compressed nerve roots). These findings support a discogenic cause of LBP. Some researchers have pointed toward muscular sprains and strains as being the predominant cause of back pain [37,38], whereas more recent opinions propose that chronic LBP can be related to other structures in the spine, such as ligaments, fascia, zygapophyseal joints, and sacroiliac joints [39].

Postmortem work by Vernon-Roberts and Pirie [40] concluded that degenerative disc disease preceded facet degenerative joint disease. They found that degenerative disc disease always was accompanied by osteoarthritis in the associated facet joints, but osteoarthritis in facet joints was minimal to absent when the corresponding disc was well preserved. This finding has led some investigators to look beyond the concept of chronic LBP as being caused by a single factor or structure. Kirkaldy-Willis and colleagues [41] championed the concept of a three-joint complex to account for a multifactorial source of back pain. They described how, in any combination, the disc and the two corresponding zygapophyseal joints can contribute to pain. Kirkaldy-Willis [42] further theorized a "myofascial cycle" that took into account emotional factors, changes in muscles, and secondary changes in the three-joint complex over time. As a result, a degenerative cascade of changes develops in the spine and progresses through three phases. An initial phase of dysfunction is followed by a second unstable phase and then finally progresses to a third phase of stabilization [43]. These concepts still await clinical validation.

More recent studies to determine the cause of chronic LBP have centered around injection procedures. Studies using discography, zygapophyseal (facet) joint injections, and sacroiliac joint injections suggest that as much as 85% of chronic LBP may be related to the discs, facet, or sacroiliac joints [44–47]. It is not clear, however, whether a response to these diagnostic blocks confirms the presence of a clinical syndrome.

Evidence exists to support the notion that LBP may be partly related to protective muscular spasm. Animal models have shown that stimulation of various structures, such as the disk, facet joint capsule, or supraspinous ligament, produces reflex multifidus muscle activity locally, which is suppressed when these structures are anesthetized [48–50]. Similarly, muscle tension in the LBP seems to increase in various experimental models, such as in experimental muscle inflammation [51]. This information supports the observation that patients who have LBP have increased muscle activity compared with asymptomatic controls during full flexion, static postures, and stress [52–56].

Finally, because LBP is so common and usually transitory, Bigos and Battié [57] and Hadler [58] question whether LBP can be called a disease at all or can fit into an injury model. Because symptom onset is typically gradual and frequently not related to accidental cause, a cumulative trauma model also may be more appropriate to explain these symptoms in workers.

Natural history of back pain

"Intermittency" was the word Rowe used to summarize back pain histories of male patients who were followed for a decade [3]. More than half of the men described acute attacks of disabling LBP that lasted 3 to 10 days and occurred at intervals from 3 months to 2 or 3 years. Between episodes, patients resumed normal activity without pain. A third investigation reported similar episodes with mild occasional backache in between. More recent work confirms that recovery in terms of pain resolution and disability is typically significant but incomplete in most patients [59–61].

In a prospective study of 49,000 Swedish workers sick-listed with LBP, 57% recovered in 1 week, 90% in 6 weeks, and 95% in 12 weeks, and 1.3% remained disabled at 1 year [59–62]. Individuals who have sciatica lose more work time than workers who have LBP only. Average lost work time per episode of LBP in other studies is typically less than 1 month [24,38,63]. The length of disability can be influenced by insurance, however. Railroad workers who sustained back injury on duty took an average of 14.9 months to return to work versus only 3.5 months for persons who injured their backs off duty [64].

Recurrence is common and occurs in as many as 60% to 85% of patients with a single prior episode of LBP [3,33,65,66]. Biering-Sorensen [67] found that the more frequently and recently a person experienced LBP, the more liable he or she is to experience LBP in the coming year regardless of age. The conflicts with Abenhaim's prospective data covering 3 years in which older workers (45–64 years old) seemed to be protected somewhat from recurrences [68]. Others point out that chronic phases of back pain occur more often than previously believed [69]. Improved fitness and specific rehabilitation are shown to influence outcome positively in patients who have LBP and sciatica [70–75]. Garcy and colleagues [76] found that workers who received workers' compensation who had previous severe and chronic disabling spinal disorders returned to work after a functional restoration program and succeeded without significantly different risks than the controls for new or recurrent back injury.

Risk factors for occupational back pain

The study of risk factors related to back problems is a key issue in industry because the ultimate goal is prevention. Literature on this topic dates back to the 1920s and reflects several work-related factors of importance, all of which can increase the load on the spine. Many risk factors, whether work related or personal, are interrelated. For instance, vibrations, static work posture, and physical fitness of the worker can contribute to pain in any one job. The true risk for any single factor is difficult to ascertain.

Personal risk factors

Personal risk factors can influence the occurrence of LBP. Because many study results are conflicting, further investigation is needed. It is also difficult to draw conclusions from many of the studies because of their case control designs. Personal risk factors are divided into risk factors that are nonmodifiable (eg, age, gender, anthropometry, genetics, psychosocial factors, and structural abnormalities) and potentially modifiable (eg, physical fitness, strength, lumbar mobility, posture, and smoking).

Genetic risk factors

In recent studies investigating LBP in populations, including monozygotic twins, genetic factors seem to have a significant effect on structural changes in the spine, including disc degeneration, herniation, and Schmorl nodes [77–79]. Battie and colleagues [77] found that although these MRI changes were significantly associated with increased spinal loading and twisting at work, they only accounted for 7% of the sample variance. Adding age accounted for a total of 16% of variability, whereas adding the genetic and early environmental factors shared by twins explained a total of 77% of the variability in the upper lumbar spine. In the lower lumbar spine the pattern of influence was similar, with genetic factors dominating, whereas half of the variability remained unexplained (Fig. 3). When the twins were discordant for sitting time at work, occupational driving, regular aerobic exercise, other sports participation, recalled back injuries, and cigarette smoking, there was no significantly associated difference in spine structural changes.

The association between genetic factors and back pain has been described by MacGregor and colleagues [80]. In a group of more than 1000 twins, including various definitions of back pain, genetic influence was demonstrated for LBP between 52% and 68%. In this study of women, however, there was also overlap between genetic association of reporting LBP and genetic

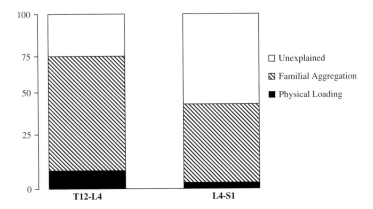

Fig. 3. Determinants of lumbar disc degeneration in the upper and lower lumbar spine in identical twins. (*Adapted from* Battie MC, Videman T, Gibbons LE, et al. 1995 Volvo Award in clinical sciences. Determinants of lumbar disc degeneration: a study relating lifetime exposures and magnetic resonance imaging findings in identical twins. Spine 1995;20(24):2601–12; with permission.)

influences on psychological well-being. Issues such as these must be investigated further to understand more clearly the role of genetics in LBP. These various twin studies suggest that genetics may have a much more powerful influence on the experience of LBP in the workplace than any other known risk factors.

Genetic variability in genes that code for structural components of the lumbar discs, such as collagen IX and aggrecan, and genes that code for cytokines, such as the interleukin-1 cluster, is also associated with lumbar disc disease and risk for sciatica [81–83].

Age and gender

LBP affects men and women in their most productive years, with the peak frequency of symptoms occurring in the age range of 30 to 55 [3,6–8, 18,33,84,85]. Recent work involving more than 29,000 people aged 12 to 41 has confirmed that LBP prevalence is significant as early as age 12 to 14 in both sexes. Prevalence rates approach adult prevalence rates by approximately age 20 (Fig. 4) [86].

Overall, men and women have an equal prevalence of LBP, with women having a slightly earlier onset and approaching adult levels approximately 1 or 2 years earlier than men [4,7,85–89]. Previous pregnancy is a risk factor for future LBP, however, and oral contraceptive use is associated with increased number of office visits for LBP [90]. Women have more back complaints in heavy physical jobs than men [91], whereas men have surgery as much as three times more often for disc herniations [25,30,85,92] and file more workers' compensation claims [12,19].

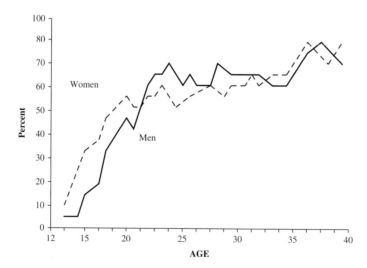

Fig. 4. The lifetime cumulative incidence of LBP for men and women aged 12 to 41. (*Adapted from* Leboeuf-Yde C, Kyvik KO. At what age does low back pain become a common problem? A study of 29,424 individuals aged 12–41 years. Spine 1998;23(2):228–34; with permission.)

The relationship between age and lumbar disc herniations is similar to that of LBP. In Spangfort's review of the literature [93], the mean age at operation for disc herniation was 40.8 years (40.7 for men and 41.0 for women). Almost all patients who undergo disc herniation surgery are between 35 and 45 years old (Fig. 5).

Anthropometry

Retrospective and prospective data generally indicate no strong correlation between body height, weight, build, or mild leg length inequality and LBP [3,7,8,67,84,85,89,94–97]. On the other hand, in a prospective study of 3020 Boeing Aircraft workers, taller men and higher weight or obese women were found to have higher risk of recurrent LBP [59,98]. No other anthropometric measures in these workers predicted initial LBP-related work absence. Tallness may predict HNP and sciatica [3,99]. Obesity is only weakly associated with LBP and is probably unlikely to have a cause-and-effect association based on monozygotic twin studies [100]. Obesity may play a role in simple LBP becoming chronic in nature, however [101]. There is no association between low birth weight and LBP in adolescents, but high birth weight is a risk factor for LBP [102].

Psychosocial factors

Earlier studies that measured psychosocial factors in patients who had LBP revealed clear associations, but study design did not allow a cause-and-effect relationship to be demonstrated [13,33,85,103–108]. These psychosocial factors include stress defined variably, depression, somatization, catastrophizing, cognitive functioning, and pain behavior [109]. Larson

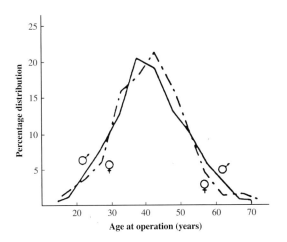

Fig. 5. Percent of distribution of operations for herniated lumbar discs by age and sex. (*From* Andersson GBJ. Epidemiology of spinal disorders. In: Frymoyer JW, editor. The adult spine: principles and practice. 3rd edition. Philadelphia: Lippincott-Raven; 1997; with permission.)

and colleagues [110] were the first to demonstrate prospectively the significant effect of depression as an independent variable on the onset of first episode of future LBP. Chronic LBP in a patient with depression seems to have an additive effect on disability [111].

Specific work-related factors associated with chronic LBP and disability include an overrepresentation of lower-ranked manual workers, a poor psychosocial work environment, increased job dissatisfaction, poor appraisal from supervisors, monotonous work, time pressures, worry over mistakes, and mental stress [33,99,103,112–114]. If cause and effect are specifically analyzed, however, perceived work load and perceived work capabilities seem to predict future back pain better than actual work load and capabilities [115,116]. In a prospective study of metal industry employees, persons with low job control had a 3.2-fold risk for subsequent hospitalization for back disorders compared with persons with high job control, and individuals with low supervisor support had a 2.9-fold risk compared with persons with high supervisor support [117].

Finally, Pincus and colleagues [118] reviewed the literature regarding psychological factors that predicted the transformation from acute to chronic LBP. They found that psychological distress, depressed mood, and, to a lesser extent, somatization predicted chronicity prospectively, whereas catastrophizing as a coping strategy also predicted chronicity.

Structural abnormalities

Several studies using twin cohorts have demonstrated the association between various structural changes in the lumbar spine and risk factors. Further detail is found in the genetic factors section. Studies of twins show that no protective or harmful effects result from lifetime leisure time endurance exercise. Power sports athletes had increased degeneration in the thoracolumbar spine compared with their twin that was disconcordant for power sport involvement [119].

Disc degeneration also is influenced by the occupation of the worker. Several studies have demonstrated that heavy physical work can accelerate the development of degeneration by up to 10 years [8,120–124]. For instance, Riihimaki and colleagues [125] found an approximately twofold increased risk for disc space narrowing in concrete workers compared with house painters. The relationship between disc degeneration regardless of the measuring tool and LBP is controversial, however. Several notable studies point out that individuals with extensive disc degeneration are more likely to have LBP [3,8,33,114,123,126–129]; others disagree [6,12,30,92, 130,131]. Buirski and colleagues [132], who compared MRI results in patients with and without LBP, found that the incidence of all noted abnormalities seemed to be equal in both groups.

LBP is more common in patients with spondylolisthesis in most studies [8,33,133–135]. The presence of spondylolysis on lumbar radiographs is associated with a higher rate of LBP in college football players versus controls (80.5% versus 32%) [136]. Spina bifida occulta [33,137] and sacralized transverse process [3] do not seem to be associated with increased incidence of LBP, however.

Physical fitness

Higher levels of physical fitness are generally believed to be protective against an occurrence of LBP in workers, as has been demonstrated in select populations. An often quoted study by Cady and colleagues [70] prospectively followed 1652 firefighters after assessing fitness based on five measures. In comparing the three fitness groups (259 high, 266 low, 1127 middle), they demonstrated a ninefold increase in back injuries in the least fit group versus the most fit group over 4 years. The least fit group, however, was of older age. Mayer and colleagues [138] followed 66 patients who had chronic back pain through a 3-week comprehensive outpatient rehabilitation program and then over the subsequent year. The treatment group had substantially less pain and dysfunction as measured by the Million analog scale, twice the return to work rate, and improved fitness measures. These studies support associations also seen in a cross-sectional study by Deyo and Tsui-Wu [139] concerning fitness and LBP. Recovery rates after an episode of acute LBP were found to be shorter in workers with improved fitness [127], whereas the persons with lowest fitness levels had the highest risk for LBP and musculoskeletal injury [140,141]. Specific exercise prescriptions for individual workers are difficult because there is disagreement concerning the best exercises [75,142] and because some studies have failed to show any effect of physical fitness on LBP occurrence [33,143,144]. Recent work by Hides and colleagues [145] showed a long-term effect of trunk muscle stabilizing exercises on LBP. They found 1-year recurrence rates of 30% versus 84% and 3-year recurrence rates of 35% versus 75% in control patients.

Leisure-time physical activities and their relationships to LBP are difficult to interpret because most studies only measure leisure activities crudely and little is known about which activities seem to be the most relevant to the back. Studies in industry are conflicting. For instance, Leino [71] followed 902 workers for 10 years and found mean exercise activity to be moderately inversely associated with back pain. This supports Kelsey's [28] earlier case-control study looking at HNP but contrasts with other similar studies [25,146].

Former elite athletes have reportedly less back pain than controls [147]. There were no clear benefits in Videman's study for vigorous exercise compared with lighter exercise and back pain findings. No acceleration of disc degeneration was found in competitive runners compared with controls. Power sport athletes had increased degeneration through the entire lumbar spine, however, whereas soccer players had increased degeneration in the lower lumbar spine compared with controls.

Workers with poor motor control may be at risk of low back injury. McGill has shown that the spine actually can buckle during minor tasks, in which a small motor error causes over-rotation of a functional spinal unit and loading of the soft tissues [148]. This is especially true with sudden unanticipated loads [149]. Endurance of the spine support muscles is also important because continuous contraction is needed to prevent buckling. McGill observed a significant variation in people's ability to hold a load with their hands and breathe deeply. It is postulated that people with decreased lung function and a greater demand on the diaphragm muscle are not able to use it to stabilize the spine (through increased intra-abdominal pressure increase) during lifting [150].

Lumbar spine mobility

Patients generally regard the ability to touch their toes (a demonstration of lumbar mobility) as a favorable sign related to low back health. Earlier retrospective studies have been supportive of this notion, showing reduced lumbar flexibility in patients with LBP [151–154] and improved flexibility with symptom relief [138,155,156]. It is arguable that the restriction in range of motion is not anatomic but more often a protective response to pain [157,158] and psychological distress [154]. Despite the absence of proof in early reports that poor mobility causes LBP, objective measures are routinely used to assess a patient's mobility. Lumbar mobility measurements also are commonly used to monitor treatment response [138,155,156,159], permanent impairment, and disability [160]. Recent prospective studies have shown no association between reduced lumbar mobility and risk for future LBP [116,131], and other studies actually have demonstrated increased lumbar flexibility associated with increased LBP [161,162].

Muscle strength

The hypothesis that poor trunk muscle strength places workers at risk for developing LBP has not been supported clearly in the literature. Although patients who have LBP reportedly have substantially less isometric and isokinetic strength versus healthy controls [96,123,163–168], some investigators noted no difference [142,169]. Most importantly, these studies do not address the possibility that LBP could cause the strength deficiency [168] instead of being a consequence of poor strength. Reimer and colleagues [170] screened 1100 prospective grocery warehouse employees for job-specific physical abilities and matched workers to appropriate jobs. They found a 51% reduction in low back injury reports over 2 years and a 20% reduction in total injury reports. These results support earlier work by Keyserling and colleagues [171], but a change in insurance during the study period may have influenced injury reporting. Chaffin and colleagues [161] similarly found an increased risk of LBP for workers whose job required strength at or above the worker's ability. Other investigators have found no correlation between trunk muscle strength and LBP prospectively [172,173]. In a prospective study with a large patient population, Battie and colleagues [143] found no correlation between isometric trunk strength and subsequent low back injuries. Workers, however, were not matched to jobs based on trunk strength. Female collegiate athletes with baseline asymmetric hip abductor and extensor strength were at higher risk of requiring future treatment for LBP. Although similar strength asymmetries existed in male collegiate athletes, no association was noted with subsequent LBP in the men [174].

Posture

Hansson and colleagues [175] studied 600 men of similar age and occupation who were separated into normals, first-time acute LBP, and chronic LBP. Lumbar lordosis as measured by spinal radiographs was found to be comparable in all groups. Similarly, other postural abnormalities, such as kyphosis and scoliosis, are not associated with LBP in general [6–8, 85,176,177] unless scoliosis is more than 80° or the scoliosis vertex is located in the lumbar spine [6]. McGill and colleagues [178] recently studied back extensor muscle fiber angle in erect standing and forward flexion postures and found that flexion changed extensor muscle angle and the ability to resist anterior shear forces. Anterior shear is highly related to risk of reporting a back injury.

Smoking

Despite a clear association between smoking and LBP, HNP, bone mineral density, rate of hip fracture, and dynamics of bone and wound healing, this association is weak [179,180]. The previously assumed cause-and-effect relationship between smoking and LBP seems to be inaccurate based on recent work comparing identical twins, only one of whom smoked. In the Danish twin study of 29,000 people, no differences were noted in the prevalence rates for LBP in the twin who smoked over his or her nonsmoking sibling [181].

Work-related risk factors

Heavy physical work

The prevalence of LBP in workers with jobs with heavy physical demands has been shown in several studies to be higher than in a matched group of workers in jobs with light physical demands. For instance, Tsai and colleagues [182] conducted a cross-sectional study of 10,350 US oil company employees. Workers identified by job title as having physically demanding jobs, such as boiler maker, mechanic, and welder, were found to have a related risk of LBP injury of 1.5. Similarly, Riihimaki and colleagues [125] prospectively followed concrete reinforcement workers and house painters for 5 years, and 60% of concrete reinforcement workers versus 47% of house painters experienced sciatica at follow-up. Concrete reinforcement workers also were significantly more likely to be granted disability than house painters (8% versus 3%). Workers' compensation claims for LBP also are more frequent in heavy manual labor jobs than in other types of work [3,183]. Others investigators, however, have reported no significant differences in LBP prevalence between light- and heavy-duty work [3,8,28].

Unfortunately, the exact amount of physical work needed to increase one's risk for LBP is unknown. These results must be interpreted with caution because the definition of heavy physical labor in various studies has been made using comparisons between jobs with high-energy demands and jobs with low-energy demands, such as sedentary work. Sedentary work still provides significant statis load to the spine.

Static work postures

It has been generally agreed upon that static sitting occupations or sedentary jobs create an increased risk for LBP [8,32,176,183–186]. A recent comprehensive review of this subject by Hartvigsen et al [187] has argued that the literature does not support an increased risk of LBP. They systematically reviewed 14 reports studying sitting at work and 21 reports on sedentary occupations. Only 8 studies were considered high quality. They concluded that regardless of study quality, most studies failed to find a positive association between sitting at work and LBP. The high-quality studies actually found a marginally negative association. They argue that a few often-quoted studies of cross-sectional design may have perpetuated this "myth" of increased LBP in static occupations.

Static standing at work may increase the risk of LBP [91,188–190]. Various flooring changes seem to decrease subjective pain [191–193] in some but not all studies [184,194,195]. Variations in the amount of standing in these studies may have influenced results.

Lifting

Several investigators have shown a clear risk of LBP in workers involved with jobs that require significant lifting tasks [8,19,28,33,176,196,197]. Injury severity rate is proportional to the bulk of the object, lifting frequency, the object location at the start of the lift, and particularly the object's weight [198]. LBP is more likely to occur when workers lift loads that exceed their physical capabilities [199]. Capabilities vary widely from worker to worker. Even isokinetic lifting strength poorly predicts subsequent LBP [173]. Some investigators have attempted to quantify what is considered a safe weight for lifting and recommended weights less than 25 to 35 pounds [31,200]. The National Institute for Occupational Safety and Health has a lifting equation that was revised in 1991 to include aspects of asymmetric lifting and less than optimal hand-container coupling and to accommodate a larger range of work situations [199]. Its purpose is to define recommended weight limits for lifting that would be safe for 99% of men and 75% of women in any particular job.

Other factors that workers must consider with lifting include the understanding that forces through the spine are actually greater in the loading phase than the lifting phase [201–203] and when arms are fatigued [204]. Excessive speed of lift may increase the risk of LBP [205], and lowering weight in contrast to lifting may be more risky [206]. The often advocated "lifting with the legs" technique is perceived as requiring more energy [207], results in higher spinal compression forces [208,209], and is less preferred by workers [210,211] than lifting with the back. A combined technique referred to as "freestyle" may be a better option [212].

The epidemiologic data concerning the use of back belts in preventing occupational LBP injuries are not sufficient to warrant general use because of low compliance, lack of efficacy, and lack of cost-effectiveness [213–215].

Twisting and bending

Twisting and bending motions clearly increase forces throughout the spine in various studies [216–219]. Frequent bending and lifting in industry is a significant cause of LBP [6,19,20,23,220]. In a case-control study of automobile assembly workers, Praemer and colleagues found that 51% of subjects were exposed to severe trunk flexion and 45% to twisting positions [63]. In this study, the odds ratio for LBP in positions of mild flexion and twisting was 7.4 (CI 1.8–29.4), with an odds ratio of 8.9 for severe flexion ≥10% of cycle time and an odds ratio of 6.1 for mild flexion. A strong increasing risk was observed with intensity and exposure and duration of exposure. Marras and colleagues [221] used a three-dimensional electrogoniometry device to study workers in 403 jobs across 48 industries to assess which factors or combination of factors correctly identified high- and low-risk jobs. They found that low back disorder risks were predicted by a combination of five occupational related factors: lifting frequency, load moment, trunk lateral velocity, trunk twisting velocity, and trunk sagittal angle. None of the factors alone predicted high risk for low back disorders. These results highlight the difficulty in assigning risks to individual movements discussed previously by other investigators [6].

Whole-body vibration

Approximately 4% to 7% of all employees in the United States, Canada, and some European countries are exposed to potentially harmful whole-body vibration [222]. LBP, early degeneration of the lumbar spine, and herniated lumbar disc are the most commonly reported musculoskeletal disorders among professional drivers. Workers in these situation are often exposed to machinery that vibrates at a fundamental frequency similar to the body's natural frequency of 4 to 6 Hz [37]. Although many studies associate whole-body vibration exposure to increased LBP [120,223–233], it still remains unclear whether this is a cause-and-effect relationship or simply a risk factor only in combination with things such as sitting, for example. Equally unclear is what constitutes a safe dosage of exposure [234]. Genetic studies like those of Battie and colleagues would suggest that the risk of accelerating degenerative disc disease from whole-body vibration exposure compared with genetic factors is negligible [77].

Summary

Significant advances have been made in our understanding of occupational LBP over the last decade, thanks in large part to a noteworthy improvement in the number and quality of prospective trials. Many previous associations between personal and work-related risk factors and LBP have been defined and may only account for a small percentage of overall risk. More recent work using large cohorts of twins confirms that genetic factors may drive a large portion of the risk factors. Unidentified factors also account for a percentage of the risk in occupational LBP.

The importance of physical fitness and spine support muscle fitness is believed to be protective against future occurrences. Our understanding of the origin of LBP also continues to advance. Clearly, psychosocial factors can play a role in increasing the risk of future LBP and in acute pain becoming chronic. Some of the psychological influence may be through a muscular pain component. There is a better understanding that LBP is a condition that begins in adolescence.

Factors that influence the natural history may minimize LBP in the future. With such high rates of prevalence and recurrence, it is becoming well established that LBP is likely an inevitable part of being human and walking on two feet. "Ascribing the symptoms of regional back pain to common usage (such as workplace exposures) is as tenable as labeling angina pectoris as a 'stair climber's chest'" [58]. It is arguable that an emphasis should be placed on resources, education, and support to allow workers to be productive regardless of whether they suffer from back pain.

Acknowledgments

I would like to thank my wife, Mary, for her steadfast devotion and love and my children, Liz, Luke, and Erik, for helping me with my homework. A personal note of thanks to Cynthia Miller for her considerable efforts in preparing the manuscript.

References

[1] Shelerud R. Epidemiology of occupational low back pain. Occup Med 1998;13(1):1–22.
[2] Department of Labor BoLS. Occupational injuries and illnesses in the United States by industry, 1990. Washington, DC: Department of Labor, Bureau of Labor Statistics; 1992.
[3] Rowe ML. Low back pain in industry: a position paper. J Occup Med 1969;11(4):161–9.

[4] Deyo RA, Tsui-Wu YJ. Descriptive epidemiology of low-back pain and its related medical care in the United States. Spine 1987;12(3):264–8.

[5] Frymoyer JW. Magnitude of the problem. Philadelphia: WB Saunders; 1966.

[6] Andersson G. Epidemiologic aspects on low back pain in industry. Spine 1981;6:53–60.

[7] Horal J. The clinical appearance of low back disorders in the city of Gothenburg, Sweden: comparisons of incapacitated probands with matched controls. Acta Orthop Scand Suppl 1969;118:1–109.

[8] Hult L. Cervical, dorsal and lumbar spinal syndromes: a field investigation of a non-selected material of 1200 workers in different occupations with special reference to disc degeneration and so-called muscular rheumatism. Acta Orthop Scand Suppl 1954;17:1–102.

[9] Verbrugge LM, Ascione FJ. Exploring the iceberg: common symptoms and how people care for them. Med Care 1987;25(6):539–69.

[10] Biering-Sorensen F. A prospective study of low back pain in a general population. III. Medical service–work consequence. Scand J Rehabil Med 1983;15(2):89–96.

[11] Snook S. Low back pain in industry. Presented at the Symposium on Idiopathic Low Back Pain. St. Louis, 1982.

[12] Spengler DM, Bigos SJ, Martin NA, et al. Back injuries in industry: a retrospective study. I. Overview and cost analysis. Spine 1986;11(3):241–5.

[13] Nachemson AL. Spinal disorders: overall impact on society and the need for orthopedic resources. Acta Orthop Scand Suppl 1991;241:17–22.

[14] Fordyce WE. Back pain, compensation, and public policy. Hanover: University Press of New England; 1985.

[15] Kelsey JL, White AA III. Epidemiology and impact of low-back pain. Spine 1980;5(2): 133–42.

[16] United States Government Printing Office. Supplemental SSS: social security statistical supplement. Washington, DC: United States Government Printing Office; 1977–1979. HE 3.3/3:979.

[17] Abenhaim L, Suissa S. Importance and economic burden of occupational back pain: a study of 2,500 cases representative of Quebec. J Occup Med 1987;29(8):670–4.

[18] Behrens V, Seligman P, Cameron L, et al. The prevalence of back pain, hand discomfort, and dermatitis in the US working population. Am J Public Health 1994;84(11):1780–5.

[19] Klein BP, Jensen RC, Sanderson LM. Assessment of workers' compensation claims for back strains/sprains. J Occup Med 1984;26(6):443–8.

[20] Johnston W. Back injuries: a problem for both workers and employers. Ohio Monitor 1982; 55:15.

[21] Kosiak M, Aurelius JR, Hartfiel WF. Backache in industry. J Occup Med 1966;8(2):51–8.

[22] Levitt S, Johnston L-T, Beyer R. The process of recovery: patterns of industrial back injury, Part 1. Ind Med Surg 1971;40:7–14.

[23] Snook SH, Campanelli RA, Hart JW. A study of three preventive approaches to low back injury. J Occup Med 1978;20(7):478–81.

[24] Spitzer W, BLeBlanc F, Dupuis M, et al. Scientific approach to the assessment and management of activity-related spinal disorders: A monograph for clinicians. Report of the Quebec Task Force on Spinal Disorders. Spine 1987;12(7 Suppl):S1–59.

[25] Heliovaara M, Knekt P, Aromaa A. Incidence and risk factors of herniated lumbar intervertebral disc or sciatica leading to hospitalization. J Chronic Dis 1987;40(3):251–8.

[26] Heliovaara M. Occupation and risk of herniated lumbar intervertebral disc or sciatica leading to hospitalization. J Chronic Dis 1987;40(3):259–64.

[27] Kelsey JL. An epidemiological study of acute herniated lumbar intervertebral discs. Rheumatol Rehabil 1975;14(3):144–59.

[28] Kelsey JL. An epidemiological study of the relationship between occupations and acute herniated lumbar intervertebral discs. Int J Epidemiol 1975;4(3):197–205.

[29] Kelsey JL, Hardy RJ. Driving of motor vehicles as a risk factor for acute herniated lumbar intervertebral disc. Am J Epidemiol 1975;102(1):63–73.

[30] Kelsey JL, Ostfeld AM. Demographic characteristics of persons with acute herniated lumbar intervertebral disc. J Chronic Dis 1975;28(1):37–50.

[31] Kelsey JL, Githens PB, O'Conner T, et al. Acute prolapsed lumbar intervertebral disc: an epidemiologic study with special reference to driving automobiles and cigarette smoking. Spine 1984;9(6):608–13.

[32] Kelsey JL, Githens PB, White AA III, et al. An epidemiologic study of lifting and twisting on the job and risk for acute prolapsed lumbar intervertebral disc. J Orthop Res 1984;2(1): 61–6.

[33] Bergquist-Ullman M, Larsson U. Acute low back pain in industry. Acta Orthop Scand 1977;170:1–117.

[34] Frymoyer JW. Occupational low back pain: assessment, treatment, and prevention. St. Louis: Mosby; 1991.

[35] Rosen JC, Frymoyer JW, Clements JH. A further look at validity of the MMPI with low back patients. J Clin Psychol 1980;36(4):994–1000.

[36] Kuslich SD, Ulstrom CL, Michael CJ. The tissue origin of low back pain and sciatica: a report of pain response to tissue stimulation during operations on the lumbar spine using local anesthesia. Orthop Clin North Am 1991;22(2):181–7.

[37] Bovenzi M. Low back pain disorders and exposure to whole-body vibration in the workplace. Semin Perinatol 1996;20(1):38–53.

[38] Wood P, Bradley E. The lumbar spine and back pain. In: Jayson M, editor. Epidemiology of back pain. London: Churchill-Livingstone; 1987. p. 1–15.

[39] Bogduk N. The sources of low back pain. Edinburgh: Churchill-Livingstone; 1992.

[40] Vernon-Roberts B, Pirie CJ. Degenerative changes in the intervertebral discs of the lumbar spine and their sequelae. Rheumatol Rehabil 1977;16(1):13–21.

[41] Kirkaldy-Willis WH, Wedge JH, Yong-Hing K, et al. Pathology and pathogenesis of lumbar spondylosis and stenosis. Spine 1978;3(4):319–28.

[42] Kirkaldy-Willis WH. Pathology and pathogenesis of low back pain. New York: Churchill-Livingstone; 1992.

[43] Kirkaldy-Willis WH, Farfan HF. Instability of the lumbar spine. Clin Orthop Relat Res 1982;(165):110–23.

[44] Maigne JY, Aivaliklis A, Pfefer F. Results of sacroiliac joint double block and value of sacroiliac pain provocation tests in 54 patients with low back pain. Spine 1996;21(16): 1889–92.

[45] Schwarzer AC, Aprill CN, Bogduk N. The sacroiliac joint in chronic low back pain. Spine 1995;20(1):31–7.

[46] Schwarzer AC, Aprill CN, Derby R, et al. Clinical features of patients with pain stemming from the lumbar zygapophysial joints: is the lumbar facet syndrome a clinical entity? Spine 1994;19(10):1132–7.

[47] Schwarzer AC, Aprill CN, Derby R, et al. The relative contributions of the disc and zygapophyseal joint in chronic low back pain. Spine 1994;19(7):801–6.

[48] Indahl A, Kaigle A, Reikeras O, et al. Electromyographic response of the porcine multifidus musculature after nerve stimulation. Spine 1995;20(24):2652–8.

[49] Stubbs M, Harris M, Solomonow M, et al. Ligamento-muscular protective reflex in the lumbar spine of the feline. J Electromyogr Kinesiol 1998;8(4):197–204.

[50] Williams M, Solomonow M, Zhou BH, et al. Multifidus spasms elicited by prolonged lumbar flexion. Spine 2000;25(22):2916–24.

[51] Johansson H, Sojka P. Pathophysiological mechanisms involved in genesis and spread of muscular tension in occupational muscle pain and in chronic musculoskeletal pain syndromes: a hypothesis. Med Hypotheses 1991;35(3):196–203.

[52] Flor H, Turk DC, Birbaumer N. Assessment of stress-related psychophysiological reactions in chronic back pain patients. J Consult Clin Psychol 1985;53(3):354–64.

[53] Ahern DK, Follick MJ, Council JR, et al. Comparison of lumbar paravertebral EMG patterns in chronic low back pain patients and non-patient controls. Pain 1988;34(2):153–60.

[54] Arena JG, Sherman RA, Bruno GM, et al. Electromyographic recordings of 5 types of low back pain subjects and non-pain controls in different positions. Pain 1989;37(1): 57–65.

[55] Sihvonen T, Partanen J, Hanninen O, et al. Electric behavior of low back muscles during lumbar pelvic rhythm in low back pain patients and healthy controls. Arch Phys Med Rehabil 1991;72(13):1080–7.

[56] Ambroz C, Scott A, Ambroz A, et al. Chronic low back pain assessment using surface electromyography. J Occup Environ Med 2000;42(6):660–9.

[57] Bigos SJ, Battie M. Industrial Low back pain: risk factors. Philadelphia: WB Saunders; 1996.

[58] Hadler NM. Back pain in the workplace: what you lift or how you lift matters far less than whether you lift or when. Spine 1997;22(9):935–40.

[59] Hestbaek L, Leboeuf-Yde C, Manniche C. Low back pain: what is the long-term course? A review of studies of general patient populations. Eur Spine J 2003;12(2):149–65.

[60] Pengel L, Herbert R, Maher C, et al. Acute low back pain: systematic review of its prognosis. BMJ 2003;327:323–34.

[61] Von Korff M, Saunders K. The course of back pain in primary care. Spine 1996;21(24): 2833–7 [discussion: 2838–9].

[62] Choler U, Larsson R, Nachemson AL, et al. Back pain. SPRI Rep 1985;188:1–100.

[63] Praemer A, Furnes S, Rice D. Musculoskeletal conditions in the United States. Presented at the American Academy of Orthopedic Surgeons. Park Ridge, IL, 1992.

[64] Sander P, Meyers J. The relationship of disability to compensation status in railroad workers. Spine 1986;11:141–3.

[65] Troup JD, Martin JW, Lloyd DC. Back pain in industry: a prospective survey. Spine 1981; 6(1):61–9.

[66] Valkenburg H, Haanen H. The epidemiology of low back pain. Presented at the American Academy of Orthopaedic Surgeons Symposium on Idiopathic Low Back Pain. St. Louis, 1982.

[67] Biering-Sorensen F. A prospective study of low back pain in a general population. I. Occurrence, recurrence and aetiology. Scand J Rehabil Med 1983;15(2):71–9.

[68] Abenhaim L, Suissa S, Rossignol M. Risk of recurrence of occupational back pain over three year follow up. Br J Ind Med 1988;45(12):829–33.

[69] Von Korff M. Studying the natural history of back pain. Spine 1994;19:2041S–6S.

[70] Cady LD, Bischoff DP, O'Connell ER, et al. Strength and fitness and subsequent back injuries in firefighters. J Occup Med 1979;21(4):269–72.

[71] Leino PI. Does leisure time physical activity prevent low back disorders? A prospective study of metal industry employees. Spine 1993;18(7):863–71.

[72] Nachemson A, Eck C, Lindstrom I, et al. Chronic low back disability can largely be prevented: a prospective randomized trial in industry. Presented at the 56th Annual Meeting of the American Academy of Orthopaedic Surgeons. Las Vegas, February 9–14, 1989.

[73] Saal JA, Saal JS. Nonoperative treatment of herniated lumbar intervertebral disc with radiculopathy: an outcome study. Spine 1989;14(4):431–7.

[74] Saal JA, Saal JS, Herzog RJ. The natural history of lumbar intervertebral disc extrusions treated nonoperatively. Spine 1990;15(7):683–6.

[75] van Tulder MW, Koes BW, Bouter LM. Conservative treatment of acute and chronic non-specific low back pain: a systematic review of randomized controlled trials of the most common interventions. Spine 1997;22(18):2128–56.

[76] Garcy P, Mayer T, Gatchel RJ. Recurrent or new injury outcomes after return to work in chronic disabling spinal disorders: tertiary prevention efficacy of functional restoration treatment. Spine 1996;21(8):952–9.

[77] Battie MC, Videman T, Gibbons LE, et al. 1995 Volvo Award in clinical sciences. Determinants of lumbar disc degeneration: a study relating lifetime exposures and magnetic resonance imaging findings in identical twins. Spine 1995;20(24):2601–12.

[78] Sambrook PN, MacGregor AJ, Spector TD. Genetic influences on cervical and lumbar disc degeneration: a magnetic resonance imaging study in twins. Arthritis Rheum 1999;42(2): 366–72.

[79] Manek N, Noponen-Hietala N, Ala-Kokko L, et al. Schmorl nodes are common, highly heritable, and an independent risk factor for back pain in healthy females: a candidate gene study of twins. Arthritis Rheum 2002;46:S374.

[80] MacGregor AJ, Andrew T, Sambrook PN, et al. Structural, psychological, and genetic influences on low back and neck pain: a study of adult female twins. Arthritis Rheum 2004; 51(2):160–7.

[81] Ala-Kokko L. Genetic risk factors for lumbar disc disease. Ann Med 2002;34(1):42–7.

[82] Paassilta P, Lohiniva J, Goring HH, et al. Identification of a novel common genetic risk factor for lumbar disk disease. JAMA 2001;285(14):1843–9.

[83] Solovieva S, Leino-Arjas P, Saarela J, et al. Possible association of interleukin 1 gene locus polymorphisms with low back pain. Pain 2004;109(1–2):8–19.

[84] Hirsch C, Jonsson B, Lewin T. Low-back symptoms in a Swedish female population. Clin Orthop Relat Res 1969;63:171–6.

[85] Svensson HO, Andersson GB. Low-back pain in 40- to 47-year-old men: work history and work environment factors. Spine 1983;8(3):272–6.

[86] Leboeuf-Yde C, Kyvik KO. At what age does low back pain become a common problem? A study of 29,424 individuals aged 12–41 years. Spine 1998;23(2):228–34.

[87] Harreby M, Kjer J, Hesselsoe G, et al. Epidemiological aspects and risk factors for low back pain in 38-year-old men and women: a 25-year prospective cohort study of 640 school children. Eur Spine J 1996;5(5):312–8.

[88] Leboeuf-Yde C, Klougart N, Lauritzen T. How common is low back pain in the Nordic population? Data from a recent study on a middle-aged general Danish population and four surveys previously conducted in the Nordic countries. Spine 1996;21(13):1518–25 [discussion: 1525–6].

[89] Svensson HO, Andersson GB, Johansson S, et al. A retrospective study of low-back pain in 38- to 64-year-old women: frequency of occurrence and impact on medical services. Spine 1988;13(5):548–52.

[90] Wreje U, Isacsson D, Aberg H. Oral contraceptives and back pain in women in a Swedish community. Int J Epidemiol 1997;26(1):71–4.

[91] Magora A. Investigation of the relation between low back pain and occupation. IMS Ind Med Surg 1970;39(12):504–10.

[92] Weber H. Lumbar disc herniation: a controlled, prospective study with ten years of observation. Spine 1983;8(2):131–40.

[93] Spangfort EV. The lumbar disc herniation: a computer-aided analysis of 2,504 operations. Acta Orthop Scand Suppl 1972;142:1–95.

[94] Ericksson K, Nemeth G, Ericksson E. Low back pain in elite cross-country skiers: a retrospective epidemiologic study. Scand J Med Sci Sport 1996;6:31–5.

[95] Manninen P, Riihimak H, Heliovaara M. Incidence and risk factors of low-back pain in middle-aged farmers. Occup Med (Lond) 1995;45(3):141–6.

[96] Pope MH, Bevins T, Wilder DG, et al. The relationship between anthropometric, postural, muscular, and mobility characteristics of males ages 18–55. Spine 1985;10(7): 644–8.

[97] Soukka A, Alaranta H, Tallroth K, et al. Leg-length inequality in people of working age: the association between mild inequality and low-back pain is questionable. Spine 1991; 16(4):429–31.

[98] Battie M, Bigos S, Fisher L, et al. Anthropometric and clinical measurements as predictors of industrial back pain complaints: a prospective study. J Spinal Discord 1990;3: 195–204.

[99] Heliovaara M, Makela M, Knekt P, et al. Determinants of sciatica and low-back pain. Spine 1991;16(6):608–14.

[100] Leboeuf-Yde C, Kyvik KO, Bruun NH. Low back pain and lifestyle. Part II. Obesity. Information from a population-based sample of 29,424 twin subjects. Spine 1999;24(8): 779–83 [discussion: 783].

[101] Leboeuf-Yde C. Body weight and low back pain: a systematic literature review of 56 journal articles reporting on 65 epidemiologic studies. Spine 2000;25(2):226–37.

[102] Hestbaek L, Leboeuf-Yde C, Kyvik KO, et al. Is low back pain in youth associated with weight at birth? A cohort study of 8000 Danish adolescents. Dan Med Bull 2003;50(2): 181–5.

[103] Cats-Baril WL, Frymoyer JW. Demographic factors associated with the prevalence of disability in the general population: analysis of the NHANES I database. Spine 1991;16(6):671–4.

[104] Dhanens T, Jarret S. MMPI pain assessment index: predictive and concurrent validity. Int J Clin Neuropsychol 1984;6:46–9.

[105] Flodmark BT, Aase G. Musculoskeletal symptoms and type A behaviour in blue collar workers. Br J Ind Med 1992;49(10):683–7.

[106] Frymoyer JW, Pope MH, Costanza M, et al. Epidemiologic studies of low back pain. Spine 1980;5:419–23.

[107] Love AW, Peck CL. The MMPI and psychological factors in chronic low back pain: a review. Pain 1987;28(1):1–12.

[108] Vallfors B. Acute, subacute and chronic low back pain: clinical symptoms, absenteeism and working environment. Scand J Rehabil Med Suppl 1985;11:1–98.

[109] Turk DC. Understanding pain sufferers: the role of cognitive processes. Spine J 2004;4(1): 1–7.

[110] Larson SL, Clark MR, Eaton WW. Depressive disorder as a long-term antecedent risk factor for incident back pain: a 13-year follow-up study from the Baltimore Epidemiological Catchment Area sample. Psychol Med 2004;34(2):211–9.

[111] Currie SR, Wang J. Chronic back pain and major depression in the general Canadian population. Pain 2004;107(1–2):54–60.

[112] Bigos SJ, Battie MC, Spengler DM, et al. A prospective study of work perceptions and psychosocial factors affecting the report of back injury. Spine 1991;16(1):1–6.

[113] Hales TR, Bernard BP. Epidemiology of work-related musculoskeletal disorders. Orthop Clin North Am 1996;27(4):679–709.

[114] Nachemson A. The lumbar spine: an orthopedic challenge. Spine 1976;1:59–71.

[115] Hultman G, Nordin M, Saraste H. Physical and psychological workload in men with and without low back pain. Scand J Rehabil Med 1995;27(1):11–7.

[116] Troup JD, Foreman TK, Baxter CE, et al. 1987 Volvo award in clinical sciences: the perception of back pain and the role of psychophysical tests of lifting capacity. Spine 1987; 12(7):645–57.

[117] Kaila-Kangas L, Kivimaki M, Riihimaki H, et al. Psychosocial factors at work as predictors of hospitalization for back disorders: a 28-year follow-up of industrial employees. Spine 2004;29(16):1823–30.

[118] Pincus T, Burton AK, Vogel S, et al. A systematic review of psychological factors as predictors of chronicity/disability in prospective cohorts of low back pain. Spine 2002;27(5): E109–20.

[119] Videman T, Battie MC, Gibbons LE, et al. Lifetime exercise and disk degeneration: an MRI study of monozygotic twins. Med Sci Sports Exerc 1997;29(10):1350–6.

[120] Barnekow-Bergkvist M, Hedberg GE, Janlert U, et al. Determinants of self-reported neck-shoulder and low back symptoms in a general population. Spine 1998;23(2):235–43.

[121] Biering-Sorensen F, Hansen FR, Schroll M, et al. The relation of spinal x-ray to low-back pain and physical activity among 60-year-old men and women. Spine 1985;10(5):445–51.

[122] Kellgren JH, Lawrence JS. Rheumatism in miners. II. X-ray study. Br J Ind Med 1952;9(3): 197–207.

[123] Lawrence JS. Disc degeneration: its frequency and relationship to symptoms. Ann Rheum Dis 1969;28(2):121–38.

[124] Wickstrom G, Hanninen K, Lehtinen M, et al. Previous back syndromes and present back symptoms in concrete reinforcement workers. Scand J Work Environ Health 1978;4 (Suppl 1):20–9.

[125] Riihimaki H, Wickstrom G, Hanninen K, et al. Predictors of sciatic pain among concrete reinforcement workers and house painters: a five-year follow-up. Scand J Work Environ Health 1989;15(6):415–23.

[126] Frymoyer J, Newberg A, Pope MH, et al. Spine radiographs in patients with low back pain. J Bone Joint Surg Am 1984;66:1048–55.

[127] Nachemson A. Towards a better understanding of low-back pain: a review of the mechanics of the lumbar disc. Rheumatol Rehabil 1975;14(3):129–43.

[128] Torgerson WR, Dotter WE. Comparative roentgenographic study of the asymptomatic and symptomatic lumbar spine. J Bone Joint Surg Am 1976;58(6):850–3.

[129] Videman T, Nurminen M, Troup JD. 1990 Volvo Award in clinical sciences: lumbar spinal pathology in cadaveric material in relation to history of back pain, occupation, and physical loading. Spine 1990;15(8):728–40.

[130] Aprill C, Bogduk N. High-intensity zone: a diagnostic sign of painful lumbar disk on magnetic resonance imaging. Br J Radiol 1992;65:361–9.

[131] Battie M, Bigos S, Fisher L, et al. The role of spinal flexibility in back pain complaints within industry: a prospective study. Spine 1990;15:768–73.

[132] Buirski G, Silberstein M. The symptomatic lumbar disc in patients with low-back pain: magnetic resonance imaging appearances in both a symptomatic and control population. Spine 1993;18(13):1808–11.

[133] Fisher F, Friedman M. Roentgenographic abnormalities in soldiers with low back pain: a comparative study. AJR Am J Roentgenol 1958;79:673–6.

[134] Magora A, Schwartz A. Relation between low back pain syndrome and x-ray findings: I. Degenerative osteoarthritis. Scand J Rehabil Med 1976;8:115–25.

[135] Wiltse LL. The effect of the common anomalies of the lumbar spine upon disc degeneration and low back pain. Orthop Clin North Am 1971;2(2):569–82.

[136] Iwamoto J, Abe H, Tsukimura Y, et al. Relationship between radiographic abnormalities of lumbar spine and incidence of low back pain in high school and college football players: a prospective study. Am J Sports Med 2004;32(3):781–6.

[137] Splithoff CA. Lumbosacral junction; roentgenographic comparison of patients with and without backaches. JAMA 1953;152(17):1610–3.

[138] Mayer TG, Gatchel RJ, Kishino N, et al. Objective assessment of spine function following industrial injury: a prospective study with comparison group and one-year follow-up. Spine 1985;10(6):482–93.

[139] Deyo R, Tsui-Wu YJ. Lifestyle and low back pain: the influence of smoking, exercise, and obesity. Clin Res 1987;35:577A.

[140] Heir T, Eide G. Age, body composition, aerobic fitness and health condition as risk factors for musculoskeletal injuries in conscripts. Scand J Med Sci Sports 1996;6(4):222–7.

[141] Jones B, Bovee M, Harris JI, et al. Intrinsic risk factors for exercise-related injuries among male and female army trainees. Am J Sport Med 1993;21:705–10.

[142] Biering-Sorensen F. Physical measurements as risk indicators for low-back trouble over a one-year period. Spine 1984;9(2):106–19.

[143] Battie M, Bigos S, Fisher L, et al. A prospective study of the role of cardiovascular risk factors and fitness in industrial back pain complaints. Spine 1989;14:141–7.

[144] Frymoyer JW, Pope MH, Clements JH, et al. Risk factors in low-back pain: an epidemiological survey. J Bone Joint Surg Am 1983;65(2):213–8.

[145] Hides JA, Jull GA, Richardson CA. Long-term effects of specific stabilizing exercises for first-episode low back pain. Spine 2001;26(11):E243–8.

[146] Riihimaki H, Tola S, Videman T, et al. Low-back pain and occupation: a cross-sectional questionnaire study of men in machine operating, dynamic physical work, and sedentary work. Spine 1989;14(2):204–9.

[147] Videman T, Sarna S, Battie MC, et al. The long-term effects of physical loading and exercise lifestyles on back-related symptoms, disability, and spinal pathology among men. Spine 1995;20(6):699–709.

[148] Cholewicki J, McGill SM. Mechanical stability of the in vivo lumbar spine: implications for injury and chronic low back pain. Clin Biomech (Bristol, Avon) 1996;11(1):1–15.

[149] Magnusson ML, Aleksiev A, Wilder DG, et al. European Spine Society: the AcroMed Prize for Spinal Research 1995. Unexpected load and asymmetric posture as etiologic factors in low back pain. Eur Spine J 1996;5(1):23–35.

[150] McGill SM, Sharratt MT, Seguin JP. Loads on spinal tissues during simultaneous lifting and ventilatory challenge. Ergonomics 1995;38(9):1772–92.

[151] Burton AK, Tillotson K, Troup J. Variation in lumbar sagittal mobility with low-back trouble. Spine 1989;14:584–90.

[152] Mayer TG, Tencer AF, Kristoferson S, et al. Use of noninvasive techniques for quantification of spinal range-of-motion in normal subjects and chronic low-back dysfunction patients. Spine 1984;9(6):588–95.

[153] Mellin G. Correlations of spinal mobility with degree of chronic low back pain after correction for age and anthropometric factors. Spine 1987;12(5):464–8.

[154] Pope MH, Rosen JC, Wilder DG, et al. The relation between biomechanical and psychological factors in patients with low-back pain. Spine 1980;5(2):173–8.

[155] Mayer T, Gatchel R, Mayer H. A prospective two-year study of functional restoration in industrial low back injury: an objective assessment procedure. JAMA 1987;258:1763–7.

[156] Mellin G. Physical therapy for chronic low back pain: correlations between spinal mobility and treatment outcome. Scand J Rehabil Med 1985;17(4):163–6.

[157] Pearcy M, Portek I, Shepherd J. The effect of low-back pain on lumbar spinal movements measured by three-dimensional X-ray analysis. Spine 1985;10(2):150–3.

[158] Stokes IA, Wilder DG, Frymoyer JW, et al. 1980 Volvo award in clinical sciences: assessment of patients with low-back pain by biplanar radiographic measurement of intervertebral motion. Spine 1981;6(3):233–40.

[159] Mayer TG. Assessment of lumbar function. Clin Orthop Relat Res 1987;221:99–109.

[160] Waddell G, Somerville D, Henderson I, et al. Objective clinical evaluation of physical impairment in chronic low back pain. Spine 1992;17(6):617–28.

[161] Chaffin DB, Herrin GD, Keyserling WM. Preemployment strength testing: an updated position. J Occup Med 1978;20(6):403–8.

[162] Howell DW. Musculoskeletal profile and incidence of musculoskeletal injuries in lightweight women rowers. Am J Sports Med 1984;12(4):278–82.

[163] Hasue M, Fujiwara M, Kikuchi S. A new method of quantitative measurement of abdominal and back muscle strength. Spine 1980;5(2):143–8.

[164] Langrana NA, Lee CK, Alexander H, et al. Quantitative assessment of back strength using isokinetic testing. Spine 1984;9(3):287–90.

[165] Malchaire JB, Masset DF. Isometric and dynamic performances of the trunk and associated factors. Spine 1995;20(15):1649–56.

[166] McNeill T, Warwick D, Andersson G, et al. Trunk strengths in attempted flexion, extension, and lateral bending in healthy subjects and patients with low-back disorders. Spine 1980;5(6):529–38.

[167] Nordgren B, Schele R, Linroth K. Evaluation and prediction of back pain during military field service. Scand J Rehabil Med 1980;12(1):1–8.

[168] Rowe ML. Preliminary statistical study of low back pain. J Occup Med 1963;5:336–41.

[169] Nachemson A, Lindh M. Measurement of abdominal and back muscle strength with and without low back pain. Scand J Rehabil Med 1969;1(2):60–3.

[170] Reimer DS, Halbrook BD, Dreyfuss PH, et al. A novel approach to preemployment worker fitness evaluations in a material-handling industry. Spine 1994;19(18):2026–32.

[171] Keyserling WM, Herrin GD, Chaffin DB. Isometric strength testing as a means of controlling medical incidents on strenuous jobs. J Occup Med 1980;22(5):332–6.

[172] Leino P, Aro S, Hasan J. Trunk muscle function and low back disorders: a ten-year follow-up study. J Chronic Dis 1987;40(4):289–96.

[173] Mostardi RA, Noe DA, Kovacik MW, et al. Isokinetic lifting strength and occupational injury: a prospective study. Spine 1992;17(2):189–93.

[174] Nadler SF, Malanga GA, Feinberg JH, et al. Relationship between hip muscle imbalance and occurrence of low back pain in collegiate athletes: a prospective study. Am J Phys Med Rehabil 2001;80(8):572–7.

[175] Hansson T, Bigos S, Beecher P, et al. The lumbar lordosis in acute and chronic low-back pain. Spine 1985;10(2):154–5.

[176] Magora A. Investigation of the relation between low back pain and occupation. Physical requirements: sitting, standing, and weight lifting. Ind Med Surg 1972;41:5–9.

[177] Redfield JT. The low back x-ray as a pre-employment screening tool in the forest products industry. J Occup Med 1971;13(5):219–26.

[178] McGill SM, Hughson RL, Parks K. Changes in lumbar lordosis modify the role of the extensor muscles. Clin Biomech (Bristol, Avon) 2000;15(10):777–80.

[179] Porter SE, Hanley EN Jr. The musculoskeletal effects of smoking. J Am Acad Orthop Surg 2001;9(1):9–17.

[180] Leboeuf-Yde C. Smoking and low back pain: a systematic literature review of 41 journal articles reporting 47 epidemiologic studies. Spine 1999;24(14):1463–70.

[181] Leboeuf-Yde C, Kyvik KO, Bruun NH. Low back pain and lifestyle. Part I. Smoking: information from a population-based sample of 29,424 twins. Spine 1998;23(20):2207–13 [discussion: 2214].

[182] Tsai SP, Gilstrap EL, Cowles SR, et al. Personal and job characteristics of musculoskeletal injuries in an industrial population. J Occup Med 1992;34(6):606–12.

[183] Jensen R. Epidemiology of work-related back pain. Top Acute Care Trauma Rehabilitation 1988;2:1–15.

[184] Rys M, Konz S. An evaluation on floor surfaces. Presented at the Proceedings of Human Factors Society 33rd Annual Meeting. Denver, CO, October 16–20, 1989.

[185] Kottke FJ. Evaluation and treatment of low back pain due to mechanical causes. Arch Phys Med Rehabil 1961;42:426–40.

[186] Kumar S. Cumulative load as a risk factor for back pain. Spine 1990;15(12):1311–6.

[187] Hartvigsen J, Leboeuf-Yde C, Lings S, et al. Is sitting-while-at-work associated with low back pain? A systematic, critical literature review. Scand J Public Health 2000;28(3):230–9.

[188] Ryan GA. The prevalence of musculo-skeletal symptoms in supermarket workers. Ergonomics 1989;32(4):359–71.

[189] Cook J, Branch TP, Baranowski TJ, et al. The effect of surgical floor mats in prolonged standing: an EMG study of the lumbar paraspinal and anterior tibialis muscles. J Biomed Eng 1993;15(3):247–50.

[190] Troussier B, Lamalle Y, Charruel C, et al. Socioeconomic incidences and prognostic factors of low back pain caused by occupational injuries among the hospital personnel of Grenoble University Hospital Center. Rev Rhum Ed Fr 1993;60(2):144–51.

[191] Redfern M, Chaffin D. Influence of flooring on standing fatigue. Hum Factors 1995;37:570–81.

[192] Macfarlane GJ, Thomas E, Papageorgiou AC, et al. Employment and physical work activities as predictors of future low back pain. Spine 1997;22(10):1143–9.

[193] Cham R, Redfern MS. Effect of flooring on standing comfort and fatigue. Hum Factors 2001;43(3):381–91.

[194] Rys M, Konz S. Carpet vs. concrete. Presented at Proceedings of Human Factors Society 32nd Annual Meeting. Santa Monica, CA, October 22–24, 1988.

[195] Lonz S, Vaandla V, Rtys M, et al. Standing on concrete vs. floor mats. In: Das B, editor. Advances in industrial ergonomics and safety. Taylor & Francis; 1990. p. 991–8.

[196] Ikata T. Statistical and dynamic studies of lesions due to overloading on the spine. Shikoku Acta Med 1965;40:262.

[197] Lloyd MH, Gauld S, Soutar CA. Epidemiologic study of back pain in miners and office workers. Spine 1986;11(2):136–40.

[198] Health NIfOSa. Work practices guide for manual lifting. Cincinnati (OH): National Institute for Occupational Safety and Health; 1981. p. 81–122.

[199] Waters TR, Putz-Anderson V, Garg A, et al. Revised NIOSH equation for the design and evaluation of manual lifting tasks. Ergonomics 1993;36(7):749–76.

[200] Chaffin DB, Park KS. A longitudinal study of low-back pain as associated with occupational weight lifting factors. Am Ind Hyg Assoc J 1973;34(12):513–25.

[201] de Looze MP, Toussaint HM, van Dieen JH, Kemper HC. Joint moments and muscle activity in the lower extremities and lower back in lifting and lowering tasks. J Biomech 1993; 26(9):1067–76.

[202] Gagnon M, Smyth G. Biomechanical exploration on dynamic modes of lifting. Ergonomics 1992;35(3):329–45.

[203] Grieve D. Dynamic characteristics of man during crouch-and-stoop-lifting. In: Nelson R, Moorehouse C, editors. Biomechanics. Baltimore: University Park Press; 1074. p. 19–29.

[204] Chen Y. Changes in lifting dynamics after localized arm fatigue. Int J Ind Ergonom 2000; 28:611–9.

[205] Lavender SA, Li YC, Andersson GB, et al. The effects of lifting speed on the peak external forward bending, lateral bending, and twisting spine moments. Ergonomics 1999;42(1): 111–25.

[206] Lariviere C, Gagnon D, Loisel P. A biomechanical comparison of lifting techniques between subjects with and without chronic low back pain during freestyle lifting and lowering tasks. Clin Biomech (Bristol, Avon) 2002;17(2):89–98.

[207] Norris C. Biomechanics of the lumbar spine. In: Norris C, editor. Back stability. Champaign (IL): Human Kinetics Publishers; 2000. p. 14–42.

[208] de Looze M, Dolan P, Kingma I, et al. Does an asymmetric straddle-legged lifting movement reduce the low-back load? Hum Mov Sci 1998;17:243–59.

[209] Dolan P, Earley M, Adams MA. Bending and compressive stresses acting on the lumbar spine during lifting activities. J Biomech 1994;27(10):1237–48.

[210] McGill S. Low back biomechanics in industry: the prevention of injury through safer lifting. In: Grabiner M, editor. Current issues in biomechanics. Champaign (IL): Human Kinetics; 1993. p. 69–120.

[211] van Dieen JH, Hoozemans MJ, Toussaint HM. Stoop or squat: a review of biomechanical studies on lifting technique. Clin Biomech (Bristol, Avon) 1999;14(10):685–96.

[212] Park K, Chaffin D. A biomechanical evaluation of two methods of manual load lifting. AIIE Transactions 1974;6:105–13.

[213] Minor SD. Use of back belts in occupational settings. Phys Ther 1996;76(4):403–8.

[214] Mitchell LV, Lawler FH, Bowen D, et al. Effectiveness and cost-effectiveness of employer-issued back belts in areas of high risk for back injury. J Occup Med 1994;36(1):90–4.

[215] Reddell CR, Congleton JJ, Dale Huchingson R, et al. An evaluation of a weightlifting belt and back injury prevention training class for airline baggage handlers. Appl Ergon 1992; 23(5):319–29.

[216] Garg A, Badger D. Maximum acceptable weights and maximum voluntary isometric strengths for asymmetric lifting. Ergonomics 1986;29(7):879–92.

[217] McGill SM. The influence of lordosis on axial trunk torque and trunk muscle myoelectric activity. Spine 1992;17(10):1187–93.

[218] Mital A, Karwowski W, Mazouz AK, et al. Prediction of maximum acceptable weight of lift in the horizontal and vertical planes using simulated job dynamic strengths. Am Ind Hyg Assoc J 1986;47(5):288–92.

[219] Schultz AB, Andersson GB, Haderspeck K, et al. Analysis and measurement of lumbar trunk loads in tasks involving bends and twists. J Biomech 1982;15(9):669–75.

[220] Lawrence JS. Rheumatism in coal miners. III. Occupational factors. Br J Ind Med 1955; 12(3):249–61.

[221] Marras WS, Lavender SA, Leurgans SE, et al. The role of dynamic three-dimensional trunk motion in occupationally-related low back disorders: the effects of workplace factors, trunk position, and trunk motion characteristics on risk of injury. Spine 1993;18(5):617–28.

[222] Association ISS. Vibration at work. Paris: Institut National De Recherche Et De Securite; 1989.

[223] Boshuizen HC, Bongers PM, Hulshof CT. Self-reported back pain in tractor drivers exposed to whole-body vibration. Int Arch Occup Environ Health 1990;62(2):109–15.

[224] Boshuizen HC, Bongers PM, Hulshof CT. Self-reported back pain in fork-lift truck and freight-container tractor drivers exposed to whole-body vibration. Spine 1992;17(1):59–65.

[225] Bovenzi M, Betta A. Low-back disorders in agricultural tractor drivers exposed to whole-body vibration and postural stress. Appl Ergon 1994;25(4):231–41.

[226] Bovenzi M, Zadini A. Self-reported low back symptoms in urban bus drivers exposed to whole-body vibration. Spine 1992;17(9):1048–59.

[227] Brendstrup T, Biering-Sorensen F. Effect of fork-lift truck driving on low-back trouble. Scand J Work Environ Health 1987;13(5):445–52.

[228] Burton AK, Tillotson KM, Symonds TL, et al. Occupational risk factors for the first-onset and subsequent course of low back trouble: a study of serving police officers. Spine 1996; 21(22):2612–20.

[229] Jonsson B, Brulin C, Ericsson B, et al. Besvar fran roriseorgagen bland skogsmaskin forare. Solna, Sweden: National Board of Occupational Safety and Health; 1983.

[230] Magnusson M, Wilder DG, Pope M, et al. Investigation of the long-term exposure to whole-body vibration: a two-country study. Eur J Phys Med Rehabil 1993;3:28–34.

[231] Burdorf A, Naaktgeboren B, de Groot HC. Occupational risk factors for low back pain among sedentary workers. J Occup Med 1993;35(12):1213–20.

[232] Schwarze S, Notbohm G, Dupuis H, et al. Dose-response relationships between whole-body vibration and lumbar disk disease: a field study on 388 drivers of different vehicles. J Sound Vib 1998;215:613–28.

[233] Xu Y, Bach E, Orhede E. Work environment and low back pain: the influence of occupational activities. Occup Environ Med 1997;54(10):741–5.

[234] Lings S, Leboeuf-Yde C. Whole-body vibration and low back pain: a systematic, critical review of the epidemiological literature 1992–1999. Int Arch Occup Environ Health 2000;73(5):290–7.

ELSEVIER
SAUNDERS

Clin Occup Environ Med
5 (3) 529–544

CLINICS IN
OCCUPATIONAL AND
ENVIRONMENTAL
MEDICINE

Prevention Strategies for Occupational Low Back Pain

Bryan D. Kaplansky, MD[a],*, Frank Y. Wei, MD[b],
Mark V. Reecer, MD[c]

[a]Summit Spine and Sports Medicine, P.C., 3828 New Vision Drive,
Fort Wayne, IN 46845, USA
[b]Southdale Office Center, 6600 France Avenue S., Edina, MN 55435, USA
[c]Fort Wayne Physical Medicine, 5750 Coventry Lane, Fort Wayne, IN 46804, USA

Back pain, the most common musculoskeletal condition affecting the working population, represents 25–40% of workers' compensation claims [1]. The resultant economic cost of occupational low back pain (LBP) is likewise over-whelming: the cost for occupational LBP in the United States has been estimated at up to $100 billion per year [1] and continues to rise [2]. In light of the enormous socioeconomic impact of occupational LBP and disability, several prevention strategies continue to be studied and implemented, including (1) education and training, (2) exercise, (3) ergonomics, (4) risk factor modification, (5) worker selection, and (6) orthotics.

There are three levels of prevention. Primary prevention involves measures to prevent the occurrence of LBP. Secondary prevention involves measures that attempt to reduce the prevalence of LBP through early detection and treatment. Tertiary prevention involves strategies that minimize the consequences of LBP by reducing chronic impairment and disability.

Most prevention programs address primary prevention of LBP in the workplace. However, there is considerable overlap among the primary, secondary, and tertiary prevention strategies for occupational LBP. For example, education and training, exercise programs, risk factor modification, and ergonomics interventions can be used at the primary, secondary, and tertiary levels of prevention.

The goals of these prevention strategies pertain to both the worker and industry. These goals include (1) reducing the incidence and prevalence

This article was originally published in Occupational Medicine: State of the Art Reviews 1998;13(1):33–45.

* Corresponding author.
E-mail address: kapbd1@comcast.net (B.D. Kaplansky).

of low back injuries, (2) reducing chronic disability and restoring function, (3) keeping the worker on the job, (4) improving productivity, and (5) reducing the socioeconomic costs of occupational LBP.

Education and training

Education and training are common strategies used in industry to prevent LBP. Education techniques range from simply providing workers with printed material about biomechanics and lifting techniques to the more comprehensive "back schools." The education of supervisors and management is considered an important aspect of secondary and tertiary prevention of LBP and disability.

Lifting techniques

Lifting is an occupational activity associated with an increased risk for LBP [3,4]. Several factors have been considered in evaluating lifting techniques, including the compressive forces on the lumbar spine, energy expenditure, ratings of perceived exertion, lifting strength, and productivity. In an effort to lessen the risk for low back injuries, numerous lifting techniques have been described and recommended [5–11].

Although a few studies have reported benefits of certain techniques based on biomechanical and physiologic data [5,6,10], there is still no consensus on the safest lifting technique with respect to the prevention of occupational LBP [8,12–14]. Prospective studies that have compared workers trained to use certain lifting techniques to those without such training have reported contradictory results with respect to LBP prevention in the workplace [15–19]. Most of the studies noted no significant differences between the trained and untrained groups. Furthermore, some commonly prescribed lifting techniques, such as the squat lifting posture, may actually be detrimental under certain working conditions [20].

While a specific lifting technique cannot be recommended, several practical recommendations can be made. Keeping the lifted object as close as possible to the center of gravity of the body is a biomechanical principle that is well supported in the literature [12,21]. Other recommendations include pivoting with the feet instead of twisting with the load, lifting in a smooth and controlled manner, and avoiding overexertion [20]. The use of mechanical aids also may prevent some forms of LBP in the workplace by reducing the load and postural stress.

Back schools

Back school programs vary but usually incorporate a group format. The more comprehensive programs educate individuals about anatomy and physiology, mechanisms of injury, the natural history of disorders, fitness, stress and pain relationships, risk factor modification, and proper posture and body mechanics for material and nonmaterial handling activities. Comprehensive back schools usually consist of 1–2 day programs, although they may last longer, and most occur at the workplace. These education programs are most frequently used at the primary level but are also incorporated at secondary and tertiary levels. The goals of education programs for workers include establishing a greater knowledge of injury prevention strategies, emphasizing the importance of compliance with treatment programs, and developing an understanding that back pain is usually benign and self-limited.

The scientific literature concerning educational programs for the prevention of LBP is contradictory. Physician-directed education about LBP in symptomatic patient appears to help increase patient compliance, reduce health care use, and increase patient satisfaction in the general population [22–24]. It also may reduce sick leave in the occupational setting [25]. However, the efficacy of structured back schools in the workplace is unproven. Controlled studies report contradictory results with respect to back school and LBP prevention [26–33]. A recent randomized, controlled study evaluated the effectiveness of an education program designed to prevent LBP injury in 4000 postal workers [34]. The education program consisted of a back school followed by three or four reinforcement sessions. The follow-up period was 5.5 years. The authors reported that the education program "did not reduce the rate of low back injuries, the median cost per injury, the time off of work per injury, or the rate of repeated injury after return to work." A meta-analysis regarding back schools noted insufficient evidence to support conclusively the use of back schools [35]. Currently, there is little evidence to support structured educational strategies to prevent LBP in the workplace.

Management training

Employers and their management staffs may play an important role in the prevention of occupational LBP. Garg and Moore described potentially effective prevention strategies that can be used by management, including a "positive acceptance" of worker-reported LBP, a company policy of encouraging workers to report all episodes of LBP, early intervention and conservative treatment, appropriate follow-up of the worker's treatment and progress, keeping the injured employee at work in some capacity, job analysis, and the enforcement of safety rules [8]. Key barriers to the secondary and tertiary prevention of occupational LBP include delays in the onset of treatment, reliance upon inappropriate decision-makers for returning an employee to work or an inadequate return to work plan, limited return to work alternatives, inappropriate use of disability determination guidelines, failure to recognize the psychosocial aspects of disability, and a lack of a coordinated effort by the employer, employee, and physician [36].

Clinical trials have underscored the importance of formulating a return to work plan during rehabilitation efforts by reporting better return-to-work rates [37] and less subsequent disability [38]. Similar beneficial effects of a return-to-work plan within the chronic pain population have been reported [39]. Hall et al. extended the philosophy of an early return to work for symptomatic patients even further by noting in a prospective study that the probability of a successful return to regular duty work increased with the recommendation of returning to work without restrictions [40]. The probability of failure increased when restrictions were outlined.

The socioeconomic implications of a delayed return to work are well-known. Most costs for occupational LBP are related to indemnity costs [2], underscoring the importance of secondary and tertiary prevention and a return-to-work strategy. This, combined with the fact that the probability of an injured worker ever returning to the job decreases as the length of time off work increases [41], has serious consequences for the system. Although it is the physician's role to determine work capacity and an appropriate return-to-work plan, industry should be a willing and able partner in this difficult process.

Exercise

Exercise programs have focused on the development of strength, flexibility, and endurance. Various types of exercise programs have been investigated, including stretching and strengthening exercises, aerobics, work simulation/conditioning, and computer-assisted training that may involve isometric, isotonic, or isokinetic methods.

The scientific literature is contradictory with respect to the effectiveness of exercise for LBP prevention in the workplace. One of the few studies that examined the efficacy of exercise for the primary prevention of LBP evaluated firefighters with no history of LBP [42]. After 4 years of observation, the authors concluded that the more physically fit firefighters clearly had lower injury rates. The same authors evaluated back-related medical costs, comparing workers with different degrees of flexibility and back strength. Firefighters with less flexible backs had medical costs seven times higher than their more flexible counterparts; those with weaker backs had a threefold increase in back-related medical costs [43].

More frequently, studies have evaluated the effectiveness of exercise for secondary and tertiary prevention of LBP. Although the findings are somewhat contradictory, exercise appears to have a beneficial effect for the prevention of LBP [44–46]. Exercising was most beneficial when customized for specific conditions [46]. The greater the intensity of the exercises, the greater the benefit to the individual [47]. Exercise was also noted to be beneficial only as long as it was practiced; discontinuation of the exercise program resulted in no sustainable benefit to the individual [44].

In addition, several controlled studies have reported the benefits of exercise for secondary and tertiary prevention of LBP, including those reporting a reduction in symptoms and a statistically significant decrease in missed work days due to low back pain [27,48,49]. A recent randomized, comparative, multicenter trial evaluated the effects of exercise in patients with LBP [50]. The 12-month supervised stretching and strengthening program was individualized, with some patients using a training apparatus. The authors reported that the exercise programs led to a significant reduction in absenteeism (75–80%). The benefit from the exercise program persisted during the subsequent unsupervised 12-month follow-up period even though compliance with the program diminished. However, other studies have reported limited benefits of exercise for LBP prevention [15,51–55].

Several studies have evaluated combined strategies for prevention of LBP. Bergquist-Ullman and Larsson divided auto workers with recent back injuries into three groups: (1) back school with active exercise, (2) active exercise with manual therapy, and (3) passive modalities [56]. There was no significant difference in the recurrences of LBP or the number of sick days due to LBP between the groups within 1 year after completing the initial treatment. However, the length of symptom duration was significantly less for the active exercise groups.

A randomized, prospective investigation by Lindstrom et al. studied Swedish auto workers with an 8-week sick leave due to subacute, nonspecific, mechanical LBP [57]. The studied group underwent a graded exercise program, back education, functional capacity measurements, and a worksite evaluation. During the 2-year follow-up, the studied group had significantly less sick leave due to LBP.

Other controlled studies have reported the benefits of combined prevention regimens [39,58,59]. Improvements included a reduction of symptoms, a reduction in recurrent LBP, improved function, and diminished sick leave or an earlier return to work.

Further controlled and randomized studies need to be performed to elucidate the value of exercise for LBP prevention. Defining which outcome parameters are most important is also of value because there are a multitude of studies with different assessment methods [60]. It appears that a higher level of fitness may provide a protective effect against low back injury and does seem to correlate with a more rapid resolution of symptoms and an earlier return to work.

Ergonomics

Ergonomics involves the study of the interaction between a worker and his environment. Job design is an ergonomic approach, the goal of which is to match the workplace with the worker. Since "overexertion" while maneuvering objects is the most common event leading to injury in the workplace [61], job design theoretically should benefit both the employee and employer by:

1. Increasing worker safety by decreasing the risk for injury,
2. Diminishing the risk for chronic symptoms/disability,
3. Keeping the worker working, matching the work task to the worker's capabilities,
4. Improving the productivity, and
5. Reducing corporate medical and disability costs.

A knowledge of risk factors for occupational LBP is the first step in an ergonomic evaluation. Static postures, heavy physical work demands, frequent bending and stooping, twisting, sudden and unexpected movements, exposure to vibration, and job tasks that involve lifting, pushing, and pulling are physical factors that are often linked to an increase in the occurrence of back pain [3,62]. Likewise, there are several psychological and social risk factors [63–68].

The next step in an ergonomics evaluation involves job analysis [69], a process that combines the study of biomechanical, physiologic, and psychophysical criteria to determine reasonable loads for workers. In addition to worker and task characteristics, the work station, equipment, materials, and the environment also are analyzed.

Various ergonomic tools, including biomechanical and psychophysical models, have been developed to facilitate the process of job analysis and job design [70–82]. Specific ergonomic design criteria based on the available models have been reported. These criteria include acceptable limits for compressive forces, strength, energy expenditure, heart rate, postural stress, and perceived stress [20]. The National Institute for Occupational Safety and Health (NIOSH) revised its 1981 [83] lifting equation in 1991 [84] in an attempt to determine recommended weight limits for workers. The revised lifting equation reflects a greater variety of lifting tasks. A lifting index or an "index of relative physical stress" was also described to protect workers from hazardous loads [84]. Despite widespread acceptance and usage of the revised NIOSH guidelines, however, there is no universally accepted method of determining a safe lifting capacity, and the equation has not been fully validated.

Despite a lack of validated assessment tools, job design is considered the most effective means of prevention for low back injuries in the workplace [20,85]. Snook et al. noted in a retrospective study that job design can reduce back injuries associated with manual handling tasks by 33% [85]. A prospective epidemiologic study evaluating nursing assistants in a nursing home noted a 50% drop in the incidence rate for back injuries after a job design program was implemented [86]. The program included mechanical aids and other interventions to reduce the physical demands of the job. The authors also reported that there were no lost or restricted work days due to back injuries after the ergonomics intervention.

Although job design may hold the most promise as a prevention strategy, there is a lack of controlled studies evaluating the efficacy of ergonomics for LBP prevention. It is still not clear how beneficial job design is with respect to reducing the incidence of low back injuries [87,88]. There are several reported possible reasons for the lack of meaningful ergonomic studies, including (1) the generally high cost of intervention, (2) lack of participation and commitment to ergonomic principles, (3) difficulty in identifying the specific ergonomic changes needed, (4) uncertainty as to what outcome parameters to use, and (5) poor study protocols [87].

Several authors have reported the importance of reducing the physical demands of the job so that they are within the physical capacity of most of the working population [11,79,80,85,89–93]. Others have argued that setting limits on lifting will have little impact on the incidence of LBP but may have a significant impact on disability by enabling the worker with low back symptoms or dysfunction to remain on the job [78,94]. Debate continues as to whether ergonomic intervention is effective at the primary prevention level for LBP or whether ergonomic efforts should focus on secondary and tertiary prevention strategies.

Risk factor modification

Several individual characteristics and their potential association with LBP have been studied, including a person's age, sex, posture, spinal mobility, strength and fitness, weight, and tobacco usage [3]. Smoking and obesity are modifiable risk factors that have been of particular interest. Both smoking [3,45,95,96] and obesity [3,45,96] have been linked to LBP in prospective and cross-sectional studies. However, other contradictory studies regarding these risk factors indicate that a definite relationship to LBP has not been established [3]. Furthermore, there is a lack of prospective trials evaluating whether modification of these risk factors alters the prevalence of LBP and disability [45].

It is unclear whether modification of risk factors can lead to prevention of LBP [45]. However, encouraging workers to improve their general health by normalizing their weight and stopping smoking is time well spent.

Worker selection

The primary goal of preemployment screening is to identify individuals who are at increased risk for low back injuries so that the potential for injury can be minimized. The three primary methods of worker selection are radiologic screening, medical history/examination, and preemployment strength testing.

The strategy of worker selection has considerable medicolegal ramifications. Preemployment clinical information cannot be used to screen out a worker who can physically perform the essential tasks of the job for which he or she is applying [97]. Nonetheless, employers continue to use the worker selection strategies described below in an effort to prevent LBP.

Radiographic screening

The use of preplacement radiography to screen out potential workers who are thought to be at greater risk for low back injuries has been controversial. Although some companies still use this method to evaluate potential employees, the practice of preplacement screening radiography has fallen out of favor. While spondylolisthesis may be a radiographic abnormality that is seen more often in persons with LBP than in asymptomatic individuals [98], most of the scientific literature reports that screening radiography is not predictive for future LBP [98–102].

The lack of predictive value for radiographs is likely multifactorial. Plain x-rays tend to correlate poorly with most low back disorders [99,101]. Symptomatic individuals frequently have normal spine x-rays while asymptomatic volunteers frequently demonstrate abnormalities on plain x-rays. X-ray findings rarely alter a clinician's treatment plan. The cost of spinal x-rays usually outweighs the potential benefits [102] that are obtained for most low back disorders. Furthermore, the cause of LBP is often multifactorial in the industrial setting [103], and in most cases, a specific anatomic etiology for LBP may be elusive even with imaging studies. For these reasons, spinal x-rays are not recommended as a screening tool to prevent LBP.

Medical history/physical examination

The preemployment clinical examination is still the most common screening technique used in industry to screen out individuals with previous back disorders [104].

One large prospective study evaluated the effectiveness of the preemployment history and physical examination as a screening method for acute industrial back pain [104]. While the authors reported risk factors for occupational LBP based on an individual's history, they found that the physical examination findings added no significant predictive value for future LBP.

An additional prospective study evaluating applicants for light duty work at a telephone company reported similar results [105]. The authors concluded that a preplacement medical evaluation for light duty assignments was not predictive for future work attendance or job performance and was not found to be cost-effective.

Preemployment strength testing

Preemployment strength testing is another controversial screening method that is still used in industry. Methods of testing strength include isometric, isokinetic, or isoinertial methods. The issue of which is the most appropriate type of test is debated in the literature [106–116]. Numerous studies have advocated the use of preemployment strength testing as a screening method to reduce low back injuries in the workplace [109,110,115,117,118]. However, numerous studies have likewise shown that preemployment strength testing is ineffective as a screening tool, whether isometric [51,112] or isokinetic and isoinertial testing methods are used [113,114,119]. In a prospective evaluation of shipyard workers, Mooney et al. found that preplacement isometric lumbar extensor strength is not a predictor of workplace injury [112]. The incidence of back injury claims was highest for the higher physical job demand classifications. There may be a risk associated with preemployment strength testing, therefore, in that it leads to the selection of certain individuals for more physically demanding work based on the erroneous assumption that their strength will protect them from subsequent back injuries [120].

Lumbar orthotics

Lumbar orthotics continue to be used in industry despite their controversial status. The theoretical biomechanical advantages of a lumbar corset include an increase in intraabdominal pressure and subsequent reduction in spinal loading during job tasks, limitation of spinal movement, and an increase in the lifting capacity for individuals. These theoretical benefits, however, are generally not supported by the most recent scientific literature [20]. Most studies have reported that intraabdominal pressure does not play a significant role in reducing the load on the spine and supporting back and abdominal musculature [20]. Furthermore, lumbar corsets do not have a significant effect on intraabdominal pressure [20].

The effect of lumbar corsets on range of motion is contradictory in the literature. Several authors have reported that lumbar orthotics reduce the gross range of motion of the lumbar spine [121–123]. Others have reported that lumbar orthotics do not have a stabilizing effect on the intervertebral mobility of the lower lumbar spine and may actually lead to a paradoxical increase in the level of intervertebral motion in certain individuals [124].

Furthermore, limited data exist on the interaction between lumbar orthotics and lifting capacity. In a study of back belts and manual lifting, McCoy et al. concluded that back belts increased a worker's perceived maximum acceptable lifting weight compared with the perceived lifting weight without the use of lumbar orthosis [125]. However, there were insufficient data to predict reliably how a worker's risk of low back injury would be affected by this change in perception. Other authors have reported that lumbar belts do not have a significant effect on lifting capacity [126].

Few clinical studies have evaluated the use of lumbar orthotics for the prevention of LBP in the workplace. A retrospective review of 1316 workers who performed lifting activities on a military base noted that back belts were only minimally effective at preventing injury [127]. Furthermore, the overall cost per injury was substantially higher for workers who had been wearing a back belt compared with those who were not wearing a back belt. The authors concluded that back belt use was not efficacious or cost-effective for prevention of low back injury.

Two controlled studies evaluated the use of lumbar orthotics. Walsh and Schwartz published a randomized observer-blinded protocol using grocery warehouse workers [128]. Three groups were evaluated: (1) those completing an education program, (2) those receiving both an education program and a lumbar corset, and (3) a control group. While there was a statistically significant decrease in lost workdays for the group that received both education and the lumbar corset, there was no significant difference with respect to the low back injury rate and productivity. It is unclear whether the reduced absenteeism was due to the education program, the lumbar corset, or a combination of the two.

Reddell also reported a controlled study evaluating baggage handlers [129]. The study groups included (1) individuals with a lumbar belt, (2) those receiving 1 hour of training, (3) those receiving both the belt and 1 hour of training, and (4) a control group. No significant difference among the groups with regard to low back injury rate or lost or restricted workdays was found.

There are potential risks for workers wearing lumbar orthotics. Long-term use of a lumbar corset may result in physical dependence and a loss of abdominal muscle tone [121]. Other investigators, however, have reported no adverse effects in terms of abdominal muscle strength from wearing lumbar orthoses [128,130,131]. An increase in low back injuries and lost workdays also has been reported in individuals who used a lumbar belt and then discontinued its use [129]. Increased worker complaints from the direct effects of the orthosis itself also have been reported [128,129]. Studies have reported that lumbar orthoses can adversely affect the cardiovascular system by increasing systolic blood pressure and heart rate [132,133]. A worker may be at even greater risk when using a lumbar orthosis because the individual may attempt to lift more weight [122] due to his or her inappropriate perception that an orthosis provides increased security.

In summary, no conclusive scientific literature is available to support the use of lumbar orthotics in the workplace. Although is is unlikely that there are any severe adverse effects from using a lumbar orthosis in healthy workers, there is no evidence to suggest that the use of lumbar orthotics is an effective prevention strategy.

Summary

Among the strategies to prevent occupational LBP, only job design/rede sign and exercise programs appear to have a protective effect; however, the studies pertaining to exercise remain contradictory, and controlled trials evaluating ergonomics interventions are lacking. Risk factor modification is beneficial from a general health perspective, but studies are contradictory with respect to its role in prevention of LBP. There is no conclusive evidence to support the use of structured education programs in the workplace, and the cost of these programs is not justified. There is no support for the use of orthotics or worker selection methods based on the available data, and these methods should not be employed in the workplace.

Despite efforts from the medical community and industry, there is little evidence that there has been a substantial impact on the prevalence of LBP and disability. Further work is needed in both occupational and non-occupational settings to determine effective prevention strategies for LBP in the future.

Acknowledgments

The authors thank Joan Burton, RN, and Leslie Kaplansky for their assistance in preparing the manuscript.

References

[1] Frymoyer JW. Cost and control of industrial musculoskeletal injuries. In: Nordin M, Andersson G, Pope M, editors. Musculoskeletal disorders in the workplace: principles and practice. Chicago: Mosby; 1997. p. 62–71.

[2] Webster BS, Snook SH. The cost of 1989 workers' compensation low back pain claims. Spine 1993;19:1111–6.

[3] Andersson GBJ. The epidemiology of spinal disorders. In: Frymoyer JW, editor. The adult spine: principles and practice. New York: Raven; 1997. p. 93–142.

[4] Andersson GBJ. Epidemiologic aspects on low back pain in industry. Spine 1981;6:53–60.

[5] Adams MA, Hutton WC. The effect of posture on the lumbar spine. J Bone Joint Surg Br 1985;67B:625–9.

[6] Anderson CK, Chaffin DB. A biomechanical evaluation of five lifting techniques. Appl Ergon 1986;17:2–8.

[7] Calliet R. Low back pain syndrome. 4th edition. Philadelphia: FA Davis; 1988.

[8] Garg A, Moore JS. Prevention strategies and the low back industry. Occup Med 1992;7: 629–40.

[9] Nachemson A. Low back pain: its etiology and treatment. Clin Med 1971;78:18–24.

[10] Parke KS, Chaffin DB. A biomechanical evaluation of two methods of manual load lifting. AIIE Trans 1974;6:105–13.

[11] Snook SH. The design of manual handling tasks. Ergonomics 1978;21:963–85.

[12] Andersson GBJ, Ortengren R, Nachemson A. Quantitative studies of back loads in lifting. Spine 1976;1:178–85.

[13] Garg A, Herrin GD. Stoop or squat: a biomechanical and metabolic evaluation. AIIE Trans 1979;11:293–302.

[14] Songcharoen P, Chotigavanich C, Thanapipatsiri S. Lumbar paraspinal compartment pressure in back muscle exercise. J Spinal Disord 1994;7:49–53.

[15] Dehlin O, Berg S, Hedenrud B, et al. Effect of physical training and ergonomic counseling on the psychological perception of work and on the subjective assessment of low back in sufficiency. Scand J Rehabil Med 1981;13:1–9.

[16] Feldstein A, Valanis B, Vollmer W, et al. The back injury prevention project pilot study: assessing the effectiveness of back attack. An injury prevention program among nurses, aides, and orderlies. J Occup Med 1993;35:114–20.

[17] Harber P, Pena L, Hsu P, et al. Personal history, training, and worksite as predictors of back pain of nurses. Am J Ind Med 1994;25:519–26.

[18] Videman T, Rauhala H, Lindstrom K, et al. Patient-handling skill, back injuries, and back pain: an intervention study in nursing. Spine 1989;14:148–56.

[19] Wood DJ. Design and evaluation of a back injury prevention program within a geriatric hospital. Spine 1987;12:77–82.

[20] Garg A. Manual material handling: the science. In: Nordin M, Andersson G, Pope M, editors. Musculoskeletal disorders in the workplace: principles and practice. Chicago: Mosby; 1997. p. 85–119.

[21] Leskinen TPJ, Stalhammar HR, Kuorinka IAA. A dynamic analysis of spinal compression with different lifting techniques. Ergonomics 1983;26:595–604.

[22] Deyo RA, Diehl AK. Patient satisfaction with medical care for low-back pain. Spine 1986; 11:28–30.

[23] Jones SL, Jones PK, Katz J. Compliance for low-back pain patients in the emergency department: a randomized trial. Spine 1988;13:553–6.

[24] Roland M, Dixon M. Randomized controlled trial of an educational booklet for patients presenting with back pain in general practice. J R Coll Gen Pract 1989;39:244–6.

[25] Indahl A, Velund L, Reikeraas O. Good prognosis for low back pain when left untampered: a randomized clinical trial. Spine 1995;20:473–7.

[26] Daltroy LH, Iversen MD, Larson MG, et al. Teaching and social support: effects on knowledge, attitudes, and behaviors to prevent low back injuries in industry. Health Educ Q 1993;20:43–62.

[27] Donchin M, Woolf O, Kaplan L, et al. Secondary prevention of low back pain: a clinical trial. Spine 1990;15:1317–20.

[28] Klaber Moffett JA, Chase SM, Portek I, et al. A controlled prospective study to evaluate the effectiveness of a back school in the relief of chronic low back pain. Spine 1986;11:120–2.

[29] Lankhorst GJ, Van de Stadt RJ, Vogelaar TW, et al. The effect of the Swedish back school in chronic idiopathic low back pain: a prospective controlled study. Scand J Rehabil Med 1983;15:141–5.

[30] Leclaire R, Esdaile JM, Suissa S, et al. Back school in a first episode of compensated acute low back pain: a clinical trial to assess efficacy and prevent relapse. Arch Phys Med Rehabil 1996;77:673–9.

[31] McCauley M. The effect of body mechanics instruction on work performance among young workers. Am J Occup Ther 1990;44:402–7.

[32] Moffett JAK, Chase SM, Portek I, et al. A controlled, prospective study to evaluate the effectiveness of a back school in the relief of chronic low back pain. Spine 1986;11: 120–2.

[33] Versloot JM, Rozeman A, van Son AM, et al. The cost-effectiveness of a back school program in industry: a longitudinal controlled field study. Spine 1992;17:22–7.

[34] Daltroy LH, Iversen MD, Larson MG, et al. A controlled trial of an educational program to prevent low back injuries. N Engl J Med 1997;337:322–8.

[35] Linton SJ, Kamwendo K. Low back schools: a critical review. Phys Ther 1987;67: 1375–83.

[36] Mitchell S, Leclair S. Building a working alliance with employers: the politics of work disability. Phys Med Rehabil Clin North Am 1992;3:647–63.

[37] Catchlove R, Cohen K. Effects of a directive return to work approach in the treatment of workman's compensation patients with chronic pain. Pain 1982;14:181–91.

[38] Sanderson PL, Todd BD, Holt GR, et al. Compensation, work status, and disability in low back pain patients. Spine 1995;20:554–6.

[39] Mayer TG, Gatchel RJ, Mayer H, et al. A prospective two-year study of functional restoration in industrial low back injury: an objective assessment procedure. JAMA 1987;258: 1763–7.

[40] Hall H, McIntosh G, Melles T, et al. Effect of discharge recommendations on outcome. Spine 1994;19:2033–7.

[41] McGill CM. Industrial back problems: control program. J Occup Med 1968;10:174–8.

[42] Cady LD, Bischoff DP, O'Connell ER, et al. Strength and fitness and subsequent back injuries in firefighters. J Occup Med 1979;21:269–72.

[43] Cady LD, Thomas PC, Karwasky RJ. Program for increasing health and physical fitness of firefighters. J Occup Med 1985;27:110–4.

[44] Dillingham TR, DeLateur BJ. Exercise for low back pain: what really works? Phys Med Rehabil State Art Rev 1995;9:697–708.

[45] Lahad A, Malter AD, Berg AO, et al. The effectiveness of four interventions for the prevention of low back pain. JAMA 1994;272:1286–91.

[46] Scheer SJ, Radack KL, O'Brien DR Jr. Randomized controlled trials in industrial low back pain relating to return to work. Part I. Acute interventions. Arch Phys Med Rehabil 1995;76(Suppl):966–73.

[47] Manniche C, Lundberg E, Christensen I, et al. Intensive dynamic back exercises for chronic low back pain: a clinical trial. Pain 1991;47:53–63.

[48] Gundewall B, Liljequist M, Hansson T. Primary prevention of back symptoms and absence from work. Spine 1993;18:587–94.

[49] Kellett DM, Kellett DA, Nordholm LA. Effects of an exercise program on sick leave due to back pain. Phys Ther 1991;71:283–93.

[50] Ljunggren AE, Weber H, Kogstad O, et al. Effect of exercise on sick leave due to low back pain: a randomized, comparative, long-term study. Spine 1997;22:1610–7.

[51] Battie MC, Bigos SJ, Fischer LD, et al. Isometric lifting strength as a predictor of industrial back pain reports. Spine 1989;14:851–6.

[52] Battie MC, Bigos SJ, Fischer LD, et al. A prospective study of the role of cardiovascular risk factors and fitness in industrial back pain complaints. Spine 1989;l4:141–7.

[53] Battie MC, Bigos SJ, Fischer LD, et al. The role of spinal flexibility in back pain complaints within industry. Spine 1990;15:769–73.

[54] Cox M, Shephard RJ, Corey P. Influence of an employee fitness program upon fitness, productivity and absenteeism. Ergonomics 1981;24:795–806.

[55] Dehlin O, Berg S, Hedenrud B, et al. Muscle training, psychological perception of work and low back symptoms in nurses aides. Scand J Rehabil Med 1978;10:201–9.

[56] Bergquist-Ullman M, Larsson U. Acute low back pain in industry. Acta Orthop Scand Suppl 1977;170:100–13.

[57] Lindstrom I, Ohlund C, Eek C, et al. The effect of graded activity on patients with subacute low back pain: a randomized prospective clinical study with an operant-conditioning behavioral approach. Phys Ther 1992;72:279–90.

[58] Linton SJ, Bradley LA, Jensen I, et al. The second prevention of low back pain: a controlled study with follow-up. Pain 1989;36:197–207.

[59] Stankovic R, Johnell O. Conservative treatment of acute low-back pain: a prospective randomized trial. McKenzie method of treatment versus patient education in "mini back school". Spine 1990;l5:120–3.

[60] Kara BE, Conrad KM. Back injury prevention interventions in the workplace: an integrative review. AAOHN J 1996;44:189–96.

[61] US Department of Labor. Survey of occupational injuries and illnesses, 1994. Washington, DC: Bureau of Labor Statistics; 1996.

[62] Magora A, Tautsein I. An investigation to the problem of sick-leave in the patient suffering from low back pain. Ind Med Surg 1969;38:398–408.

[63] Bigos SJ, Battie MC, Spengler DM, et al. A prospective study of industrial work perceptions and psychosocial factors affecting the report of back injury. Spine 1991;16:1–6.

[64] Bongers PM, deWinter DR, Kompier MAJ, et al. Psychosocial factors at work and musculoskeletal disease. Scand J Work Environ Health 1993;19:297–312.

[65] Gatchel RJ, Polatin PB, Mayer TG. The dominant role of psychosocial risk factors in the development of chronic low back pain disability. Spine 1995;20:2702–9.

[66] Ingelgard A, Karlsson H, Nonas K, et al. Psychosocial and physical work environment factors at three workplaces dealing with materials handling. Int J Ind Ergon 1996;17:209–20.

[67] Papageorgiou AC, MacFarlane GJ, Thomas E, et al. Psychosocial factors in the workplace: do they predict new episodes of low back pain? Spine 1997;22:1137–42.

[68] Symonds TL, Burton AK, Tillotson KM, et al. Do attitudes and beliefs influence work loss due to low back trouble? Occup Med 1996;46:25–32.

[69] Scheer SJ, Mital A. Ergonomics. Arch Phys Med Rehabil 1997;78(Suppl):36–45.

[70] Genaidy A, Al-Shedi A, Shell RL. Ergonomic risk assessment: preliminary guidelines for analysis of repetition, force and posture. J Hum Ergol (Tokyo) 1993;22:45–55.

[71] Herrin GD, Jaraiedi M, Anderson CK. Prediction of overexertion injuries using biomechanical and psychophysical models. Am Ind Hyg Assoc J 1986;47:322–30.

[72] Juul-Kristensen B, Fallentin N, Ekdahl C. Criteria for classification of posture in repetitive work by observation methods: a review. Int J Ind Ergon 1997;19:397–411.

[73] Kumar S. Isolated planar trunk strength and mobility measurement for the normal and impaired backs. Part I. The devices. Int J Ind Ergon 1996;17:81–90.

[74] Kumar S. Trunk strength and mobility measurement for the normal and impaired backs. Part II. Protocol, software logic, and sample results. Int J Ind Ergon 1996;17:91–101.

[75] Kumar S. Isolated planar trunk strength measurements in normals. Part III. Results and database. Int J Ind Ergon 1996;17:103–11.

[76] Lee K, Waikar A, Aghaazadch F. Maximum acceptable weight of lift for side and back lifting. J Hum Ergol (Tokyo) 1990;19:3–11.

[77] Liles DH, et al. A job severity index for the evaluation and control of lifting injury. Hum Factors 1984;26:683–94.

[78] Snook SH. Psychophysical considerations in permissible loads. Ergonomics 1985;28: 327–30.

[79] Snook SH, Irvine CH, Bass SF. Maximum weights and work loads acceptable to male industrial workers: a study of lifting, lowering, pushing, pulling, carrying, and walking tasks. Am Ind Hyg Assoc J 1970;31:579–86.

[80] Snook SH, Ciriello VM. Maximum weights and work loads acceptable to female workers. J Occup Med 1974;16:527–34.

[81] Straker LM. Work-associated back problems: measurement problems. J Soc Occup Med 1991;41:41–4.

[82] Straker LM, Stevenson MG, Twomey LT. A comparison of risk assessment of single and combination manual handling tasks. I. Maximum acceptable weight measures. Ergonomics 1996;39:128–40.

[83] National Institute for Occupational Safety and Health. In: Work practices guide for manual lifting. Washington, DC: US Department of Health and Human Services, National Technical Information Service; 1981. p. 82.

[84] Waters TR, Putz-Anderson V, Garg A, et al. Revised NIOSH equation for the design and evaluation of manual lifting tasks. Ergonomics 1993;36:749–76.

[85] Snook SH, Campanelli RA, Hart JW. A study of three preventative approaches to low back injury. J Occup Med 1978;20:478–81.

[86] Garg A, Owen B. Reducing back stress to nursing personnel: an ergonomic intervention in a nursing home. Ergonomics 1992;35:1353–75.

[87] Frank JW, Kerr MS, Brooker AS, et al. Disability resulting from occupational low back pain. Part I. What do we know about primary prevention? A review of the scientific evidence on prevention before disability begins. Spine 1996;21:2908–17.

[88] Frank JW, Kerr MS, Brooker AS, et al. Disability resulting from occupational low back pain. Part II. What do we know about secondary prevention? A review of the scientific evidence on prevention after disability begins. Spine 1996;21:2918–29.

[89] Bink B. The physical working capacity in relation to working time and age. Ergonomics 1962;5:25–8.

[90] Chaffin DB, Andersson G. Occupational biomechanics. New York: Wiley; 1991.

[91] Chavalitsakulchai P, Shahnavaz H. Ergonomics method for prevention of the musculoskeletal discomforts among female industrial workers: physical characteristics and work factors. J Hum Ergol (Tokyo) 1993;22:95–113.

[92] Garg A, Chaffin DB, Herrin GD. Predictions of metabolic rates of manual materials handling jobs. Am Ind Hyg Assoc J 1978;39:661–74.

[93] Mital A. Are manual lifting weight limits based on the physiological approach realistic and practical? In: Asfour SS, editor. Trends in ergonomics/human factors. New York: Elsevier; 1987.

[94] Rowe ML. Low back disability in industry: updated position. J Occup Med 1971;13:476–8.

[95] Boshuizen HC, Verbeek AM, Broersen JPJ, et al. Do smokers get more back pain? Spine 1993;18:35–40.

[96] Deyo RA, Bass JE. Lifestyle and low-back pain: the influence of smoking and obesity. Spine 1989;14:501–6.

[97] Americans With Disabilities Act of 1990. Pub L No. 101–336, 104 Stat 327.

[98] Gibson ES. The value of preplacement screening radiography of the low back. Occup Med 1988;3:91–107.

[99] Bigos SJ, Hansson T, Castillo RN, et al. The value of pre-employment roentgenographs for predicting acute back injury claims and chronic back pain disability. Clin Orthop 1992;283: 124–9.

[100] Gibson ES, Martin MD, Terry CY. Incidence of low back pain and pre-placement x-ray screening. J Occup Med 1980;22:515.

[101] LaRocca H, Macnab I. Value of pre-employment radiographic assessment of the lumbar spine. Ind Med 1970;39:253–8.

[102] Rowe ML. Are routine spine films on workers in industry cost- or risk-benefit effective? J Occup Med 1992;24:41–3.

[103] Bigos SJ, Battie MC, Spengler DM, et al. A longitudinal, prospective study of industrial back injury reporting. Clin Orthop 1992;279:21–34.

[104] Bigos SJ, Battie MC, Fisher LD, et al. A prospective evaluation of preemployment screening methods for acute industrial back pain. Spine 1992;17:922–6.

[105] Alexander RW, Brennan JC, Maida AS, et al. The value of preplacement medical examinations for nonhazardous light duty work. J Occup Med 1977;19:107–12.

[106] Beimborn DS, Morrissey MC. A review of the literature related to trunk muscle performance. Spine 1987;13:655–60.

[107] Delitto A, Rose SJ, Crandell CE, et al. Reliability of isokinetic measurements of trunk muscle performance. Spine 1991;16:800–3.

[108] Graves JE, Pollack ML, Carpenter DM, et al. Quantitative assessment of full range of motion isometric lumbar extension strength. Spine 1990;15:289–98.

[109] Keyserling WM. Strength testing as a method of evaluating ability to perform strenuous work. In: Stanton-Hicks M, Boas R, editors. Chronic low back pain. New York: Raven Press; 1982. p. 149–56.

[110] Keyserling VM, Herrin GD, Chaffin DB. Isometric strength testing as a means of controlling medical incidents on strenuous jobs. J Occup Med 1980;22:332–6.

[111] Langrana NA, Lee CK, Alexander H, et al. Quantitative assessment of back strength using isokinetic testing. Spine 1984;9:287–90.

[112] Mooney V, Kenney K, Leggett S, et al. Relationship of lumbar strength in shipyard workers to workplace injury claims. Spine 1996;21:2001–5.

[113] Newton M, Thow M, Somerville D, et al. Trunk strength testing with iso-machines. Part 2. Experimental evaluation of the Cybex II Back Testing System in normal subjects and patients with chronic low back pain. Spine 1993;18:812–24.

[114] Newton M, Waddell G. Trunk strength testing with iso-machines. Part 1. Review of a decade of scientific evidence. Spine 1993;18:801–11.

[115] Reimer DS, Halbrook BD, Dreyfuss PH, et al. A novel approach to pre-employment worker fitness evaluations in a material-handling industry. Spine 1994;19:2026–32.

[116] Smith SS, Mayer TG, Gatchel RJ, et al. Quantification of lumbar function: Part 1. Isometric and multispeed isokinetic trunk strength measures in sagittal and axial planes in normal subjects. Spine 1985;10:757–64.

[117] Chaffin DB. Human strength capability and low-back pain. J Occup Med 1974;16:248–54.

[118] Chaffin DB, Herrin GD, Keyserling WM. Preemployment strength testing: an updated position. J Occup Med 1978;20:403–8.

[119] Dueker JA, Ritchie SM, Knox TJ, et al. Isokinetic trunk testing and employment. J Occup Med 1994;36:42–8.

[120] Magnusson M. Point of view. Spine 1996;21:2005.

[121] Grew ND, Deane G. The physical effect of lumbar spinal supports. Prosthet Orthop Int 1982;6:79–87.

[122] Lantz SA, Schultz AB. Lumbar spine orthosis wearing. I. Restriction of gross body motions. Spine 1986;11:834–7.

[123] Perry J. The use of external support in the treatment of low-back pain. J Bone Joint Surg Am 1970;52A:1440–2.

[124] Axelsson P, Johnsson R. Effect of lumbar orthosis on intervertebral mobility: a roentgen stereophotogrametric analysis. Spine 1992;17:678–81.

[125] McCoy MA, Congleton JJ, Johnson WC. The role of lifting belts in manual lifting. Int J Ind Ergon 1988;2:259–66.

[126] Woodhouse ML, Heinen J, Shall L, et al. Selected isokinetic lifting parameters of adult male athletes utilizing lumbar/sacral supports. J Orthop Sports Phys Ther 1990;11:467–73.

[127] Mitchell LV, Lawler FH, Bowen D, et al. Effectiveness and cost-effectiveness of employer-issued back belts in areas of high risk for back injury. J Occup Med 1994;36:90–4.

[128] Walsh NE, Schwartz RK. The influence of prophylactic orthoses on abdominal strength and low back injury in the workplace. Am J Phys Med Rehabil 1990;69:245–50.

[129] Reddell CR, Congleton JJ, Hunchingston RD, et al. An evaluation of a weightlifting belt and back injury prevention training class for airline baggage handlers. Appl Ergon 1992; 23:319–29.

[130] Holmstrom E, Moritz U. Effect of lumbar belts on trunk muscle strength and endurance: a follow-up study of construction workers. J Spinal Disord 1992;5:260–6.

[131] McGill CM, Norman RW, Sharratt MT. The effect of an abdominal belt on trunk muscle activity and intra-abdominal pressure during squat lifts. Ergonomics 1990;33:147–60.

[132] Hunter GR, McGuirk J, Mitrano N, et al. The effects of a weight training belt on blood pressure during exercise. J Appl Sport Sci Res 1989;3:13–8.

[133] Rafacz W, McGill SM. Wearing an abdominal belt increases diastolic blood pressure. J Occup Environ Med 1989;38:925–7.

ELSEVIER
SAUNDERS

Clin Occup Environ Med
5 (3) 545–569

CLINICS IN
OCCUPATIONAL AND
ENVIRONMENTAL
MEDICINE

Occupational Low Back Pain

Todd P. Stitik, MD*, Michael Y. Chang, DO, Joshua Levy, DO, Scott F. Nadler, DO

University Rehabilitation Associates, 90 Bergen Street, Suite 3100, Newark, NJ 07103, USA

Low back injury is one of the most common conditions in the workplace [1,2]. The causes are multifactorial and must be sought during the physician's examination [3]. Failure to perform a comprehensive history and physical examination ultimately can lead to treatment failure and injury recurrence [4,5]. Geraci has described the ramifications of taking a nonspecific history and physical; the resultant chain reaction often has a negative effect on treatment and outcome. A comprehensive history and physical may help clinicians to differentiate organic and nonorganic causes of low back pain. Different diagnoses need specific rather than generalized treatment programs. Teaching clinicians the nuances of the history and physical examination in a setting with an injured worker is the goal of this article.

History

Because of many issues related to the workers' compensation system, injured workers with low back pain can present formidable challenges to clinicians. To help meet this challenge, physicians may need to tailor their usual approach to patients with low back pain. Certain aspects of each of the general categories of a patient's history must be particularly emphasized and explored in some detail. Although the following discussion pertains mainly to the patient history during the first office visit, many of the same questions must be posed during follow-up visits.

Portions of this article are reprinted from Nadler S, Stitik T. Occupational low back pain: history and physical examination. Occupational Medicine: State of the Art Reviews 1998; 13(1):61–81.

* Corresponding author.

E-mail address: dunneCL@umdnj.edu (T.P. Stitik).

doi:10.1016/j.coem.2006.05.001   *occmed.theclinics.com*

The chief complaint

The chief complaint is generally a simple recounting of a patient's symptoms in his or her own words. Physicians should encourage patients to be as specific as possible. Specificity helps set the tone for the rest of the history and the physical examination. With respect to low back pain, the area being reported by the patient as causing pain must be described thoroughly, because "pain in the low back" can have completely different meanings for patients and physicians [6]. Even in the chief complaint, the physician is searching for clues that suggest the presence of psychosocial factors that may delay a patient's eventual recovery [7–9]. Such clues include an emphasis on vague complaints of pain rather than on specific symptoms [10]. Terminology that suggests a large emotional component to a patient's pain includes pain descriptions such as excruciating, devastating, killing, unbearable, and intolerable [6]. Once this specific complaint has been relayed adequately in as objective and detailed a manner as possible, one can move onto the history of current illness.

History of current illness

The physician should determine as accurately as possible if the low back pain is clearly caused by a work-related injury or a non–work-related injury or is simply the manifestation of an underlying illness [11]. This judgment is often difficult because many low back injuries occur gradually and without any identifiable precipitating cause [12]. It is also difficult to correlate the level of pain with a suspected severity of trauma unless there is an associated bony fracture. A detailed mechanism of injury can assist in the clarification of the work association, help establish the diagnosis and provide treatment suggestions, and assist with the suggestions for later prevention. In questioning a patient, the physician should not convey a verbal or nonverbal message of disbelief of the patient's association between the pain and work. A feeling of mistrust may develop that probably will make it more difficult to treat the patient. Vagueness on the part of the patient with respect to symptom onset, however, should alert the physician that the injury may not be related to work. According to Battie [13], the public may perceive nonspecific back pain as work related regardless of whether this association truly exists. A worker's belief of potential recompense also predicts disability from low back pain [14,15].

In terms of actual symptoms, vagueness—especially with regard to pain intensity—can greatly and perhaps inappropriately influence a physician's decision regarding a patient's ability to return to work [16]. Pain location must be described, but a patient is not always able to pinpoint it, especially in cases in which a mesodermal structure, such as muscle, ligament, periosteum, capsule, or annulus fibrosis, is the pain generator. Pain from these structures, called sclerotomal pain, can be diffuse. In contrast, although pain that follows a nerve root pattern (radicular pain) is typically more demarcated than sclerotomal pain, it also can have significant overlap [17].

In obtaining a detailed history, one should avoid questions that lead a patient to conclude that he or she has a specific diagnosis. Naming a specific diagnosis early is risky because a higher rate of prolonged disability has been noted in patients who have been labeled with a specific diagnosis at the initial evaluation [4]. Workers who have occupationally related low back pain might use this information to influence treatment and return-to-work decisions at future visits. For example, a worker might make an effort to become further educated about a particular disorder and then report symptoms of the condition during follow-up office visits. When discussing a patient's symptoms, the physician should ask general questions about the characteristics of the pain (Table 1).

In a nonacute injury, a determination that nothing can relieve the pain should alert the physician to the possibility of a nonmechanical cause (eg, tumor or infection) or psychosocial factors that may be influencing the patient's pain perception [18,19]. This line of reasoning might be invalid in workers who are acutely injured and are experiencing low back pain, however. These patients may find it difficult to identify a comfortable position.

Although a detailed history is important, by itself it is probably insufficient to make an accurate diagnosis in patients with low back pain. Andersson and Deyo [17] examined the sensitivity and specificity of various aspects of a patient's history in patients with documented lumbar herniated discs. None of the individual clinical indicators had a high enough predictive value to yield sufficient diagnostic accuracy. For example, although the sensitivity (0.98) and specificity (0.88) of sciatica were good for disc herniation, the positive predictive value was low because the prevalence of disc herniation was low. The rate of false-positive results based on the presence or absence of sciatica is poor [17]. Kosteljanetz and colleagues [20] reported that the sensitivity for paresthesia was 47% and the specificity was 18%. The subjective complaint of weakness has not been studied in sufficient detail to allow calculation of sensitivity or specificity [17].

During the history of current illness and the review of systems section of the history, one should be on the lookout for "red flags" that suggest a possible underlying serious condition. Red flags include night pain, particularly that which awakens the patient from sleep, associated febrile episodes, unexplained weight loss, bilateral sciatic-type pain, a feeling of saddle anesthesia, and new onset of bowel, bladder (especially urinary retention), or sexual dysfunction [21]. Sexual dysfunction, however, can be caused by low back pain during attempted sexual intercourse. Pain that awakens a patient is often associated with an invasive vertebral lesion, such as a metastatic or primary tumor; associated febrile episodes suggest a disc space infection or osteomyelitis; and bilateral sciatica-type pain and new onset of bowel, bladder, or sexual dysfunction suggest the possibility of cauda equina syndrome [21]. Because of the serious nature of cauda equina syndrome, it is always

Table 1
Low back pain symptoms

Pain characteristics	Examples	Comment
Frequency	Constant, intermittent, rare, nighttime	Suspect possible underlying malignancy if prominent night pain
Location	Primarily in the leg or buttock	Suggestive of radiculopathy
Referral pattern	Into buttocks, to the knees, down into the foot	Any can represent radiculopathy, but prominent leg pain with referral past the knee is most suggestive; the particular pattern of true radicular pain referral can provide insight into the involved nerve root level
Quality	Sharp, dull, numbing	Examiner may want to quantify on a scale from 1–10, with 10 being the worst pain ever felt by the individual
Factors that increase or decrease pain	Ambulation, body position, Valsalva maneuvers, medications	Leg pain with ambulation should suggest the possibility of true vascular claudication or pseudoclaudication (ambulatory radicular pain or neurogenic claudication [pseudoclaudication]) caused by spinal stenosis; seated position (eg, driving a car) and pain with flexion usually is the worst for discogenic pain; exacerbation with extension suggests posterior element etiology, such as the facet joints
Red flags	Change in bowel, bladder, or sexual function; bilateral sciatic-type pain	Cauda equina syndrome
	Night pain that awakens the patient; unexplained weight loss	Locally invasive or metastatic malignancy
	Failure of bed rest to relieve pain	Underlying systemic disease
	Associated febrile illness	Disc space infection or osteomyelitis

important for physicians to question patients regarding the presence of bowel or bladder dysfunction, even in the absence of sciatic pain. Another sensitive, although nonspecific, finding for an underlying systemic disease is the failure of bed rest to relieve pain [21]. Even in the absence of other red flags, insidious onset of low back pain portends a worse prognosis than acute onset of symptoms [22].

Past medical and surgical history

An understanding of a patient's general medical status helps clinicians rationally plan treatment with respect to medications and possible physical therapy. Understanding details about previous episodes of low back pain helps physicians to understand patient perception of the current injury and the potential course of recovery. One precautionary note is that patients infrequently believe that they have a previous history of a herniated disc based on a doctor's comment concerning a previous radiograph that revealed disc space narrowing. Such patients must be questioned in more detail regarding their signs and symptoms along with the actual evaluation they underwent that led to the diagnosis of a herniated disc. In contrast, patients without a prior history of low back pain may need additional time for explanations about low back pain in general and specific details about treatment, prognosis, and prophylaxis [10].

For patients with a baseline level of chronic low back pain, it becomes important to establish their usual baseline level of pain. Understanding this level may help clinicians gauge the severity of the most recent exacerbation. The physician must state early in the evaluation that the realistic treatment goal is to return the patient to the previous baseline level of symptoms and function. Information about the past treatment history is useful so that the clinician can avoid trying previously unsuccessful approaches and can consider using approaches that provided some pain relief. The past treatment history should include previous recorded responses on visual analog scales or pain diagrams and previous responses to medications, modalities, and therapy. One caution before concluding that a patient does not respond to physical therapy is to consider the quality of the physical therapy [23,24]. Previous physical therapy may have been unsuccessful because it was predominately a passive, modality-based rather than active therapeutic exercise program [25]. A nonorganic cause for pain should be considered when patients report that all treatment approaches make their pain worse and that their pain is always rated 10/10. Other important factors in patients with more chronic low back pain include a history of emergency room visits and hospital admissions for low back pain exacerbations. These occurrences may imply a more serious previous injury or simply that a patient has a poor perception of pain.

Physicians also should ask about litigation on the part of the patient against the workplace or as part of a motor vehicle accident or medical malpractice suit. This question is particularly relevant in workers with low back injuries because they tend to have more claims than workers without back injury claims [26]. Patients involved in litigation are influenced by various incentives that are counterproductive to prompt symptom resolution, including advice from their attorney, compensated time off from work, and the possibility of receiving permanent disability payments. These patients are difficult to treat because they (1) might not admit to symptomatic improvement, (2) continue to ask for extensive diagnostic testing, and (3) place more value on surgical intervention than rehabilitation [27,28].

Any previous history of cancer should be elicited because it raises the probability that pain is caused by an underlying malignancy. Patients without a clear history of an occupational low back injury but who have a previous history of cancer are believed to have such high specificity (0.98) for cancer that their low back pain should be considered as having a malignant origin until proven otherwise [21]. Other symptoms that raise suspicion for serious pathologic conditions include pain unrelieved with bed rest, symptoms that last longer than 1 month, and failure to improve with previous conservative therapy.

Two other important pieces of information include a history of a recent infection, particularly of the genitourinary tract, and a history of long-term treatment with corticosteroids. A recent urinary tract infection may raise suspicion that an underlying spinal infection is the cause of the low back pain if there is no clear history of a work-related event and the patient has other systemic complaints, such as fever and nausea [21]. Long-term treatment with corticosteroids, regardless of whether there is a known associated history of osteoporosis, raises the possibility of an underlying compression fracture, particularly in an older worker. A history of degenerative joint disease affecting peripheral joints should raise the possibility of lumbar spinal stenosis.

Family history

To help diagnose rare cases of underlying spondyloarthropathy in patients, physicians should question patients regarding any family history of connective tissue disorders. Patients with spondyloarthropathies may present with low back pain that seems to be related to a work injury. For example, ankylosing spondylitis should be considered in young men with atypical low back pain that is not clearly related to an occupational injury or obvious occupational risk factor. This is especially true if there is a family history of low back pain in male relatives beginning at an early age and if a patient has morning stiffness and improvement with exercise and the pain has been present for at least 3 months [21]. Disc degeneration previously has been shown to have a strong familial influence [29].

Social history

The vocational component of a worker's social history is a crucial part of the history that must not be overlooked. Because some experts believe that work return is the single most effective treatment that can be given to a worker with a low back injury [30–32], details regarding a patient's job are of prime importance. Job-related factors have been shown to predict patient outcome, but most are not related to the physical demands of the job. Specifically, it has been reported that an injured worker's negative evaluation by an employer within 6 months of the injury was the factor most predictive of patient outcome. In contrast, personal empathetic communication from a supervisor to an injured worker was found to be helpful [33]. A job description is often helpful but is not always available to a physician.

Physicians often must rely on a job description provided by the worker, which may not always be accurate. If a patient seems to be unduly concerned about the number of days of work that will be missed as a result of the injury, the physician should question the worker about the employee-supervisor relationship. The worker may be afraid of losing his or her job or, conversely, may want to miss work in retaliation against a supervisor. In some instances, a worker is simply a conscientious individual who generally does not want to miss work. Discrepancies between what a worker reports with respect to job responsibility and the written job description may lead to the need for a meeting among a supervisor, employee, and the physician to review the details. Involving a case manager may be helpful during these deliberations; the case manager can help to negotiate job-related factors, particularly with respect to work return and possible job modifications.

Taking a social history offers physicians an opportunity to perform a risk assessment of a worker's job. Certain jobs are believed to put a worker at an increased risk for low back injuries [22], including repetitive jobs, such as assembly line work, and jobs that involve standing, twisting, vibration, and heavy work [34]. Job tasks such as lifting and material handling also may cause back injuries at a greater frequency than do slip-and-fall accidents [22]. Specific job-related biomechanical risk factors, such as lifting frequency, load moment, trunk lateral velocity, trunk twisting velocity, and trunk sagittal angle, have been found to predict medium- and high-risk occupational low back pain [35]. Masset and Malchaire [36] found no association between low back pain and the workload, postures, trunk movements, and exposure to whole body vibrations. There was a correlation between low back pain and heavy efforts of the shoulders and prolonged vehicle driving. Some workers have more than one job and do not necessarily volunteer this information unless specifically asked. Information about a second job can help physicians to better predict the outcome and more rationally develop a treatment strategy.

In addition to work-related information, the social history provides an opportunity to glean other important information. For example, one can get a sense of a patient's general level of life-related stress, which has been shown to influence outcome [22]. The social history also includes a history of cigarette smoking, which is a risk factor for low back pain [37,38]. A history of intravenous drug abuse should prompt consideration of an underlying spinal infection as the cause of low back pain [21].

Information about recreational and exercise activities also may be of use. An MRI study of 115 male identical twin pairs with lifetime discordance in suspected environmental risk factors for disc degeneration showed that a heavier occupational and leisure time exposure to lifting was associated with greater disc degeneration in the upper lumbar levels [29]. A history of weight training in an otherwise sedentary worker who complains of back pain should raise one's suspicion that the pain is perhaps more avocationally than vocationally related. Another study showed that among a group of firefighters, a high level of cardiovascular fitness played a role in decreasing the frequency of low back injuries [39]. Whether this finding translates to other types of workers is unknown, but questions pertaining to a patient's level of physical fitness may be useful when strategies for injury prophylaxis are discussed. Injured workers' perceived physical capacity also may be valuable. A study of 2891 British workers revealed that the perceived ability was more predictive of low back injury and directly measured capacity [40].

Finally, education level has been mentioned as a factor that affects a patient's chances of a successful outcome. Specifically, achieving less than a high school degree is believed to serve as a red flag for the 10% to 20% of cases that are less likely to have a good outcome [41].

Review of systems

Similar to the history of current illness portion of the examination, one must be alert during the general review of systems for clues such as unexplained weight loss and night sweats, which suggest the presence of underlying systemic illnesses. Fever has been found to be a somewhat less sensitive indicator of an underlying spinal infection than was hoped [21].

Other aspects of the systems review also have relevance to the cause and treatment of low back pain. The presence of peripheral joint swelling, particularly if it is symmetrical, can serve as a marker for an underlying rheumatologic condition, such as rheumatoid arthritis. Women who have low back pain of unclear origin should be questioned about menstrual cycle irregularities, because there may be a gynecologic component to their pain. Underlying coronary artery disease can be diagnosed by the physician who elicits a history of chest pain with exertion or other anginal equivalents. In these patients, it may be critical to perform a stress test before starting a physical therapy program. One also may want to enquire about signs and symptoms of an underlying depression, such as anhedonia and ongoing changes in sleep pattern or appetite. Early discovery and treatment can avoid delay in a worker's recovery.

Physical examination

The physical examination should be performed in a sequential pattern to avoid missing key elements (Box 1), but it should be tailored to the individual to further delineate organic and nonorganic pathologic conditions. The physical examination should be used as an extension of the historical evaluation [42].

Inspection

The examiner must begin the evaluation by inspecting not only the involved area but also confluent regions of the spine. The inspection should

---

Box 1. Sequential pattern of physical examination

Inspection
Range of motion
Palpation
Flexibility
Neurologic assessment
    Strength
    Sensation
    Reflexes
Provocative maneuvers
Nonorganic signs

---

include an assessment of shoulder, scapula, iliac crest, and greater trochanteric height (Fig. 1) and an assessment for asymmetry in paraspinal fullness. The curves of the spinal column should be evaluated in anteroposterior and lateral planes, and any increased or decreased kyphosis or scoliosis should be documented (Fig. 2). Scoliosis by itself is not a risk factor for the development of low back pain until the curve approaches 80° [43].

Range of motion

The motion of the lumbar spine must be assessed in all planes, including flexion, extension, side bending, and rotation. A key measurement is lumbar flexion because it is composed of true lumbar motion along with a large pelvic component. Caillet [6] demonstrated that the initial 45° of trunk flexion is essentially the reversal of lumbar lordosis and that the remainder of the motion is a result of pelvic rotation. It is important to document not only that the individual flexes forward to the floor but also that there has been

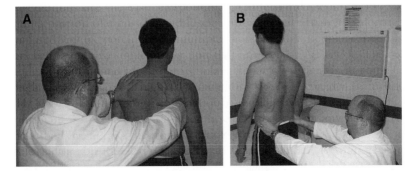

Fig. 1. Inspection. (*A*) Assessment of shoulder height. (*B*) Assessment of iliac crest height.

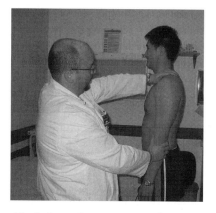

Fig. 2. Inspection: assessment of posture.

a reversal of the lordosis. Flexible individuals may be able to flex forward fully using pelvic rotation and no lumbar motion. In the documentation of lumbar motion, the clinician must standardize the examination to allow comparison at future visits.

Various methods have been described for general use. A simple measurement of fingertip distance to the floor in flexion or fingertip to knee joint line in side bending can be helpful. This method is subject to great variation and is especially affected by the flexibility of the lower extremities [44]. Schober [45] developed a test of lumbar motion by measuring 10 cm proximal to the posterior superior iliac spine (PSIS) and recording the difference in flexion. Macrae and Wright [46] modified Schober's technique by measuring 5 cm below the PSIS. The modified Schober flexion test is a simple office maneuver in which the examiner measures and marks 10 cm above and 5 cm below the PSIS (Fig. 3). The injured worker is asked to bend forward fully, and the initial marks are remeasured. Normally, individuals should have more than a 5-cm increase from the previously measured mark in full flexion, and these measurements have shown good overall reliability [44,46–49]. Van Adrichem and van der Korst [50] identified the so-called modified-modified Schober, measuring 15 cm proximal to the PSIS. This technique can be used readily to quantify changes in motion.

The inclinometer method, in which more specialized equipment is required, can be a useful tool for motion measurement (Fig. 4). An inclinometer is a handheld, circular, fluid-filled disc with a weighted gravity pendulum that remains oriented in the vertical direction. The inclinometer technique usually requires two inclinometers, one placed on the sacrum to measure hip motion and the other placed on the first lumbar vertebra to measure hip and a lumbar range. The lumbar range of motion is estimated as the difference in the two measurements. Sauer and colleagues [51] demonstrated high reliability using the inclinometer in the measurement of lumbar

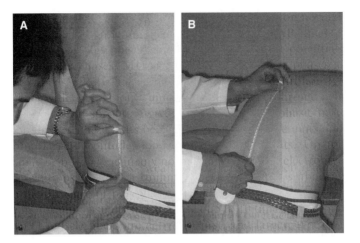

Fig. 3. Range of motion. (*A*) Modified Schober technique (neutral standing). (*B*) Modified Schober technique (full flexion).

flexion and at less reliability and extension. Others have failed to show high reliability of the inclinometer method. Williams and colleagues [52] reported interrater reliability coefficients of 0.72 for flexion and 0.76 for extension using the modified-modified Schober; the double inclinometer was 0.60 for flexion and 0.48 for extension.

Finally, during linear motion testing, the clinician must be aware of possible sources of error in measurement, including improper technique, poor standardization, the effects of stretching, or simply the time of day. Ensink

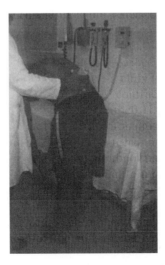

Fig. 4. Range of motion: inclinometer technique.

and colleagues [53] demonstrated a significant improvement in lumbar range using various techniques to compare measurements taken in the morning and afternoon. Range of motion testing can be a valuable tool to quantify recovery but must be used in concert with a complete physical examination [54]. The examiner must remember that a decreased range of motion in an asymptomatic individual does not predict low back pain.

Palpation

Palpation is an essential part of the examination. The clinician must palpate the region and surrounding areas and note the tissue symmetry from side to side, presence of tenderness, and compliance of the tissues. The osseous structures should be palpated for any tenderness or reproduction of pain. A trigger point is a region of muscle that has a band-like quality, produces a twitch response when palpated, and causes pain to radiate distant from its location [55]. The presence of these trigger points should be documented along with specific radiation pattern. A more detailed osteopathic palpation examination can be performed, palpating the region over the transverse processes in neutral, flexed, and extended planes to evaluate for symmetry (Fig. 5). Deyo and colleagues [21] described tenderness in the soft tissue of the low back as having poor reproducibility and low specificity; vertebral tenderness was nonspecific but suggested spinal infection. While palpating the lumbar spine area, the clinician must not forget to palpate the thoracic spine and the pelvic girdle region, including the gluteus maximus, gluteus medius, piriformis, and tensor fascia lata, because irritation of the structures also can cause symptoms of sciatica.

Flexibility

Inflexibility of the musculature about the pelvis has a direct result on the mechanics of the lumbosacral spine. Increased tightness of the hamstrings or gluteus maximus can cause a posterior tilt to the pelvis and reduce lumbar lordosis, whereas tightness of the anteriorly situated rectus femoris and

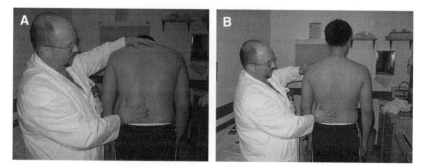

Fig. 5. Palpation. (*A*) Neutral position. (*B*) Full flexion.

iliopsoas causes an increase in lumbar lordosis by tilting the pelvis anteriorly. Both of these effects cause increased force to be distributed to the lumbar spine and set in motion postural changes in the cervical and thoracic spines. Esola and colleagues [56] strongly correlated poor hamstring flexibility with a history of low back pain. Kajala and colleagues [57] previously demonstrated hip flexor tightness as the one factor associated with low back pain in school-aged children. The rectus femoris is assessed via the Ely test, in which the prone patient has the knee maximally flexed approximating the ankle to the buttocks (Fig. 6). A true-positive test result is indicated by the elevation of the buttocks from the table, although inability to touch the ankle to the buttocks also may be used (measure and compare the distance to the buttocks for both legs). The Thomas test assesses iliopsoas flexibility. In the supine position, the opposite hip is flexed into the chest to evaluate for elevation of the nonflexed thigh off the table, which would indicate inflexibility (Fig. 7). Posteriorly, the hamstrings are assessed via a passive straight-leg raise or the popliteal angle. The hip is flexed to 90° and the knee is extended. A perpendicular line is drawn to the axis of rotation of the knee and the angle assessed (Fig. 8). Excessive hamstring inflexibility is indicated by the increasing size of this angle. The clinician must assess carefully for inflexibility, evaluating for asymmetry or reproduction of pain.

Neurologic assessment

The assessment of strength, sensation, and reflexes is essential in the evaluation of patients. An attempt should be made to identify whether a true

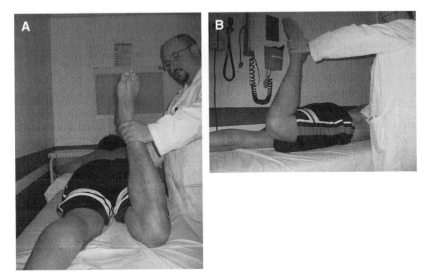

Fig. 6. Flexibility. (*A*) Normal Ely test (flexibility of rectus femoris). (*B*) Positive Ely test.

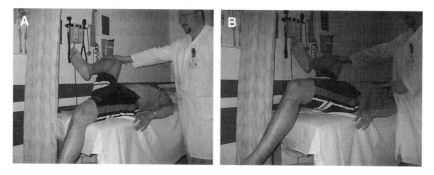

Fig. 7. Flexibility. (*A*) Normal Thomas test (flexibility of iliopsoas). (*B*) Positive Thomas test.

dermatomal and myotomal pattern is present, especially in the face of a suspected herniated nucleus pulposus. It is rare for more than one root to be involved at the same time except in the face of acute injury. Deyo and colleagues [21] emphasized the need to perform ankle and great toe dorsiflexion strength along with the complete sensory examination and ankle reflexes. This small portion of the examination should identify most disc herniation, which most commonly occurs at the L5-S1 level [58]. The strength examination should include the assessment of hip flexors (L1-3), quadriceps (L2-4), tibialis anterior (L4), extensor houses longus (L5), and the gastrocnemius/soleus (S1). The latter muscle group should be assessed via the performance of ten toe raises or the ability to ambulate on toes. Static manual testing should be avoided because significant weakness can be missed (Fig. 9). Proximal muscles, including the gluteus medius (L5), gluteus maximus (S1), and abdominal musculature, are helpful for the neurologic assessment and serve as key trunk/pelvis stabilizing muscles for heavy manual laborers. This sensory examination should cover the bilateral lower limbs to evaluate for true dermatomal loss or a more regional "stocking" pattern. These regions should include the distal thigh (L3), medial leg (L4), lateral leg (L5), and

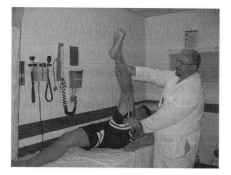

Fig. 8. Flexibility: assessment of popliteal angle (flexibility of hamstrings).

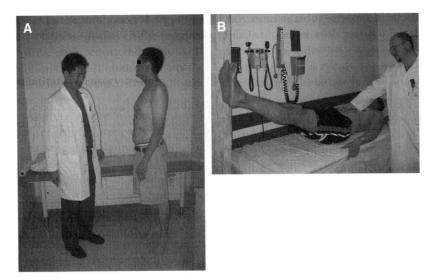

Fig. 9. Strength. (*A*) Heel walking (tibialis anterior muscle). (*B*) Poor abdominal strength with failure to maintain lumbar kyphosis.

calf (S1) along with consistent patterns of loss in the foot, medial malleolus (L4), dorsum of foot (L5), and lateral malleolus (S1) (Fig. 10). Finally, muscle stretch reflexes should be performed at the Achilles (S1), patella (L4), and medial hamstrings (L5) (Fig. 11). The latter can be performed in the side-lying position with the leg that is to be assessed positioned down and flexed approximately 30°.

Provocative maneuvers

Various tests or maneuvers can be performed to get additional information from that already described. In identifying lower lumbosacral nerve root pathology from a herniated nucleus pulposus or other compressive source, many variations of the straight-leg raise test can be performed. The classic straight-leg raise test is indicated as positive when the supine light is elevated between the angle of 30° and 70° and pain is reproduced down the posterior thigh below the knee (Fig. 12) [59]. Pain beyond 70° is not believed to be caused by nerve root tension and may indicate sacroiliac joint dysfunction. Pain below 30° is believed to be nonphysiologic [60]. The straight-leg raise test can be further improved by different variations, including the ankle dorsiflexion test, the bowstring test, or the Linder maneuver (Fig. 13) [61,62]. The ankle dorsiflexion test, or Braggard's sign, involves elevating the leg to the point of pain provocation, dropping the leg down to a nonpainful range, and subsequently dorsiflexing the ipsilateral ankle, which increases tension in the sciatic nerve distribution [62]. The bowstring test similarly involves decreasing the elevation angle to a nonpainful

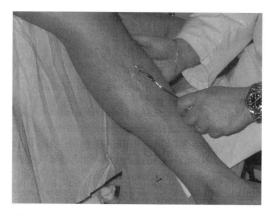

Fig. 10. Sensory evaluation with Wartenberg wheel.

position and then applying direct pressure to the ipsilateral popliteal fossa. The Linder maneuver uses neck flexion in combination with the elevated leg to elevate intrathecal pressure [62].

The crossed straight-leg raise test has been described as the most specific test for nerve root pathology resulting from a disc herniation [63]. The test involves the elevation of the noninvolved leg, which reproduces pain on the involved side below the knee. Supik and Broom [64] identified a 90% sensitivity rate with the straight-leg test in identifying the disc herniation; the bowstring test was 70% sensitive. The crossed straight-leg raise was highly

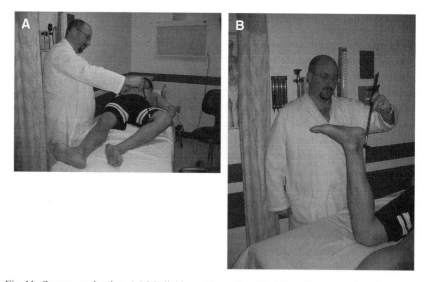

Fig. 11. Sensory evaluation. (*A*) Medial hamstring reflex. (*B*) Alternative method to elicit Achilles reflex.

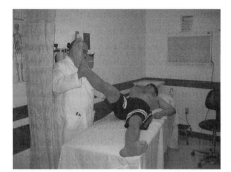

Fig. 12. Provocative maneuver: straight-leg raise, positive at 30° to 70°.

specific although present only 21% of the time. The reverse straight-leg raise test, or femoral stretch test, can be useful for identifying upper lumbar nerve root pathology (Fig. 14). Estridge and colleagues [65] demonstrated a strong correlation with L3-4 disc herniation and positive femoral stretch test. This test is best performed in the prone patient, flexing the knee to 90° and lifting the thigh. Pain is reproduced in the femoral nerve distribution, occasionally into the groin and medial lower leg.

Provocative maneuvers for sacroiliac joint dysfunction also have been described [62]. The most commonly used test is the Patrick maneuver, or FABER (flexion, abduction and external rotation) test (Fig. 15). Each hip is individually flexed, abducted, and externally rotated while pressure is placed on the opposite anterior superior iliac spine. Pain reproduced ipsilaterally in the groin may indicate degenerative joint disease of the hip, and pain reproduced either ipsilaterally or contralaterally indicates sacroiliac joint dysfunction [66]. Gaenslen's maneuver is performed in the supine patient, flexing the contralateral leg and dropping the ipsilateral leg off the table. Pain is reproduced in the region of the sacroiliac joint on the dropped leg side if joint dysfunction is present (Fig. 16). Distraction, compression, rocking, and posterior shear are other tests that are used to identify

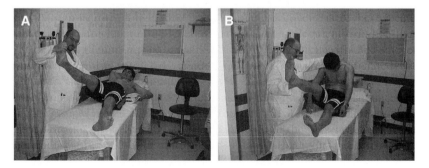

Fig. 13. Provocative maneuvers. (*A*) Ankle dorsiflexion test. (*B*) Linder maneuver.

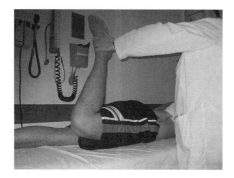

Fig. 14. Provocative maneuver: reverse straight-leg raise test.

sacroiliac joint pathology (Fig. 17) [61]. Laslett and Williams [67] demonstrated good reliability of distraction, compression, posterior shear, and Gaenslen's maneuver when performed in combination. Studies using sacroiliac joint injection block techniques demonstrated an overall poor predictive value for pain diagrams along with many of the physical tests for the sacroiliac joint [68]. Other tests more specifically used for sacroiliac or lumbopelvic motion testing include the standing and seated flexion test and the Gillette test [62]. The standing and seated flexion tests are performed with the clinician palpating just inferiorly to the PSIS. When the patient flexes forward, smooth equal motion of the PSIS should be observed. Hypomobility of the iliosacral or sacroiliac joint is identified by one PSIS elevating more proximally. In the Gillette test, a variant that assesses sacroiliac joint motion, the examiner palpates the anteroposterior lateral PSIS regions. Failure of the PSIS to descend with hip flexion to 90° implies motion abnormality. Dreyfuss and Dreyer [69] reported that up to 20% of asymptomatic individuals had positive findings in one or more of those tests. Motion test results must be used cautiously in diagnosing injured workers with sacroiliac joint dysfunction.

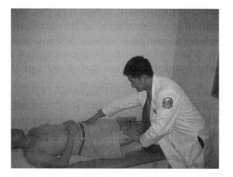

Fig. 15. Patrick maneuver, also called the flexion, abduction, external rotation (FABER) test.

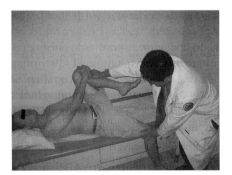

Fig. 16. Gaenslen's maneuver.

Nonorganic signs

Waddell and colleagues [70] initially described the use of provocative maneuvers to identify individuals who have physical findings without anatomic cause. They further identified a significant psychological overlay that consisted of hypochondriasis, hysteria, and depression in patients who tested positive on more than three of five of their maneuvers. The acronym DO REST is used to identify the five nonorganic signs: distraction, overreaction, regionalization, simulation, and tenderness. Distraction is a term applied to the performance of the seated straight-leg raise test in individuals with a positive supine straight-leg raise. This test purportedly should produce positive results in affected individuals; if not, then the cause of pain is considered

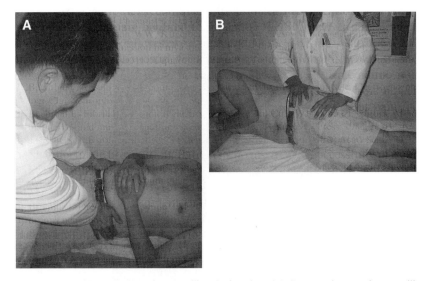

Fig. 17. (A) Rocking maneuver for sacroiliac dysfunction. (B) Compression test for sacroiliac dysfunction.

nonorganic (Fig. 18). Geraci [71] cautioned against the distracted straight-leg raise as biomechanically unequal to the supine straight-leg raise. He contended that the slump test, which combined the seated straight-leg raise with neck flexion, is a better destruction test (Fig. 19). Overreaction and excessive tenderness are considered nonorganic signs during the physical examination when they are out of proportion to what would normally be expected. One must be cautious, however, when using the nonorganic label, especially during the early, acute stages of back injury.

Consider an individual's previous response to painful stimuli. The examiner must be aware of the ethnic variations of the expression of pain; otherwise, a patient could be falsely labeled [72–74]. Regionalization identifies a motor and sensory examination that follows no true myotomal or dermatomal pattern. Most cases of herniated nucleus pulposus affect only one root; rarely, two may be involved. Nonorganic regionalization occurs in patients who describe stocking-glove or hemisensory deficits. Other neurologic conditions may need to be considered, such as peripheral neuropathy and mononeuropathy multiplex, when a regional pattern of loss is noted. Strength may be more regionally weakened in the face of acute pain, which must be quantified. The simulation test is performed with the patient standing or seated. Head compression is performed lightly and does not result in increased pressure in the lumbosacral spine (Fig. 20). The simulation test result is positive if pain is reproduced in the lumbosacral spine or leg. Variations of these tests, including shoulder compression and seated trunk rotation, may improve accuracy. The Hoover test may be performed to assess a patient's voluntary effort (Fig. 21). The patient's heels are cupped by the clinician, and the patient is instructed to individually raise his or her legs. Increased pressure should be felt on the untested cupped heel if true volition is provided; genuine effort causes opposite leg extension to stabilize the pelvis [62]. Most importantly, the clinician must be aware that positive nonorganic signs do not necessarily imply that the patient is malingering. A malingering patient may be highly motivated and highly educated, however;

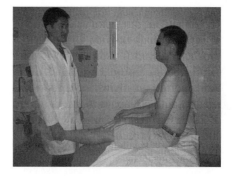

Fig. 18. Nonorganic sign: seated straight-leg raise test.

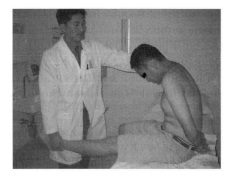

Fig. 19. Nonorganic sign: slump test.

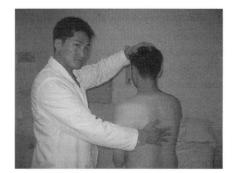

Fig. 20. Nonorganic sign: simulation/head compression test.

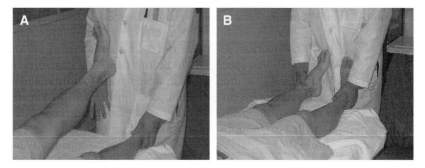

Fig. 21. Hoover test.

accordingly, repeated testing and numerous questions in combination with the rest of the evaluation will improve reliability.

Summary

The main goal of the history and physical examination is to try to establish the correct diagnosis that will result in a directed treatment plan. Most treatment failures may not be a result of the often cited psychological factors but instead may be diagnostic and treatment errors. The history and physical examination may be the first important clue that underlying issues or the root of the problem. Andersson and Deyo [17] reported that the history and physical had a low diagnostic accuracy when taken individually. Combining the results of both parts along with the use of repeated testing significantly improves the reliability of the evaluation. The history and physical examination must be used as the important first steps in treating injured workers. Further outcome research is needed to understand better the implications of a poorly performed evaluation. In the meantime, we must continue to educate students, residents in training, fellows, and our peers of the great importance of a properly performed history and physical examination. This comprehensive evaluation must take into account the multitude of psychosocial factors that ultimately affect proper diagnosis and treatment.

References

[1] Krause N, Rugulies R, Ragland DR, et al. Physical workload, ergonomic problems, and incidence of low back injury: a 7.5-year prospective study of San Francisco transit operators. Am J Ind Med 2004;46(6):570–85.

[2] Peek-Asa C, McArthur DL, Kraus JF. Incidence of acute low-back injury among older workers in a cohort of material handlers. J Occup Environ Hyg 2004;1(8):551–7.

[3] Wasiak R, Verma S, Pransky G, et al. Risk factors for recurrent episodes of care and work disability: case of low back pain. J Occup Environ Med 2004;46(1):68–76.

[4] Abenheim L, Rossignol M, Gobeille D, et al. The prognostic consequences in the making of the initial medical diagnosis of work-related back injuries. Spine 1995;20:791–5.

[5] Rossignol M, Lortie M, Ledoux E. Comparison of spinal health indicators in predicting spinal status in a 1 year longitudinal study. Spine 1993;18:54–60.

[6] Caillet R. Low back pain syndrome. 4th edition. Philadelphia: FA Davis; 1988.

[7] Cakmak A, Yucel B, Ozyalcn SN, et al. The frequency and associated factors of low back pain among a younger population in Turkey. Spine 2004;29(14):1567–72.

[8] Krause N, Dasinger LK, Deegan LJ, et al. Psychosocial job factors and return-to-work after compensated low back injury: a disability phase-specific analysis. Am J Ind Med 2001;40(4): 374–92.

[9] Selander J, Marnetoft SU, Bergroth A, et al. Return to work following vocational rehabilitation for neck, back and shoulder problems: risk factors reviewed. Disabil Rehabil 2002; 24(14):704–12.

[10] Bigos SJ, Andary MT. The practitioner's guide to the industrial back problem. Part I. Helping the patient with the symptoms and pathology. Semin Spine Surg 1992;4:42–54.

[11] Murphy PL, Volinn E. Is occupational low back pain on the rise? Spine 1999;24(7):691–7.

[12] Saunders HD, Stultz MR, Saunders R, et al. Back injury prevention. In: Key GL, editor. Industrial therapy. St. Louis (MO): Mosby; 1995. p. 125–47.

[13] Battie MC. Minimizing the impact of back pain: workplace strategies. Semin Spine Surg 1992;14:20–8.

[14] Gross DP, Battie MC. Work-related recovery expectations and the prognosis of chronic low back pain within a workers' compensation setting. J Occup Environ Med 2005;47(4):428–33.

[15] Frymoyer JW, Cats-Baril W. Predictors of low back pain disability. Clin Orthop 1987;221: 90–7.

[16] Hall H, McIntosh G, Melles T, et al. Effect of discharge recommendations on outcome. Spine 1994;19:2033–7.

[17] Andersson GB, Deyo RA. History and physical examination in patients with herniated lumbar discs. Spine 1996;21(24 Suppl):10–8.

[18] Holmberg S, Thelin A, Stiernstrom EL, et al. Psychosocial factors and low back pain, consultations, and sick leave among farmers and rural referents: a population-based study. J Occup Environ Med 2004;46(9):993–8.

[19] Pincus T, Vlaeyen JW, Kendall NA, et al. Cognitive-behavioral therapy and psychosocial factors in low back pain: directions for the future. Spine 2002;27(5):E133–8.

[20] Kosteljanetz M, Bang F, Schmidt-Olsen S. The clinical significance of straight leg raising (Lasegue's sign) in the diagnosis of prolapsed lumbar disc. Spine 1988;13:393–5.

[21] Deyo RA, Ranville J, Kent DL. What can the history and physical tell us about low back pain? JAMA 1992;268:760–5.

[22] Bigos SJ, Spengler DM, Martin NA, et al. Back injuries in industry: a retrospective study. II. Injury factors. Spine 1986;11:246–51.

[23] Bekkering GE, Hendriks HJ, van Tulder MW, et al. Effect on the process of care of an active strategy to implement clinical guidelines on physiotherapy for low back pain: a cluster randomised controlled trial. Qual Saf Health Care 2005;14(2):107–12.

[24] Helmhout PH, Harts CC, Staal JB, et al. Comparison of a high-intensity and a low-intensity lumbar extensor training program as minimal intervention treatment in low back pain: a randomized trial. Eur Spine J 2004;13(6):537–47.

[25] Jette DU, Jette AM. Physical therapy and health outcomes in patients with spinal impairments. Phys Ther 1996;76:930–44.

[26] Spengler DM, Bigos SJ, Martin NA, et al. Back injuries in industry: a retrospective study: I. Overview and cost analysis. Spine 1986;11:241–5.

[27] Hodges SD, Humphreys SC, Eck JC, et al. Predicting factors of successful recovery from lumbar spine surgery among workers' compensation patients. J Am Osteopath Assoc 2001;101(2):78–83.

[28] Tait RC, Chibnall JT. Work injury management of refractory low back pain: relations with ethnicity, legal representation and diagnosis. Pain 2001;91(1–2):47–56.

[29] Battie MC, Videman T, Gibbons LE, et al. Determinants of lumbar disc degeneration: a study relating lifetime exposures and magnetic resonance imaging findings in identical twins. Spine 1995;20:2601–12.

[30] Quebec Task Force Study. Scientific approach to the assessment and management of activity related spinal disorders. Spine 1987;12:1–59.

[31] Evans TH, Mayer TG, Gatchel RJ. Recurrent disabling work-related spinal disorders after prior injury claims in a chronic low back pain population. Spine J 2001;1(3): 183–9.

[32] Fishbain DA, Cutler RB, Rosomoff HL, et al. Prediction of "intent", "discrepancy with intent", and "discrepancy with nonintent" for the patient with chronic pain to return to work after treatment at a pain facility. Clin J Pain 1999;15(2):141–50.

[33] Wood DJ. Design and evaluation of a back injury prevention program within a geriatric hospital. Spine 1987;12:77–82.

[34] Rohrer MH, Santos-Eggiman B, Paccaud F, et al. Epidemiologic study of LBP in 1398 Swiss conscripts between 1985 and 1992. Eur Spine J 1994;3:2–7.

[35] Marras WS. Biomechanical risk factors for occupationally related low back disorders. Ergonomics 1995;38:377–410.

[36] Masset D, Malchaire J. Low back pain. Epidemiologic aspects and work related factors in the steel industry. Spine 1994;19:143–6.

[37] Manninen P, Riihimak H, Heliovaara M. Incidence and risk factors of low back pain in middle-aged farmers. Occup Med 1995;45:141–6.

[38] Oleske DM, Neelakantan J, Andersson GB, et al. Factors affecting recovery from work-related, low back disorders in autoworkers. Arch Phys Med Rehabil 2004;85(8):1362–4.

[39] Cady LD, Thomas PC, Karwasky RJ, et al. Program for increasing health and physical fitness of fire-fighters. J Occup Med 1985;27:110–4.

[40] Troup JDG, Foreman TK, Baxter CE, et al. The perception of the back pain and the role of psychophysical tests of lifting capacity. Spine 1987;12:645–57.

[41] Leonard JW. Low back pain clinical evaluation and treatment. In: O'Young B, Young MA, Stiens SA, editors. PM&R secrets. Philadelphia: Hanley & Belfus; 1997. p. 304–9.

[42] Young S, Aprill C, Laslett M. Correlation of clinical examination characteristics with three sources of chronic low back pain. Spine J 2003;3(6):460–5.

[43] Jackson RP, Simmons EH, Stripinis D. Incidence and severity of back pain in adult idiopathic scoliosis. Spine 1983;8:749–56.

[44] Merritt JL, McLean TJ, Erickson RP. Measurement of trunk flexibility in normal subjects: reproducibility of three clinical methods. Mayo Clin Proc 1986;61:192–7.

[45] Schober P. Lendenwirbelsaule und kreuzschmerzen. Munch Med Wochenschr 1937;84: 336–8.

[46] Macrae IF, Wright V. Measurement of back movement. Ann Rheum Dis 1969;28:584–9.

[47] Beattie P, Rothstein JM, Lamb RL. Reliability of the attraction method for measuring lumbar spine backward bending. Phys Ther 1987;67:364–9.

[48] Fitzgerald GK, Wynveen KJ, Rheault W, et al. Objective assessment with establishment of normal values for lumbar spinal range of motion. Phys Ther 1983;63:1776–81.

[49] Reynolds PMG. Measurement of spinal mobility: a comparison of three methods. Rheumatol Rehabil 1975;14:180–5.

[50] van Adrichem JAM, van der Korst JK. Assessment of the flexibility of the lumbar spine: a pilot study in children and adolescents. Scand J Rheumatol 1973;2:87–91.

[51] Sauer PM, Ensink FB, Frese K, et al. Lumbar range of motion: reliability and validity of the inclinometer technique in the clinical measurement of trunk flexibility. Spine 1996;21: 1332–8.

[52] Williams R, Binkley J, Block R, et al. Reliability of the Modified-Modified Schober and double inclinometer methods for measuring lumbar flexion extension. Phys Ther 1993;73: 26–37.

[53] Ensink FB, Saur FM, Frese K, et al. Lumbar range of motion: influence of time of day and individual factors on measurement. Spine 1996;21:1339–43.

[54] Hamaoui A, Do MC, Bouisset S. Postural sway increase in low back pain subjects is not related to reduced spine range of motion. Neurosci Lett 2004;357(2):135–8.

[55] Hsieh CY, Hong CZ, Adams AH, et al. Interexaminer reliability of the palpation of trigger points in the trunk and lower limb muscles. Arch Phys Med Rehabil 2000;81(3):258–64.

[56] Esola MA, McClure PW, Fitzgerald GK, et al. Analysis of lumbar spine and hip motion during forward bending in subjects with and without history of low back pain. Spine 1996;21: 71–8.

[57] Kujala UM, Salminen JL, Taimela S, et al. Subject characteristics and low back pain in young athletes and nonathletes. Med Sci Sports Exerc 1992;24:627–32.

[58] Kortelainen P, Puranen J, Korvisto E, et al. Symptoms and signs of sciatica and their relation to the localization of the lumbar disc herniation. Spine 1985;10:88–92.

[59] Hunt DG, Zuberbier OA, Kozlowski AJ, et al. Reliability of the lumbar flexion, lumbar extension, and passive straight leg raise test in normal populations embedded within a complete physical examination. Spine 2001;26(24):2714–8.

[60] Fahrni WH. Observations on straight leg raising with special reference to nerve root adhesions. Can J Surg 1966;9:44–8.

[61] Cram RH. A sign of sciatic nerve root pressure. J Bone Joint Surg Br 1953;35B:192–4.

[62] Magee DJ. Orthopedic physical assessment. Philadelphia: WB Saunders; 1992.

[63] Hudgins WR. The crossed straight leg raising test: a diagnostic sign of herniated disc. J Occup Med 1979;21:407–8.

[64] Supik LF, Broom MJ. Sciatic tension signs and lumbar disc herniation. Spine 1994;19: 1066–9.

[65] Estridge MN, Rouhe A, Johnson NG. The femoral stretching test: a valuable sign in diagnosing upper lumbar disc herniations. J Neurosurg 1982;57:813–7.

[66] Beetham WP, Polley HF, Slocumb CH, et al. Physical examination of the joints. Philadelphia: WB Saunders; 1965.

[67] Laslett M, Williams M. The reliability of selected pain provocation tests for sacroiliac pathology. Spine 1994;19:1243–9.

[68] Dreyfuss P, Michaelson M, Pauza K, et al. The value of the medical history and physical examination in diagnosing sacroiliac joint pain. Spine 1996;21:2594–602.

[69] Dreyfuss P, Dreyer S. Positive sacroiliac screening tests in asymptomatic adults. Spine 1994; 19:1138–43.

[70] Waddell G, McCulloch JA, Kummel E, et al. Non-organic physical signs in low back pain. Spine 1980;5:117–25.

[71] Geraci MC. Validation of physical examination: cervical and lumbar spine. Assoc Acad Phys Prog 1997;254–65.

[72] Nelson DV, Novy DM, Averill PM, et al. Ethnic comparability of the MMPI in pain patients. J Clin Psychol 1996;52:485–97.

[73] Bigos SJ, Spengler DM, Martin NA, et al. Back injuries in industry: a retrospective study: III. Employee-related factors. Spine 1986;11:252–6.

[74] Nachemson AL. Adult scoliosis and back pain. Spine 1979;4:513–7.

**ELSEVIER
SAUNDERS**

Clin Occup Environ Med
5 (3) 571–589

CLINICS IN
OCCUPATIONAL AND
ENVIRONMENTAL
MEDICINE

Diagnosis of Low Back Pain:
Role of Imaging Studies

Randolph B. Russo, MD[a,b,*]

[a]*Orthopaedic Associates of Grand Rapids, PC, 750 East Beltline NE,
Suite 301, Grand Rapids, MI 49525, USA*
[b]*Department of Physical Medicine and Rehabilitation,
Michigan State University, East Lansing, MI 48824, USA*

Radiographic evaluation of the lumbar spine has seen invaluable advances over the past two decades. Enhancement of neuroimaging techniques and better imaging-related research have played important roles in improved identification of pain generators in the lumbar spine.

With the advancement of imaging techniques comes expansion of treatment methods. Awareness of asymptomatic findings by practitioners is imperative to avoid exposure to unnecessary treatment. Because of the high prevalence of spinal pathology in the asymptomatic population, practitioners must correlate nonspecific lumbar pain carefully with the results of imaging studies. False-positive rates of commonly used imaging studies have been reported [1–4]. Understanding the limitations of imaging studies permits better identification of patients who may benefit from more invasive interventions. Appropriate use of radiographic evaluation is mandatory in the practice of cost-effective medicine. Decisions regarding obtaining imaging studies must be based on whether they will influence patient management.

There are few areas in medicine in which a simple adjustment in practice habits can reduce medical costs substantially. The use of imaging must be dictated by the history and physical examination. Early use of imaging can mislead physicians into making decisions on the basis of results and labeling patients with incorrect diagnoses while the true pain generator remains unrecognized.

Approximately 70% of North Americans experience low back pain during their lifetime, with most of them demonstrating improvement within 2 to

---

Portions of this article originally appeared in Russo R, Cook P. Diagnosis of low back pain: role of imaging studies. Occupational Medicine: State of the Reviews 1998;13(1):83–96.

* Department of Physical Medicine and Rehabilitation, Michigan State University, 750 East Beltline NE, Suite 301, Grand Rapids, MI 49525.

E-mail address: rrusso@oagr.com

4 weeks [5]. The use of early radiographic evaluation is often unnecessary for uncomplicated acute low back injuries. Select patient populations have been identified for early evaluation. If the following red flags are associated with the pain, spinal imaging is indicated: possible fracture, neoplasm, infection, and cauda equina syndrome. High suspicion for the presence of one of these entities should prompt more formal evaluation of the spine. This article provides an overview of the commonly used diagnostic procedures in the evaluation of lumbar spine disorders.

Standard radiographs

Plain radiographs, or x-rays, continue to be the initial step in the diagnostic evaluation of lumbar spine pain. They provide low radiation exposure, low cost, and noninvasive evaluation of the osseous architecture but reveal little concerning the soft tissue anatomy. Standard screen film radiography is rapidly being replaced by digital/computed radiography at many centers.

Generally, only two views are necessary in the evaluation of the low back: anteroposterior (AP) and full lateral. Scavone and colleagues [6] studied the diagnostic value of alternate views and obtained unique information on only 2.4% of the oblique and spot lateral views. Spondylolysis and a congenital facet fusion were the only missed diagnoses on AP and lateral films. It was recommended that oblique and spot lateral views be eliminated from routine lumbar spine series. Elimination of these views reduces cost by as much as 40% and radiation exposure by almost 50%. Clinical judgment must be used in the at-risk population.

After review of standard radiographs it was found that nearly 75% of plain radiographs provided no useful information in more than 1000 lumbosacral spine radiographic studies [7]. In patients with a history of minor trauma, no fractures were noted except in elderly women with osteoporosis. Follow-up radiographs of the lumbosacral spine also were found to be overused and demonstrated no interval changes in approximately 65% of patients. In radiographs with changes, 32% were follow-up postoperative films, fracture films, or films that demonstrated some progression of degenerative changes. Only two new significant findings were uncovered, which were metastatic lesions. Correlation of clinical information, however, was not provided. A thorough understanding of the appropriate use of lumbar radiography can have significant financial implications. Liang and Komaroff [8] suggested that the risks and costs of the initial visit radiographic evaluation of patients with acute low back pain do not justify the relatively small potential benefit. It is useful when ordering films to ask which radiologic findings will change the treatment and what the probability is that they will be present.

Common radiographic views

On an AP image (Fig. 1), the spinous processes are shown as teardrop-like structures in the midline. Following them cephalad to caudal provides

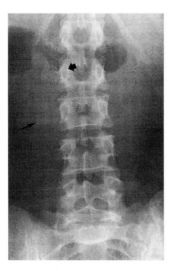

Fig. 1. Normal AP view of the lumbar spine. Thin arrow points to a transverse process and the short arrow to a pedicle. (*From* Russo R, Cook P. Diagnosis of low back pain: role of imaging studies. Phys Med Rehab 1999;13:427–42; with permission.)

information on alignment of the spine. The upper lumbar zygoapophyseal (facet) joints lie in the vertical plane, whereas the more caudal joints, L4-5 and especially L5-S1, frequently are oblique and poorly visualized. Sclerosis and tropism often can be observed on this view. The pedicles are seen end-on and appear as round, hypodense areas with a cortical rim of bone. Metastatic disease to the spine often can affect the pedicle, with loss of visualization on the AP view (known as the "winking owl" sign). Widening of the interpedicular space may suggest an expansile lesion or a burst fracture injury after trauma. Transverse processes are seen as lateral projections from the middle of each vertebral body and can fracture with trauma. Inclusion of the sacroiliac joints and hip joints on the AP image provides valuable diagnostic information concerning osteoarthritic changes and a potential source of referred pain to the low back area or pelvis. Including these areas may reduce the need for additional imaging.

The lateral view demonstrates the association between vertebral bodies and provides information concerning the intervertebral disc spaces. Moving cephalad to caudad, the disc spaces become larger, except for the variable L5-S1 interspace. Spondylolisthesis is best seen on this view. The spot lateral view may be necessary if adequate visualization of the L5-S 1 interspace is not appreciated on the full lateral view.

Oblique views should not be included on routine series. When completed, they provide information concerning the facet joints and pars interarticularis. The oblique view demonstrates the appearance of a "Scottie dog": the transverse process is the nose, the pedicle forms the eye, the inferior articular facet represents the front leg, and the superior articular facet is the ear. The pars interarticularis, which is the portion of the lamina that lies between the facets, forms the dog's neck (Fig. 2). Disruption of the pars interarticularis is demonstrated as a bony separation resembling a collar on the Scottie dog's neck, which indicates spondylolysis.

A multitude of findings can be evident on plain radiographs, but few are clinically significant. The prevalence of radiographic changes increases with age. Lumbar spondylosis (disc space narrowing, spur formation, and marginal sclerosis) was observed in 95% of adults autopsied by age 50. A similarly aged group of living patients demonstrated degenerative changes on 87% of their radiographs [9].

Guidelines for lumbar spine radiography

Because of the high incidence of lumbar pain, several sources have provided guidelines for the use of lumbar spine radiography. Radiographic evaluation is unnecessary in patients whose low back pain is less than 7 weeks' duration or is improving with treatment, unless one of the following exceptions is noted [10]:

1. Age >65 years
2. History suggests high risk of osteoporosis with minor trauma or injury of sufficient force to cause fracture

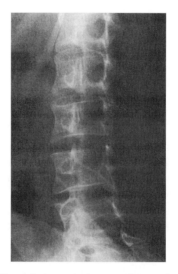

Fig. 2. Normal oblique radiograph demonstrates several examples of a "Scottie dog." (*From* Russo R, Cook P. Diagnosis of low back pain: role of imaging studies. Phys Med Rehab 1999;13:427–42; with permission.)

3. Persistent sensory deficit or significant motor deficit
4. Progressive pain despite adequate treatment
5. Rest pain or pain worse at night
6. Fever, chills, unexplained weight loss
7. Previous lumbar surgery of fracture
8. Recurrent back pain with no radiograph in the past 2 years
9. A patient unable to give a reliable history
10. Severe psychological or social circumstances

This list is meant as a guide for ordering radiographs and must be combined with clinical impressions before proceeding with radiographic evaluation.

The Public Health Services' Agency for Health Care Policy and Research released its clinical practice guidelines for acute low back problems in adults in 1994. They included a section on criteria for standard radiographic use [11]. The rationale for its preparation was to limit overtreatment and overuse of services. In response to these radiographic recommendations, a group of investigators modified the practice guidelines and implemented them with a group of physicians in Canada. Following the modifications, which included deletion of age-related indications and modifying radiographic recommendations in patients with previous cancer, they found a 74% reduction of radiograph use compared with that resulting from an adherence to the Agency for Health Care Policy and Research guidelines. A similar sensitivity for detecting serious abnormalities was observed in the two groups [12]. Plain radiographs frequently demonstrate abnormal findings of uncertain clinical significance. Correlation of radiographic findings with clinical evaluation is imperative when caring for patients with low back injuries.

Bone scintigraphy

Bone scintigraphy, or bone scanning, is a nuclear medicine imaging technique that is used in the evaluation of metabolic activity within bone. Bone is composed of balanced osteoblastic and osteoclastic activity, which results in continuous bone remodeling. Interruption of this normal balance can demonstrate abnormalities detected by scintigraphy. Bone scintigraphy uses a radioisotope, most commonly technetium-99m, that is injected intravenously and allowed to circulate throughout the body. Radiation is emitted by this tracer in proportion to its attachment to the target structures. A scintillation camera detects the emission of gamma rays. Normal imaging is performed within 2 to 4 hours of the injection (Fig. 3A). Images also can be completed immediately (vascular phase) or, occasionally, at 24 hours to evaluate residual increased bone activity. Increased osteoblastic activity appears as a hot spot, whereas loss of blood flow to bone or interruption of metabolic activity results in decreased activity on the scan, or a cold spot [13,14].

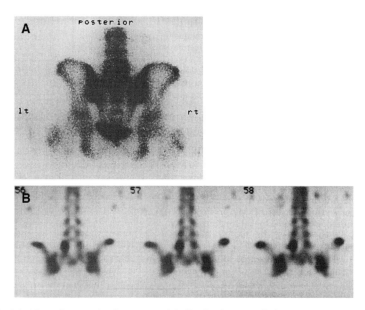

Fig. 3. (*A*), Normal appearing bone scan. (*B*), Single photon emission computed tomography imaging after the above bone scan demonstrates an obvious right L5 abnormality. (*From* Russo R, Cook P. Diagnosis of low back pain: role of imaging studies. Occup Med 1998;13:83–96; with permission.)

Elevated osteoblastic activity can be seen with osteomyelitis, discitis, degenerative arthritis, and tumors and after fractures. One notable exception is multiple myeloma, in which a normal scan is often observed. Areas such as the sacroiliac joints, growth plates, calvaria, acromioclavicular joints, axial spine, and pelvis (particularly the iliac wings) can show increased uptake despite the lack of a pathologic lesion.

Scintigraphy is valuable for persistent posttraumatic pain, especially for suspected pars interarticularis stress fractures, which may go undetected on standard radiography. The bone scan can show positive results within 3 days of a fracture. Relative dating of a fracture can be documented by the absence of increased activity, indicating that the injury is old [13]. Addition of single photon emission CT to scintigraphy has improved precision tremendously [14]. Single photon emission CT imaging helps to further localize a bone scan abnormality and can identify subtle tracer uptake that the bone scan may not have demonstrated clearly (Fig. 3B).

Recognition of osteomyelitis may lag 10 to 14 days on plain radiographs, whereas a bone scan may show positive results within 1 day [15]. Indium-111 and gallium-67 citrate are two alternative radionuclides that are used to complement technetium in the evaluation of osteomyelitis [14]. Scintigraphy is a highly sensitive imaging modality with low specificity. It may be helpful in the evaluation of a significantly degenerated joint, provide information on the acuity of a fracture, and be helpful in the identification of rheumatologic disorders, tumors, and infections.

CT

CT was the first noninvasive means to provide a detailed evaluation of the osseous and soft tissue structures of the lumbosacral spine. CT provides valuable images of the pathology associated with spinal stenosis, infections, facet and sacroiliac joint arthritis, fractures, and neoplasms. The CT system consists of an x-ray tube housed in a circular scanning gantry, image sensors, and a computerized data processing unit. The computer formulates an image from data collected as the x-ray tube rotates, which provides an axial image or "slice" of varying thickness (Fig. 4) [14]. With the ability to reformat, coronal or sagittal images can be added for improved diagnostic accuracy.

Like other radiographic studies, CT presents potential pitfalls if used in isolation from the patient's clinical evaluation. Wiesel and colleagues [4] identified false-positive rates in the asymptomatic population. In a group of 52 asymptomatic individuals, 35% demonstrated abnormal lumbar spine CT scans. Approximately 20% of the abnormalities were found in persons aged 40 years and younger and 50% in persons aged 40 years and older. Herniated nucleus pulposus represented 20% of the abnormalities. The importance of these results is that a clinically irrelevant CT abnormality is identified in approximately one of three patients. All findings on neuroradiographic evaluation must be correlated clinically before any aggressive interventions are undertaken.

The use of CT in identifying herniated nucleus pulposus has been compared with the use of myelography and MRI. Comparing CT and myelography to surgical findings showed that myelographic evaluation was

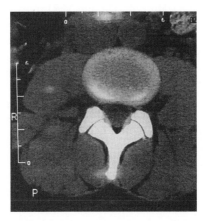

Fig. 4. CT: axial image of a normal intervertebral disc. (*From* Russo R, Cook P. Diagnosis of low back pain: role of imaging studies. Occup Med 1998;13:83–96; with permission.)

more accurate than CT in the diagnosis of herniated nucleus pulposus (83% versus 72%) and spinal stenosis (93% versus 89%) [16]. No clinical correlation was reported in this study, however. The combined use of CT and myelography exceeds the diagnostic ability of either alone [17]. Combined imaging demonstrates delineation of the edge of the thecal sac and can identify the pathologic process that may be causing impaired filling of the spinal nerve root [18]. Myelograms of the lumbar spine must be followed with a CT scan through areas of pathology. Compared with MRI, one study found CT to be nearly equal for accuracy in the diagnosis of herniated nucleus pulposus causing nerve compression [19]. In a separate study, CT myelography was found to be inferior to MRI [20]. Improved CT resolution with newer software has allowed better anatomic evaluation on sagittal and coronal reconstructions. Updated diagnostic study comparisons have not been completed. In this author's experience, MRI is a better initial evaluation.

CT provides a noninvasive tool for evaluation of the lumbosacral spine, with its major limitation being radiation exposure and cost. Like the other neuroimaging modalities, CT has a high false-positive rate, which must be considered when correlating radiographic to clinical findings.

Myelography

Before the 1970s, myelography was the only imaging modality that provided information concerning nerve root compression. With the advent of CT and MRI, its use has dropped precipitously. Given the availability of less invasive tests of equal sensitivity, its primary use has been relegated to presurgical investigation of lumbar spine disorders and disorders that are poorly visualized on CT or MRI, including severe degenerative scoliosis.

Myelography, however, continues to be the only dynamic neuroimaging study that allows visualization of the entire spinal column (Fig. 5). With the advent and greater availability of dynamic MRI, however, this may change. Its major drawbacks include radiation exposure and invasive nature. False-positive rates have been documented and are consistent with the other neuroimaging tests of the lumbar spine. Several investigators have compared the use of the myelogram with CT and MRI [18–20]. The results have varied when comparing each of these modalities. All found MRI to be at least equal to or more accurate than CT myelography. One small series found MRI and CT to be better than a myelogram alone [21]. Although it is unlikely that the myelogram will be replaced completely, its role will remain limited. A lumbar myelogram invariably should be followed with CT to improve the diagnostic accuracy.

Lumbar discography

No diagnostic study stimulates more professional differences than the use of lumbar discography for the evaluation of discogenic low back pain. It

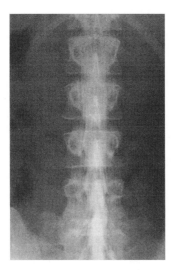

Fig. 5. Anteroposterior myelogram demonstrates small extradural defect between L4 and L5 on the right. (*From* Russo R, Cook P. Diagnosis of low back pain: role of imaging studies. Phys Med Rehab 1999;13:427–42; with permission.)

remains the only imaging modality that allows correlation of radiographic findings and a patient's clinical symptoms. The procedure involves a needle placed posterolaterally within the intervertebral disc space. Nonionic contrast is then injected into the disc to evaluate its morphology and, most importantly, the associated pain response (Fig. 6). Readers are referred to other sources for a more detailed description of the procedure.

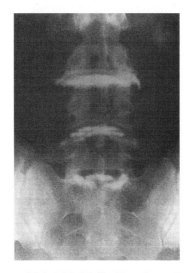

Fig. 6. Three-level discogram: L3-4, L4-5, L5-S1. (*From* Russo R, Cook P. Diagnosis of low back pain: role of imaging studies. Occup Med 1998;13:83–96; with permission.)

Intervertebral disc injections date back to the early to mid 1900s, when Schmorl first evaluated cadaveric discs [22]. Several publications have reported on intervertebral disc injections since his first report [23,24]. A dramatic rise in the use of discography has occurred with the advent of new technologies for the treatment of discogenic low back pain. Holt's finding of a 37% false-positive rate on lumbar discography sparked significant concerns regarding the use of discography. Significant methodologic flaws were present, and serious challenges to the conclusions have arisen [25].

One of the earliest works that demonstrated support for discography was the 0% false-positive rate identified by Walsh and colleagues [26]. Significant shortcomings were present, including small sample size ($n = 10$), use of asymptomatic men, and a bias for young men aged 18 to 32 years old.

Decreased nuclear signal intensity on the T2-weighted MRI images indicates water content loss within an intervertebral disc [27–29]. Internal disc disruption was proposed by H.V. Crock in 1970 [30]. He used it to describe the pathologic change of the internal structure of the disc. More recently described are high-intensity zones, which are seen as increased signal intensities within the posterior annular fibers (Fig. 7) [31–33]. The degenerative changes are found in symptomatic and asymptomatic populations. Plain radiography, myelography, nuclear imaging, and CT scan with or without contrast are unable to detect internal disc disruption. MRI is less sensitive and specific than discography for determining whether intervertebral disc degeneration is symptomatic [6,32,34]. Carragee and colleagues [35] found that the presence of a high-intensity zone does not reliably indicate the

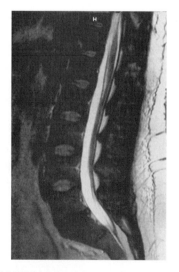

Fig. 7. T2-weighted sagittal MRI high-intensity zone in posterior annular fibers of the L5-S1 intervertebral disc. (*From* Russo R, Cook P. Diagnosis of low back pain: role of imaging studies. Phys Med Rehab 1999;13:427–42; with permission.)

presence of symptomatic internal disc disruption. Recent presentation by Dr. Carragee at the annual meeting of the International Society for the Study of the Lumbar Spine, which is yet unpublished in a scientific journal, revealed significant shortcomings for the use of discography on accurately detecting discogenic low back pain [36].

Lumbar discography remains unique in its ability to determine symptomatic disc degeneration. The provocation of concordant pain is the most important aspect of discography.

MRI

MRI, the newest neurodiagnostic imaging modality, provides an exceptional noninvasive means of evaluating the lumbosacral spine without radiation exposure. Evaluation of the lumbar spine has changed dramatically since its availability in the mid 1980s. Resolution of soft tissue abnormalities and life-threatening pathology, such as neoplasms and infections, has improved tremendously.

In general, the basis for MRI is the re-emission of an absorbed radiofrequency signal by exposure of tissue to a strong magnetic field. Atomic nuclei, once placed within this field, realign along the directions of that field, deviating from their usual random state. Energy is absorbed by the nuclei from the radiofrequency pulse, which causes their orientation in the magnetic field. When the radiofrequency is removed, the nuclei change from a high- to low-energy state, releasing energy. This energy is recorded as an electrical signal, which provides data from which images are derived. The strength of radiowaves, proton concentration, and relaxation time (time nuclei require to return to a state of relaxation) combine to determine the image that is produced.

Relaxation times are referred to as T1 and T2. It is possible to enhance the differences between these by the use of different varieties of radiofrequency pulses. High signal intensity is depicted as a bright (white) area; conversely, a dark (black) area is described as a low signal intensity. On T2-weighted images, the cerebrospinal fluid appears white, similar to a myelogram appearance. Different orthogonal planes can be used for evaluating the lumbar spine. Sagittal and axial imaging planes are the most commonly used and provide adequate visualization of the structures in question. Sagittal images are obtained with a slice thickness of 4 to 5 mm and a field of view of approximately 25 cm (Fig. 8A). This thickness allows visualization of the entire lumbar spine and lowermost thoracic spine, inclusive of the conus medullaris. Five-millimeter thick axial images are obtained through at least the lowest three intervertebral disc spaces, the disc space that correlates with clinical symptoms, or any level that demonstrates abnormalities on sagittal images (Fig. 8B). An alternate technique involves noncontiguous angled slices centered through each lumbar disc space for screening purposes [13,14,27].

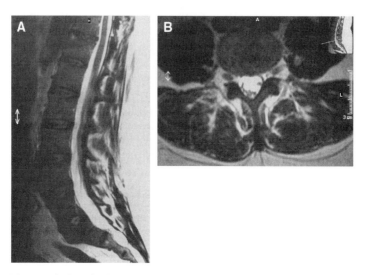

Fig. 8. (*A*) Normal T2 sagittal MRI except for small Schmorl's node abnormality in the superior end plate of T12 vertebral body. (*B*) Normal T2 axial image. (*From* Russo R, Cook P. Diagnosis of low back pain: role of imaging studies. Phys Med Rehab 1999;13:427–42; with permission.)

MRI is the preferred imaging modality for degenerative disc disease, intraspinal tumors, spinal infections, syringomyelia, cord infarction, multiple sclerosis, and intermedullary tumors [13,37–40]. Limitations of its use include high expense, regional variations for availability (rapidly becoming less of a problem), length of scan time, claustrophobia of patients (less problematic with new open-air MRI machines), and contraindications because of ferrous-containing substances. High sensitivity for detecting asymptomatic pathology, although not a true limitation, is an important consideration in patient management.

Several classification schemes can be used to describe the extension of intervertebral disc material beyond the posterior borders of the vertebral end plates [27,29]. Examples are as follows [27,41]: (1) Disc bulge, which is a symmetrical extension of disc tissue beyond the edges of the vertebral end plates (50%–100% disc circumference) (Fig. 9). A disc bulge may be a normal variant or a response to loading, or it may be associated with advanced disc degeneration. (2) Simple disc herniation, which is disc material contained by the outermost, longitudinal annular fibers (Sharpey's fibers) that is seen on the sagittal MR image as an intact margin of low or absent signal at the periphery of the disc. Many clinicians refer to this as a disc protrusion (Fig. 10). (3) Extruded disc herniation, which is a herniated fragment that penetrates through a tear in the outer annular fibers and may extend through the posterior longitudinal ligament. Continuity remains between the herniated fragment and the central disc material, with the stalk being thinner than the herniated portion of disc (Fig. 11). (4) Sequestered disc

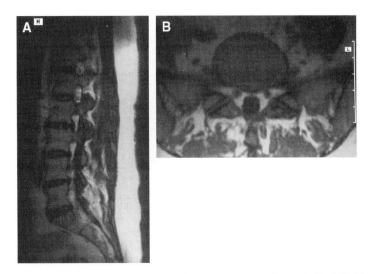

Fig. 9. Disc bulge on T2 sagittal (*A*) and T1 axial (*B*) MRI. (*From* Russo R, Cook P. Diagnosis of low back pain: role of imaging studies. Phys Med Rehab 1999;13:427–42; with permission.)

herniation, which occurs when the herniated fragment, sometimes referred to as a "free fragment," no longer maintains a connection with the central disc material (Fig. 12).

The false-positive rates for lumbosacral MRI have been well documented [1,3]. Jensen and colleagues [3] found a disc protrusion in 27% of asymptomatic individuals and a disc bulge in 52%. Only 36% were found to

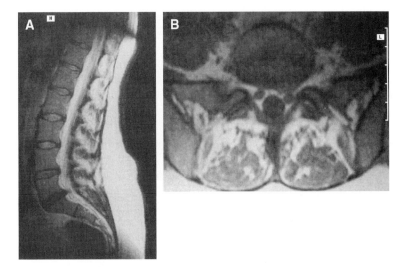

Fig. 10. T2 sagittal (*A*) and T1 axial (*B*) images of simple disc herniation or disc protrusion. (*From* Russo R, Cook P. Diagnosis of low back pain: role of imaging studies. Phys Med Rehab 1999;13:427–42; with permission.)

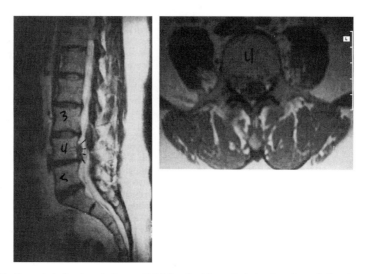

Fig. 11. Extruded disc herniation at L4-5 level with cephalad migration of disc fragments. (*From* Russo R, Cook P. Diagnosis of low back pain: role of imaging studies. Phys Med Rehab 1999;13:427–42; with permission.)

have normal-appearing intervertebral discs at all five lumbar levels. On MRI evaluations of an asymptomatic population, Boden and colleagues [1] found a herniated nucleus pulposus in 20% of individuals younger than 60 years and in 36% of persons older than 60 years. Given these numbers and the prevalence of low back pain, the MRI findings of a disc bulge or protrusion

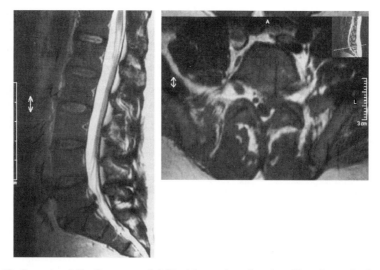

Fig. 12. Sequestered disc fragment at L5-S1 with superior migration. (*From* Russo R, Cook P. Diagnosis of low back pain: role of imaging studies. Phys Med Rehab 1999;13:427–42; with permission.)

often lack clinical significance. It is imperative to correlate the clinical picture, history, and physical examination with the radiographic findings.

MRI has been compared with CT in the evaluation of herniated nucleus pulposus causing nerve compression. The results demonstrated nearly equal diagnostic accuracy of each imaging modality [19]. This finding conflicts with studies that compare MRI and combined CT myelography, which is supposedly more sensitive than standard CT [17]. Forristall and colleagues [20] demonstrated a much greater accuracy of MRI over a contrast-enhanced CT scan for the identification of lumbar disc herniation. The difference was a 90.3% accuracy compared with surgical findings for MRI versus a 77.4% correlation with CT myelography. In light of these discrepancies, further studies are necessary to better compare and define the use of CT and MRI. MRI is an exceptional imaging modality for the lumbar spine. Its major limitations continue to be cost and false-positive findings.

Degenerative disc disease

MR scanning is exceptionally sensitive for demonstrating intervertebral disc degenerative changes. Most adults demonstrate some component of degenerative changes regardless of symptoms. A decrease in signal intensity within the intervertebral disc on T2-weighted images seems to be the earliest evidence of degeneration. In cadaveric spines, Yu and colleagues [42,43] demonstrated correlation between all discs with decreased T2 signal on MRI and radial tears or fissuring of the outer disc annular fibers. Secondary signs of more advanced degeneration include loss of disc height, disc bulging, and vertebral endplate osteophytic spurs. Vertebral body changes also have been identified in association with degenerative spine disease. The most commonly described changes occur within the adjacent vertebra of a degenerated disc. These peridiscal changes have been classified by Modic and colleagues [44,45]. They used the following classification to describe the changes.

Preplacement radiography

The use of pre-employment radiography is controversial. Several attempts to identify its use have been completed, but because of methodologic flaws, clear recommendations have not been established. Radiographic diagnoses, such as spina bifida occulta, sacralization or lumbarization, spondylolysis, spondylolisthesis, scoliosis, degenerative disc disease, facet joint abnormalities, and osteoporosis, have been correlated with the incidence of low back pain. Degenerative disc disease and spondylolisthesis are the two diagnoses that have been demonstrated more often in persons with back pain than in persons without [46–50].

Several investigators have evaluated the use of screening radiographs in the industrial population [51,52]. Although significant methodologic problems were associated with these studies, some general observations can be made. The two studies with the longest observation periods revealed no significant differences between individuals with and without radiologic abnormalities [51]. Others have shown that individuals with radiographic findings may have an increased severity of low back pain but not necessarily an increased incidence [52].

Gibson [51] performed a comprehensive review of the literature on preplacement screening radiography. The two diagnoses found to demonstrate the strongest association between back pain and radiographic findings—degenerative disc disease and spondylolisthesis—have been evaluated. Although degenerative disc disease disease would have a high prevalence on radiographs, screening evaluations would eliminate many potential employees who might never develop lumbar pain. Conversely, spondylolisthesis, would be found in a small percentage of individuals. Screening would expose a large number of persons to radiation, and many persons with positive findings also would be unlikely to develop pain.

Preplacement screening is not a common practice. The literature possesses numerous methodologic flaws, and a single randomized, controlled trial does not exist. Based on the available literature, screening radiography of the lumbar spine has little value in industry.

Ultrasound

The use of ultrasound for musculoskeletal applications has expanded considerably in recent years. Indications include the evaluation of soft tissue masses, ligamentous/tendon tears, articular disorders, and bone abnormalities. The use in the lumbar spine has not been established and is not a regularly used diagnostic technique.

Summary

The identification of the pain generator in acute low back pain can be challenging. Earlier reports showed only a 10% to 20% ability to identify a precise pathoanatomic diagnosis [53,54]. Imaging studies can be a valuable addition to a thorough history and physical examination in the diagnostic process. Injudicious ordering of radiographic tests increases the likelihood of a false-positive result and potential misdiagnosis, however. This article has supported the concept that in acute low back pain, spinal imaging is often unnecessary except in cases in which there is clinical suspicion of a "red flag" disease entity. Standard radiographs of the lumbar spine frequently reveal abnormal findings without clinical significance. Appropriate use guidelines have been outlined. The advanced imaging techniques, including CT, myelography, and MRI, also are expensive and have a high incidence of false-positive findings. Discography continues to be a fiercely debated diagnostic study. Imaging studies should be reserved for cases in which, in the physician's judgment, the results would affect patient management. The appropriate study should be chosen based on what the practitioner expects to find. Once the study has been obtained, the results must be correlated with the clinical presentation. This is particularly important for decisions that concern the use of more invasive treatment methods and return to more normal functional activities.

References

[1] Boden SD, Davis DO, Dina TS, et al. Abnormal magnetic-resonance scans of the lumbar spine in asymptomatic subjects: a prospective investigation. J Bone Joint Surg Am 1990; 72A:403–8.

[2] Hitselberger WE, Witten RM. Abnormal myelograms in asymptomatic patients. J Neurosurg 1968;28:204–6.

[3] Jensen MC, Brant-Zawadzki MN, Obuchowski N. Magnetic resonance imaging of the lumbar spine in people without back pain. N Engl J Med 1994;331:69–73.

[4] Wiesel SW, Tsourmas N, Feffer HL, et al. A study of computer assisted tomography. I. The incidence of positive CT scans in an asymptomatic group of patients. Spine 1984;9:549–51.

[5] Frymoyer JW, Pope MH, Clements JH, et al. Risk factors in low back pain. J Bone Joint Surg Am 1983;65A:213–8.

[6] Scavone JG, Latshaw RF, Widener WA. Anteroposterior and lateral radiographs: an adequate lumbar spine examination. Am J Radiol 1991;136:715–7.

[7] Scavone JC, Latshaw RF, Rohrar GV. Use of lumbar spine films: statistical evaluation at a university teaching hospital. JAMA 1981;246:1105–8.

[8] Liang M, Komaroff AL. Roentgenograms in primary care patients with acute low back pain: a cost-effective analysis. Arch Intern Med 1982;142:1108–12.

[9] Witt I, Vestergaard A, Rosenklint A. A comparative analysis of x-ray findings of the lumbar spine in patients with and without pain. Spine 1984;9:298–300.

[10] Simmons ED Jr, Guyer RD, Graham-Smith A, et al. X-ray assessment for patients with low back pain. In: Contemporary concepts in spine care. Rosemont (IL): North American Spine Society; 1993.

[11] Bigos S, Bowyer O, Braen G, et al. Acute low back problems in adults. Clinical practice guidelines. No. 14. AHCPR publication 95–0642. Rockville (MD): Agency for Health Care Policy and Research; 1994.

[12] Suarez-Almazor M, et al. Back pain guideline could cause excessive use of x-rays. Jt Letter 1997;3(1):4HAU997.

[13] Borenstein D, Wiesel S, Boden S. Low back pain: medical diagnosis and comprehensive management. 2nd edition. Philadelphia: WB Saunders; 1995. p. 109–30.

[14] Greenspan A. Orthopedic radiology: a practical approach. 2nd edition. New York: Raven Press; 1992. p. 2.1–2.11.

[15] Handmaker H, Leonards R. The bone scan in inflammatory osseous disease. Semin Nucl Med 1976;6:95–105.

[16] Bell GR, Rothman RH, Booth RE, et al. A study of computer-assisted tomography. II. Comparisons of metrizamide myelography and computed tomography in the diagnosis of herniated lumbar disc and spinal stenosis. Spine 1984;9:552–6.

[17] Williams AL, Haughton VM, Syvertsen A. Computed tomography in the diagnosis of herniated nucleus pulposus. Radiology 1980;135:95–9.

[18] Voelker JL, Mealey J Jr, Eskridge JM, et al. Metrizamide-enhanced computed tomography as an adjunct to metrizamide myelography in the evaluation of lumbar disc herniation and spondylosis. Neurosurgery 1987;20:379–84.

[19] Thornbury JR, Fryback DG, Turski PA, et al. Disk-caused nerve compression in patients with acute low-back pain: diagnosis with MRI, CT myelography, and plain CT. Radiology 1992;186:731–8.

[20] Forristall RM, Marsh HO, Pay NT. Magnetic resonance imaging and contrast CT of the lumbar spine: comparison of diagnostic methods and correlation with surgical findings. Spine 1988;13:1049–54.

[21] Modic MT, Masaryk T, Boumphrey F, et al. Lumbar herniated disk disease and canal stenosis: prospective evaluation by surface coil MR, CT and myelography. AJR Am J Roentgenol 1986;147:757–65.

[22] Falco F. Lumbar spine injection procedures in the management of low back pain. Occup Med 1998;13:121–49.

[23] Hirsch C. Attempt to diagnose the level of disc lesion clinically by disc puncture. Acta Orthop Scand 1948;18:131–40.

[24] Lindblom K. Diagnostic puncture of the intervertebral discs in sciatica. Acta Orthop Scand 1948;17:231–9.

[25] Holt E. The question of lumbar discography. J Bone Joint Surg Am 1968;50A:720–6.

[26] Walsh TR, Weinstein JN, Spratt KF, et al. Lumbar discography in normal subjects: a controlled, prospective study. J Bone Joint Surg Am 1990;72A:1081–8.

[27] Maravilla K, Cohen W. MRI atlas of the spine. New York: Raven Press; 1991. p. 197–206.

[28] Panagiotacopulos ND, Pope MH, Krag MH, et al. Water content in human intervertebral discs. Part I. Measurements by magnetic resonance imaging. Spine 1987;12:912–7.

[29] Schneiderman G, Flannigan B, Kingston S, et al. Magnetic resonance imaging in the diagnosis of disc degeneration: correlation with discography. Spine 1987;12:276–81.

[30] Crock HV. A reappraisal of intervertebral disc lesions. Med J Aust 1970;1:983–9.

[31] Aprill C, Bogduk N. High-intensity zone: a diagnostic sign of painful lumbar disc on magnetic resonance imaging. Br J Radiol 1992;65:361–9.

[32] Horton WC, Daftari TK. Which disc as visualized by magnetic resonance imaging is actually a source of pain? A correlation between magnetic resonance imaging and discography. Spine 1992;17:5164–71.

[33] Ricketson R, Simmons JW, Hauser BO. The prolapsed intervertebral disc: the high-intensity zone with discography correlation. Spine 1996;21:2758–62.

[34] Zucherman J, Derby R, Hsu K, et al. Normal magnetic resonance imaging with abnormal discography. Spine 1988;13:1355–9.

[35] Carragee EJ, Paragioudakis SJ, Khurana S. 2000 Volvo Award winner in clinical studies: lumbar high-intensity zone and discography in subjects without low back problems. Spine 2000;25(23):2987–92.

[36] Carragee EJ, et al. Clinical outcome after solid ALIF for presumed lumbar "discogenic" pain in highly selected patients: an indirect indication of diagnostic failure of discography. The Back Letter 2005;19.

[37] Kattapuram SV, Khurana JS, Scott JA, et al. Negative scintigraphy with positive magnetic resonance imaging in bone metastases. Skeletal Radiol 1990;19:113–6.

[38] Modic MT, Feiglin DH, Piraino DW, et al. Vertebral osteomyelitis: assessment using MR. Radiology 1985;157:157–66.

[39] Sze G, Krol G, Zimmerman RD, et al. Malignant extradural spinal tumors: MR imaging with gadolinium-DTPA. Radiology 1988;167:217–23.

[40] Modic MT, Pavlicek W, Weinstein MA, et al. Magnetic resonance imaging of intervertebral disk disease: clinical and pulse sequence considerations. Radiology 1985;152:103–11.

[41] Fardon DF, Milette PC. Nomenclature and classification of lumbar disc pathology: recommendations of the Combined Task Forces of the North American Spine Radiology and American Society of Neuroradiology. Spine 2001;26(5):E93–113.

[42] Yu S, Haughton VM, Sether LA, et al. Criteria for classifying normal and degenerated lumbar intervertebral disks. Radiology 1989;170:523–6.

[43] Yu S, Sether LA, Ho PSP, et al. Tears of the annulus fibrosus: correlation between MR and pathologic findings in cadavers. AJNR Am J Neuroradiol 1988;9:367–70.

[44] Modic MT, Stenberg PM, Ross JS, et al. Degenerative disk disease: assessment of changes in vertebral body marrow with MR imaging. Radiology 1988;166:193–9.

[45] Modic MT, Masaryk TJ, Ross JS, et al. Imaging of degenerative disk disease. Radiology 1988;168:177–86.
[46] Biering-Sorenson F, Hansen FR, Schroll M, et al. The relation of spinal x-rays to low back pain and physical activity among 60-year-old men and women. Spine 1985;10:445–51.
[47] Jackson DW, Wiltse LL, Cirincione RJ. Spondylolysis in the female gymnasts. Clin Orthop 1976;117:68–73.
[48] Magora A, Schwartz A. Relationship between low back pain and x-ray changes. IV. Lysis and olisthesis. Scand J Rehabil Med 1980;12:47–52.
[49] Magora A, Schwartz A. Relation between the low back pain syndrome and x-ray findings. III. Spina bifida occulta. Scand J Rehabil Med 1980;12:9–15.
[50] Magora A, Schwartz A. Relation between the low back pain syndrome and x-ray findings. II. Transitional vertebrae. Scand J Rehabil Med 1978;10:135–45.
[51] Gibson ES. Occupational back pain. Spine J 1988;3:91–107.
[52] Leggo C, Mathiason H. Preliminary results of a pre-placement back x-ray program for state traffic officers. J Occup Med 1973;15:973–6.
[53] Frymoyer JW. Back pain and sciatica. N Engl J Med 1988;318:291–300.
[54] Nachemson AL. Advances in low back pain. Clin Orthop 1985;200:266–78.

ELSEVIER
SAUNDERS

Clin Occup Environ Med
5 (3) 591–613

CLINICS IN
OCCUPATIONAL AND
ENVIRONMENTAL
MEDICINE

The Role of Electrodiagnosis in the Evaluation of Low Back Pain

Gregory J. Mulford, MD[a],*, Stephen J. Cohen, MD[b]

[a]Atlantic Health, 95 Mount Kemble Avenue, Morristown, NJ 07960, USA
[b]University of Medicine and Dentistry of New Jersey,
30 Bergen Street, Newark, NJ 07101, USA

It is well established that numerous structures may be damaged in individuals who present with the complaint of low back pain. The significant challenge for clinicians is to determine the cause of the patient's symptoms by identifying the symptom generators as precisely and accurately as possible. Only after a specific and accurate diagnosis is made can a focused, specific, and appropriate treatment plan be implemented. Electrodiagnostic testing can be an important component of the diagnostic assessment of individuals with low back pain. Electrodiagnostic studies provide useful information on the physiologic and functional status of the nervous system. This information complements imaging studies such as radiographs, CT, and MRI, which give information on the status and integrity of anatomic structures [1]. It is important to note that neither electrodiagnostic nor imaging studies are able to verify or quantify the presence or absence of pain. Pain is a complex, subjective, and multifactorial phenomenon for which there is no definitive or "gold standard" diagnostic test. Electrodiagnostic studies are a useful component of a thorough, rational, and objective assessment when an individual presents with complaints of numbness, sensory disturbance, weakness, pain, cramping, or loss of function.

There is no substitute for a thorough history and physical examination in the evaluation of individuals who present with complaints of low back pain. The relevant findings on the history and physical should be the basis on which a differential diagnosis is established [2]. Only after formulating an appropriate differential diagnosis, as supported by relevant findings from the history and physical examination, should additional diagnostic studies be considered [3]. The routine performance of any test or battery of tests is inappropriate and should be discouraged. If a clinician suspects that

---

* Corresponding author.
E-mail address: Gregory.Mulford@Atlantichealth.org (G.J. Mulford).

1526-0046/06/$ - see front matter © 2006 Elsevier Inc. All rights reserved.
doi:10.1016/j.coem.2006.05.002
occmed.theclinics.com

mechanical structures have been injured and if the test results will affect the course of treatment, then imaging studies may be indicated. If, on the other hand, an injured individual has complaints or physical findings that suggest abnormalities of nervous system function, then electrodiagnostic consultation is appropriate. It is important to emphasize the complementary nature of imaging tests and electrodiagnostic studies. For example, an MRI that demonstrates a disc herniation provides little information on the presence or absence of radiculopathy (nerve root injury). Conversely, electrodiagnostic studies that identify the presence of radiculopathy, plexopathy, or peripheral neuropathy do not determine whether a specific structural abnormality is causing or contributing to the electrophysiologic abnormalities. It is frequently helpful for imaging and electrodiagnostic studies to be performed to develop a clearer understanding of all of the pathologic structural and physiologic processes that may be present and contributing to an individual's clinical condition.

Symptoms of numbness, weakness, sensory disturbance, or pain may be the result of injury to neurologic structures, and physical signs of atrophy, weakness not caused by painful inhibition of muscle contraction, disordered sensation, or abnormal reflexes may indicate neuropathic abnormalities and justify the performance of electrodiagnostic studies [4]. Not all individuals with such complaints or findings require electrodiagnostic testing. Only when the test results will help guide further diagnostic evaluation, establish a definitive diagnosis, determine optimal treatment, or aid in prognostication should electrodiagnostic evaluation be considered.

If a treating clinician suspects that there may be injury to or abnormalities of the nervous system based on relevant information obtained by the history or physical examination, then referral for electrodiagnostic consultation is appropriate. The electrodiagnostic consultant also should obtain an appropriate history and perform a physical examination, because they are essential in determining which specific electrodiagnostic tests are most appropriate and useful in any particular clinical situation [3]. The failure of the electrodiagnostic consultant to examine a patient adequately only leads to the performance of unnecessary or inappropriate tests and diminishes the value of the electrodiagnostic consultation. For this reason, the physician who is responsible for the electrodiagnostic testing always should examine the patient personally and either perform the testing directly or directly oversee the technician who performs the studies. The practice of routinely performing a standard battery of tests regardless of the clinical situation also is inappropriate and should be avoided.

Electrodiagnostic medicine consultations should be performed by physicians who, by virtue of their education, training, credentialing, and experience, are qualified to practice electrodiagnostic medicine [5]. To arrive at an accurate diagnosis, the electrodiagnostic medicine consultant must be intimately involved in obtaining and reviewing the relevant history and physical examination, performing the studies, and interpreting the data. Performing and, most importantly, interpreting electrodiagnostic studies comprises all aspects of the practice of medicine, including establishing a diagnosis and making recommendations on diagnosis, treatment, and prognosis. A quality electrodiagnostic consultation and report should include each of these components. Performing tests and reporting data without interpreting the electrophysiologic findings in the context of the clinical picture is of limited value and is discouraged.

Electrodiagnostic studies assist in assessing the function of central and peripheral nervous system structures. Electrodiagnostic studies commonly used to evaluate function of peripheral nervous system elements, such as nerve roots, cervical and lumbosacral plexus, and peripheral nerves, include nerve conduction studies (NCSs), late responses (F-waves and H-reflexes), needle electromyography examination (NEE), and somatosensory evoked potentials (SSEPs). Quantitative sensory testing (QST) and surface EMG are less commonly used electrophysiologic techniques and are discussed only briefly. Studies such as electroencephalography, visual evoked potentials, and brainstem auditory evoked responses offer useful information regarding the functional status of the brain or brainstem and are not addressed in this text.

Nerve conduction studies

NCSs are a valuable means of assessing the functional status of peripheral motor and sensory nerves [6]. NCSs evaluate the ability of a peripheral nerve to transmit an electric signal. Motor NCSs are performed by using a stimulator to apply an electrical stimulus to a peripheral motor nerve and using surface or needle electrode recorders to obtain a compound motor action potential (CMAP) response from a distal muscle supplied by that particular motor nerve. In a similar fashion, sensory NCSs are performed by electrically stimulating a peripheral sensory nerve and recording a sensory nerve action potential (SNAP) directly from the peripheral sensory nerve branch.

Electrophysiologic parameters that are commonly measured include the amplitude of the CMAP or SNAP, distal motor or sensory onset latency, peak sensory latency, and nerve conduction velocity (Figs. 1–4) Onset latency is a measure of time from the stimulus to the initial CMAP or SNAP response and is an indicator of the fastest conducting fibers. Similarly, peak latency measures from the stimulus to the peak of the CMAP or SNAP response. These parameters are used to evaluate the functional status of peripheral nerve axon and myelin structures. In general, decreases in CMAP or SNAP amplitude suggest the presence of axonal damage or conduction block, and prolongation of distal latency or decreases in conduction velocity imply some element of demyelination [7].

NCSs offer the ability to assist in categorizing the type and severity of peripheral nerve injuries (Table 1) [3,8]. A mild nerve injury may result in a neuropraxia, which is defined as a mild and temporary failure of nerve

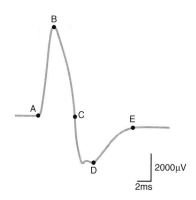

Fig. 1. Thenar muscle CMAP. Example of a typical CMAP recorded from the thenar eminence after median nerve excitation at the wrist. The time represented by the segment A-B is referred to as the rise time, whereas A-C is the duration of the negative spike. Segment A-E represents the duration of the total potential. The amplitude of A-B is the baseline-to-peak magnitude of the potential, whereas B-D is the peak-to-peak amplitude. That portion of the CMAP between A-C and C-E each constitutes one phase of this biphasic potential. The latency of point A is the onset latency, whereas point B represents the peak latency. (*Adapted from* Dumitru D. Electrodiagnostic medicine. Philadelphia: Hanley & Belfus; 1995; with permission.)

conduction without disruption of the nerve axons or architecture. A neuropraxia is usually identified by a normal amplitude response when stimulating distal to the site of injury and a reduced or absent response when stimulating proximally. Slowing of conduction velocity across the injured nerve segment

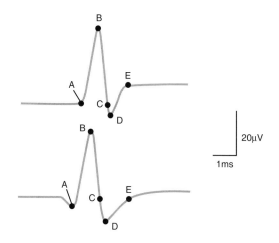

Fig. 2. Antidromic median SNAP recorded from the third digit. The same descriptions noted in Fig. 1 for the potential's various segments apply to this SNAP. In the upper trace, a bipolar recording montage (both recording electrodes on the third digit) is shown. The lower trace depicts the result of relocating the reference (E-2) electrode to the fifth digit, resulting in a referential recording montage and an initially positive triphasic SNAP. (*Adapted from* Dumitru D. Electrodiagnostic medicine. Philadelphia: Hanley & Belfus; 1995; with permission.)

M WAVE

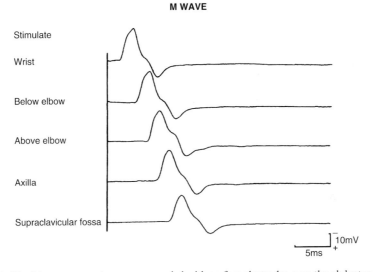

Fig. 3. The M wave, or motor wave, recorded with surface electrodes over the abductor digiti quinti elicited by electric stimulation of the ulnar nerve at several levels. The M wave is a compound action potential evoked from a muscle by a single electric stimulus to its motor nerve. The latency, commonly called the motor latency or distal latency, is the latency (ms) to the onset of the first phase of the M wave. The amplitude (mV) is the baseline-to-peak amplitude of the first phase (*From* American Association of Electrodiagnostic Medicine. Glossary of terms in clinical electromyography. Muscle Nerve 1987;10(8S):G1–60; with permission.)

also may be present. A more significant focal nerve injury that results in axonal damage is called an axonotmesis. With this type of nerve injury, NCSs classically demonstrate decreased amplitudes when stimulating proximal and distal to the site of nerve injury. In a neurotmesis (the most severe degree of nerve injury), motor and sensory conduction responses are usually completely unobtainable. With neuropraxic nerve injuries, there is little structural damage to the axons or myelin sheaths of the affected nerves and there is only a partial and temporary decrease in the ability of the nerve to conduct electric signals across the affected segment. Axonal damage and death occur with axonotmesis injuries, and the prognosis and rate of recovery are significantly worse for axonotmesis injuries than for neuropraxic injuries. In injuries that result in neurotmesis, damage occurs to the endoneurium, perineurium, and epineurium in addition to the nerve axons and myelin sheaths. Prognosis for nerve recovery is much less favorable for neurotmesis injuries because of the presence of such severe damage to the ultrastructural and architectural elements of the peripheral nerve. It may be difficult to differentiate between these various degrees of nerve injury with NCSs alone, and needle electromyography is helpful in further differentiating between neuropraxia, axonotmesis, and neurotmesis.

NCSs may have limited value in the assessment of radiculopathies for numerous reasons. Most radiculopathies are caused by disc protrusions or

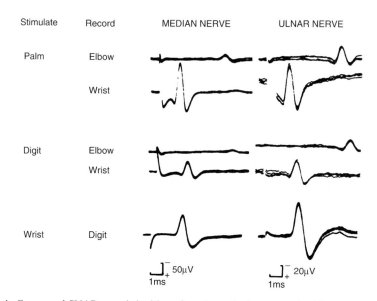

Fig. 4. Compound SNAP recorded with surface electrodes in a normal subject. A compound nerve action potential is considered to have been evoked from afferent fiber if the recording electrodes detect activity in only a sensory nerve or in a sensory branch of mixed curve. The compound SNAP has been referred to as the sensory response of sensory potential. (*From* American Association of Electrodiagnostic Medicine. Glossary of terms in clinical electromyography. Muscle Nerve 1987;10(8S):G1–60; with permission.)

spondylosis that affects only a few motor or sensory fibers, which may not cause an appreciable drop in CMAP or SNAP amplitudes or conduction velocities on NCSs. Pain and paresthesias are transmitted through C-type sensory fibers, which are not detectable with routine NCSs. The cell bodies of sensory nerves reside in the dorsal root ganglion, located in the neural formina. This location is typically protected from compression in radiculopathies and distal sensory axons remain intact, which results in normal SNAPs on NCSs [9]. Any abnormalities of sensory nerve function should raise the possibility of a lesion distal to the dorsal root ganglion and should lead the electrodiagnostic consultant to search diligently for the possibility of a brachial plexopathy or peripheral nerve pathology [3].

NCSs are an excellent way to evaluate peripheral nerve function. Their true value is in evaluating patients with suspected lumbosacral radiculopathy is in assessing peripheral nerve and plexus function and determining whether a more diffuse or distal neuropathic process is present [3]. It has been postulated that any insult to a nerve makes that nerve more susceptible to subsequent injury, which makes the dual diagnosis of peripheral neuropathy and lumbar radiculopathy a distinct possibility [10]. This diagnosis may lead to a confusing clinical picture, so meticulous technique, careful scrutiny of the data obtained, and a broader sense of a patient's clinical picture are always required when performing electrodiagnostic testing.

Table 1
Sunderland and Seddon classification and degrees of peripheral nerve injury

	First degree	Second degree	Third degree	Fourth degree	Fifth degree
	Neurapraxia	Axonotmesis		Neurotmesis	
Electrophysiology	Conduction block		Axonal loss		
Pathology	Segmental demyelination	Loss of axons, with intact supporting structures	Loss of axons, with disrupted endoneurium	Loss of axons, with disrupted endoneurium and perineurium	Loss of axons, with distion of all supporting structures (discontinuous)
Prognosis	Excellent, recovery is usually complete in 2–3 mo	Slow recovery; depends on sprouting and reinnervation	Protracted and recovery may fail because of misdirected axonal sprouts	Unlikely without surgical repair	Impossible without surgical repair

Late responses

H-reflexes, F-waves, and A-waves are typically referred to as late responses. They are secondary, or late, responses that are observed several milliseconds after the direct CMAP response when stimulating a peripheral motor nerve [3]. F-waves provide a means of indirectly evaluating motor nerve conduction proximally at the root level and have been used for more than two decades in the evaluation of radiculopathies. F-waves are recorded by stimulating a peripheral motor nerve with a supramaximal stimulus and recording the action potential that travels along the alpha motor neuron. These waves have much smaller, more variable amplitudes and longer latencies than the CMAP, generally occurring between 25 and 35 milliseconds when stimulating the upper extremity at the wrists and between 50 and 60 milliseconds when stimulating the lower extremity at the ankles [11]. F-waves are believed to represent a "backfiring" of the anterior horn cell and are not a true reflex arc. The latency, amplitude, and shape vary in size from one stimulation to the next. The shortest reproducible response, or minimal latency, is the most widely measured component and represents the conduction time along the largest diameter motor fibers in the stimulated nerve. Other parameters that are sometimes measured include F-wave amplitude, mean latency, extent of latency scatter or "chronodispersion," and persistence of the F-wave response [11–13].

Initially thought to be valuable in detecting proximal peripheral nervous system lesions, such as radiculopathies, the usefulness of F-waves is somewhat limited because they do not detect sensory lesions and abnormalities are often redundant with needle EMG abnormalities [14,15]. If the lesion is small enough, the minimal latency may not be prolonged significantly enough to be detected as abnormal, particularly if some of the fastest conducting fibers are spared [16]. Consequently, F-waves occasionally can be normal even in patients with unequivocal radiculopathies. For these reasons the routine performance of F-wave responses on all peripheral motor nerves in the electrodiagnostic evaluation of radiculopathies is difficult to justify.

A-waves, sometimes referred to as axon reflexes, are nonreflex, monosynaptic responses that may occur between the CMAP and F-wave when performing F-wave studies. Unlike the variable latency of the F-wave, which is obtained with a supramaximal stimulus, the A-wave has a constant latency and is usually elicited with a submaximal stimulus. It represents a backfiring response from collateral sprouting of a proximal portion of the motor nerve and is believed to be a pathologic response that may be seen in radiculopathies, plexopathies, peripheral neuropathies, and motor neuron disease [3].

The H-reflex, first described by Hoffman, is a CMAP that arises through the electrical activation of a monosynaptic reflex arc involving sensory afferent and motor efferent pathways [14,17]. It is most commonly used in assessing S1 fibers in the lower extremities and is elicited by stimulating the tibial nerve in the popliteal fossa with a long duration, low intensity stimulus, and recording over the gastrocnemius-soleus muscles. Parameters that are frequently measured and used to diagnose radiculopathies include side-to-side comparisons of latencies or amplitudes [18–20].

The H-reflex is sensitive—but not specific—for S1 radiculopathies [21]. Because90% to 95% of lumbosacral radiculopathies are at the L5 or S1 level, the H-reflex is valuable in distinguishing S1 from L5 radiculopathies [20]. It is important to note that an abnormal H-reflex alone is not synonymous with a radiculopathy, because the reflex is mediated over a long pathway and abnormalities may be caused by pathology anywhere along its course including the peripheral nerve, plexus, or nerve roots [22]. H-reflexes may be abnormal with advancing age, particularly over age 60, obesity, inadequate penetration of the electrical stimulus, and prior back surgeries [21].

Needle electromyography examination

NEE involves the insertion of a sterile monopolar or concentric needle electrode directly into skeletal muscle and allows the examiner to evaluate the muscle's electrical activity. It is a diagnostic procedure that directly evaluates the electrical properties of skeletal muscle membranes. It is the oldest electrophysiologic method used to evaluate patients with suspected radiculopathies and is still the single most useful electrodiagnostic procedure, having a higher diagnostic yield than other techniques [14,23,24]. The NEE is generally performed in several steps: insertional activity, examination of muscles at rest for spontaneous activity, minimal to moderate muscle contraction, information synthesis, and impression formation.

Needle insertion into normal muscle gives rise to brief bursts of electrical activity, because muscle fibers are mechanically stimulated or injured by the penetrating needle [25–27]. These bursts are called insertional activity and usually last less than 300 msec after needle movement [28]. Increased insertional activity is defined as any electrical activity that persists longer than 300 msec and is seen in the presence of motor axonal damage, denervation, and myopathy. Fibrotic muscle produces decreased insertional activity.

In normal muscles, no electrical activity is seen at rest except when the needle is near the endplate region at the neuromuscular junction. Miniature endplate potentials are recognized by their low amplitudes (10–50 μV) and characteristic sounds like that of a seashell held close to the ear. Endplate spikes are potentials that are 100 to 200 μV that fire irregularly at 5 to 50 pulses per second and constitute normal endplate activity [25]. Endplate spikes have an initial negative deflection, which signifies that they are being generated from directly under the needle at the neuromuscular junction. They are commonly seen in conjunction with miniature endplate potentials. These potentials are believed to be caused by the spontaneous release of acetylcholine from the presynaptic nerve terminal across the neuromuscular junction [29–31]. These normal findings, which can cause an increase in patient discomfort, may be incorrectly mistaken for abnormal spontaneous activity by the inexperienced electromyographer.

When a single muscle fiber spontaneously depolarizes, a muscle-fiber action potential is generated. They can vary in morphology in the form of fibrillation potentials, positive sharp waves, and complex repetitive discharges, but all are forms of abnormal spontaneous activity arising from abnormal muscle generators. Positive sharp waves and fibrillation potentials are the most common forms of abnormal spontaneous activity seen on NEE, and both are generally believed to represent muscle membrane instability and the spontaneous depolarization of a single muscle fiber [3]. Positive sharp waves usually fire at regular rates between 0.5 and 10 Hz (occasionally up to 30 Hz), demonstrate a classic "popping" sound or "dull thud," and have a characteristic morphology of an initial positive (downward) deflection followed by a slower return to baseline (Fig. 5). Fibrillation potentials also have an initial positive deflection, a sharp return to baseline with a biphasic or triphasic morphology, amplitudes of 20 to 1000 μV, firing rates of up to 20 per second, and a high-pitched sound described as "rain on a tin roof" (Fig. 6). The initial positive deflection, slower rate of firing, and more regular rhythm generally help to differentiate abnormal fibrillation potentials from normal endplate spikes (Fig. 7). Positive sharp waves and fibrillation potentials may be recorded in neurogenic and myopathic diseases. They typically develop within 1 to 3 weeks after nerve injury and take longer to appear in muscles more distal to the site of nerve injury. In radiculopathies, such membrane instability may be seen in the

POSITIVE SHARP WAVE

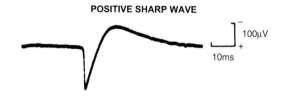

100μV

10ms

TRAIN OF POSITIVE SHARP WAVES

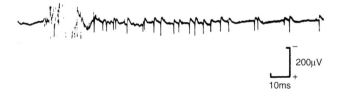

200μV

10ms

Fig. 5. A positive sharp wave is a biphasic action potential initiated by needle movement and recurring in a uniform, regular pattern. A "train" of such waves can be recorded from a damaged area of fibrillating muscle fibers. This is one of the hallmarks of axonal degeneration. (*From* American Association of Electrodiagnostic Medicine. Glossary of terms in clinical electromyography. Muscle Nerve 1987;10(8S):G1–60; with permission.)

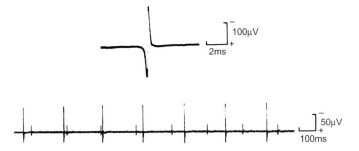

Fig. 6. Fibrillation potential. A fibrillation potential is the electric activity associated with a spontaneously contracting (fibrillating) muscle fiber. This is one of the hallmarks of axonal degeneration. (*From* American Association of Electrodiagnostic Medicine. Glossary of terms in clinical electromyography. Muscle Nerve 1987;10(8S):G1–60; with permission.)

paraspinal muscles within 7 to 10 days and in the corresponding myotomal limb muscles in approximately 21 days after nerve root injury [3,32–34]. As the process continues to evolve over time and becomes a more chronic condition, amplitudes of positive sharp waves and fibrillation potentials fall.

Complex repetitive discharges are sometimes called bizarre, high frequency, or pseudomyotonic discharges. They are generated when one muscle fiber depolarizes and, through ephaptic transmission, spreads to neighboring denervated muscle fibers, subsequently causing their depolarization. They fire regularly at frequencies up to 150 times per second, start and stop abruptly, and often sound like heavy machinery or an idling motorcycle. They have been associated with chronic radiculopathies and neuropathies and motor neuron disease and myopathies [35]. Myotonic discharges also may be seen in chronic radiculopathy or peripheral neuropathy and have a characteristic sound much like a dive bomber. Myotonic discharges demonstrate a waxing and waning of the amplitude and firing rate of the spontaneously discharging single muscle fibers generating the potentials [36].

Abnormal spontaneous potentials that arise from the motor neuron or axonal generators are fasciculation potentials and myokymic discharges. Fasciculations are the visible, spontaneous intermittent contractions seen within a portion of a muscle, and fasciculation potentials are the electrically summated voltage potentials of multiple spontaneously depolarizing muscle fibers belonging to a single motor unit that are seen on NEE [37]. Their amplitude, duration, and phases are similar to that of normal motor units, although they discharge irregularly and more slowly, typically from 0.1 to 10 Hz [38]. Voluntary motor unit action potentials (MUAPs) conversely begin firing at 4 to 5 Hz [39]. Fasciculations can be seen in any disorder that affects the lower motor neurons, including radiculopathies and polyneuropathies, although they are classically associated with amyotrophic lateral sclerosis. Most normal individuals have some degree of fasciculations, called benign fasciculations, so the electromyographer must be vigilant in

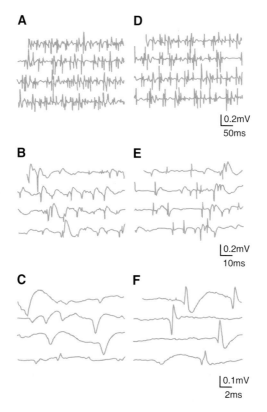

Fig. 7. Spontaneous single fiber activity of the paraspinal muscle in a 40-year-old man with radiculopathy, which consisted of positive sharp waves (*A–C*) and fibrillation potentials (*D–F*).

examining for additional evidence of denervation when fasciculation potentials are observed on NEE. Myokymic discharges, usually seen in association with visible rippling movements of the skin (myokymia) represent bursts of normal appearing motor units with interburst intervals of silence in a semirhythmic pattern [40]. Myokymic discharges often sound like the sputtering of a low-powered motorboat engine. Myokymic discharges, which represent groups of motor units, may be distinguished from complex repetitive discharges, which represent groups of single muscle fibers [41]. Typically they do not start and stop abruptly and the MUAPs of each burst of motor units are variable, unlike complex repetitive discharges, which usually start and stop abruptly and have consistent morphologies of each burst. Myokymic discharges may be seen in segmental patterns in chronic radiculopathies [42].

MUAP recruitment pattern and morphology can be evaluated during minimal to moderate muscle contraction. MUAP amplitudes normally range from several hundred microvolts to a few millivolts when testing is performed with a concentric needle and are often substantially greater when using a monopolar needle electrode. MUAP duration normally varies from 5 to 15 msec [25]. The number of phases of a MUAP equals the number of baseline crossings plus 1, and normal motor unit potentials usually have four or fewer phases. MUAPs with more than four phases are designated as polyphasic. Polyphasia is a measure of how synchronously different muscle fibers within one motor unit are firing [25]. In chronic neuropathic conditions, collateral sprouting gives rise to small polyphasic motor units. As time progresses, these units become larger, polyphasic units and eventually become large amplitude, long duration motor units. Up to 20% of MUAPs may be polyphasic in any normal muscle, so the electromyographer should be cautious about determining whether a study is abnormal based solely on the presence of polyphasic MUAPs.

Single motor units usually fire at a rate of 5 to 10 times per second [43,44]. Small, type I muscle fibers are activated first, and larger, type II units are recruited later during stronger voluntary contractions [45]. Abnormalities of motor units firing rates may occur at the onset of nerve injury, long before abnormal spontaneous activity develops, giving the first clue that neuronal damage may have occurred [17,46]. Considerable experience is needed to be able to recognize more subtle changes in MUAP firing patterns [47]. At just perceptible levels of muscle contraction, when motor unit firing begins, the needle electrode records from one to three single motor units. At this low level of muscle activation, MUAP morphology, onset firing rates, and recruitment firing rates can be assessed best [48]. Neuronal damage results in a decrease in the number of MUAPs contracting, seen as a decrease in recruitment pattern and an incomplete interference pattern. Objective analysis of interference and recruitment patterns can be difficult secondary to lack of patient effort or pain during the attempted muscle contraction. Normally, by the time a motor unit is firing at a rate of 10 Hz, a second motor unit begins firing, and when the first unit reaches a firing rate of approximately 15 Hz a third motor unit becomes activated. Single motor units firing at rates of more than 20 Hz are abnormal [48]. Under these normal conditions, the recruitment ratio, defined as the firing rate of the fastest motor unit divided by the total number of motor units firing, is 3. In pathologic states with reduced numbers of normally contracting motor units, single motor units often fire at rates of more than 20 Hz, and recruitment ratios are more than 5 [3]. For example, if a motor unit is firing at 20 Hz when the second motor unit begins firing, the recruitment ratio is 20/2 or 10, which is abnormal. In situations with mild abnormalities and minimal weakness, recruitment may be normal at minimal to moderate levels of contraction. The electromyographer should increase gradually the force of muscle contraction to allow recruitment of high-threshold motor units that may be firing at abnormally high rates [48].

NEE is useful in the evaluation of patients with suspected radiculopathies, plexopathies, or peripheral neuropathies and is most useful in determining the presence of motor axon loss [49]. Root level localization, the degree of axonal loss, and chronicity of the injury may be ascertained from a thorough NEE. Careful muscle selection is essential in determining whether the location of a nerve injury lies at the level of the nerve root, plexus, or peripheral nerve. Determination of the exact muscles evaluated on NEE depends on the differential diagnosis and the innervation of the various muscles sampled. In radiculopathies, NEE abnormalities are seen in a myotomal distribution in the form of increased insertional activity, abnormal spontaneous activity, reduced recruitment of motor units, or changes in MUAP amplitudes, morphology, and duration [21].

NEE of the paraspinal muscles is necessary for a proper assessment of radiculopathy, because abnormalities are often detected in these muscles. Depending on the time course of the injury, reinnervation to the paraspinal muscles already may have occurred, or the pathology may involve only anterior ramus fibers, sparing the posterior ramus fibers that innervated the paraspinal muscles. Precise localization of a specific nerve root involved in a radiculopathy is difficult to determine based on the presence of paraspinal abnormalities alone because of the overlapping innervation of most paraspinal muscles. Identifying the specific abnormal nerve root is most accurately accomplished by finding abnormalities in limb muscles in a myotomal distribution. It is important to sample limb muscles supplied by the nerve roots in question and muscles supplied by nerve roots above and below. A study result is said to be positive if abnormalities are present in two or more muscles receiving innervation from the same nerve root, preferably from different peripheral nerves [47]. Although the primary innervation of many muscles remains debatable, myotomal maps are helpful as approximate guides (Table 2).

A detailed review of the literature failed to identify any studies that support the routine performance of bilateral needle EMG or NCSs in the standard evaluation of the individual with low back pain. Only when bilateral

Table 2
Minimal screen needle electromyographic examination

Lower extremity	
Muscle	Root level
Lumbosacral paraspinal muscles	L1–S1
Quadriceps femoris	L2, L3, L4
Gluteus medius	L4, L5, S1
Tibialis anterior	L4, L5, S1
Peroneus longus	L5, S1
Medial gastrocnemius	S1, S2
Lateral gastrocnemius	L5, S1, S2
Extensor hallucis longus	L5, S1

Additional muscles should be investigated should the diagnosis be unclear. In the paraspinal regions, the root designations refer to the bony level that should be examined (ie, the multifidi muscle layer).

symptoms or signs are present or when multilevel abnormalities are documented on the symptomatic side is there a good chance that bilateral disease is present. There seems to be little justification for the routine performance of bilateral studies in patients who present with unilateral complaints when electrophysiologic findings are normal in the symptomatic extremity.

Spinal nerve root stimulation

It is possible to directly stimulate the spinal nerve roots using an EMG needle as the stimulating cathode, [50,51] although spinal nerve root stimulation is infrequently performed in the evaluation of lumbosacral radiculopathy. Limitations to this method include its relatively invasive and uncomfortable nature, risk of injury to spinal or neurovascular structures, difficulty in determining the exact site of neural stimulation, and potential for technical factors to result in abnormal side-to-side results thereby producing false positive findings.

Somatosensory evoked potentials

SSEPs have been used to evaluate the function of peripheral and central sensory pathways [47]. They are elicited by electrical stimulation of an accessible mixed or cutaneous nerve or of the skin in the territory of a particular nerve or nerve root and are conceptualized as NCSs over a relatively long portion of the peripheral and central nervous systems [3]. They are helpful in evaluating patients with suspected sensory root lesions because they provide a means of studying sensory function in proximal portions of the peripheral nervous system. Limitations to their use include the potential masking of any focal slowing of conduction by the long distance between the site of peripheral stimulation and the site at which the response is recorded. Focal conduction block in some fibers may be undetected because conduction in the unaffected fibers generates a normal response. Precise localization of a lesion also is limited. SSEP abnormalities provide little clue to the nature or age of a lesion involving the sensory pathways. Normal individuals may have up to 70% variation of amplitude between one trial and another for the same nerve or from one side to the other [52,53]. With proper technique and preparation, SSEPs are no more difficult to obtain than routine peripheral sensory NCSs. Waveforms can be recorded from the peripheral nerve, spinal cord, or sensory cortex after peripheral stimulation of a sensory nerve, mixed nerve, or dermatomal location (Fig. 8). Standard locations for electrode placement have been recommended by the American Electroencephalographic Society. Short-latency responses are defined as waveforms that occur within approximately 25 msec of the stimulus in normal persons and within approximately 50 msec after lower extremity stimulation [54,55].

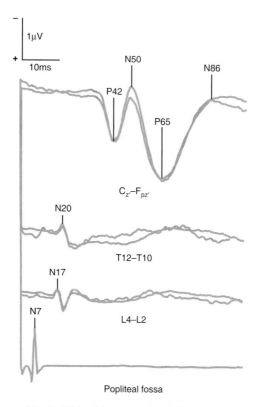

Fig. 8. Right tibial nerve stimulation (ankle).

Dermatomal/segmental SSEPs (Table 3) are relatively easy to perform but remain controversial in the diagnosis of nerve root injury, and there are questions regarding the sensitivity and specificity of these studies [14,21,53,56–61]. The diagnostic yield of SSEPs seems to be somewhat

Table 3
Upper extremity dermatomal/segmental somatosensory evoked potentials

Nerve	Cord	Trunk	Segment	Latency ($n = 20$)
Musculocutaneous	Lateral	Upper	C6	17.4 ± 1.2
Median (digit 1)	Lateral	Upper	C6	22.5 ± 1.1*
Median (digits 2 and 3)	Lateral	Middle	C7	21.2 ± 1.2
Superficial radial (digit 1)	Posterior	Upper	C6	22.5 ± 1.1*
Ulnar (digit 5)	Medial	Lower	C8	22.5 ± 1.1

Modified from Eisen A, Hoirch M. Electrodiagnostic evaluation of radiculopathies and plexopathies using somatosensory evoked potentials. Electroencephalogr Clin Neurophysiol 1982;36(Suppl):349–57; Eisen A. The use of somatosensory evoked potentials for the evaluation of the peripheral nervous system. Neurol Clin 1988;6:825–38.

higher in the lumbosacral region [60,62,63], but controversies on the usefulness of these studies in the diagnosis of radiculopathy still exist [64,65].

Quantitative sensory testing

Lesions that involve small, unmyelinated sensory fibers or occur proximal to the dorsal root ganglion may go undetected by NCSs, EMG, and SSEP techniques, which evaluate only the large-diameter, myelinated motor and sensory fibers [3]. Various QST methods theoretically offer means by which different sensory nerve populations can be evaluated [66,67]. Controlled, prospective studies using QST in the evaluation of acute neuromusculoskeletal injuries are lacking, and controversy still exists regarding the usefulness of QST [68]; however, QST seems to hold promise in the evaluation of individuals who present with sensory complaints and pain. A recent article demonstrated 80% positive QST results but a lack of correlation between changes in pain scores and sensory test results in a group of patients with clinical radiculopathy after treatment with epidural steroid injections [69]. A statistically significant correlation between MRI findings and QST was noted in a group of patients with signs and symptoms of cervical and lumbosacral intervertebral disc disease [62]. Other studies identified changes in QST findings after spinal anesthesia [70–72]. Although the literature raises intriguing possibilities regarding the potential use of this technology in the clinical setting and the Texas Workers' Compensation Commission recently incorporated QST measures into their spinal treatment guidelines [3], it is the author's opinion that there seems to be insufficient clinical research to support its routine use in the standard evaluation of patients with low back injuries. Additional well-designed, prospective clinical studies evaluating the usefulness and efficacy of QST are necessary before they are incorporated into the routine electrodiagnostic evaluation of neuromusculoskeletal injuries.

Surface electromyography

Surface EMG refers to recording of electrophysiologic signals from skeletal muscles using surface recording electrodes. Summated muscle electrical activity is observed when muscles are activated or contracting. A technology review approved by the American Association of Electrodiagnostic Medicine and endorsed by the American Academy of Physical Medicine and Rehabilitation in 1995 concluded that there are no clinical indications for the use of surface EMG in the diagnosis and treatment of disorders of nerve or muscle [73]. Surface EMG studies are more routinely used as components of gait and motion analysis and have considerable potential in the evaluation of movement, ergonomics, and kinesiology. Currently, there seems to be little evidence to support their use in the routine diagnostic evaluation of acute radiculopathy, plexopathy, peripheral nerve injury, or other acute neuro-musculoskeletal injury [74].

Indications for electrodiagnostic evaluation

In the past decade there have been significant technologic advancements in diagnostic imaging studies and therapeutic techniques designed to treat patients with low back pain. Because of the high prevalence of low back pain, however, it is not recommended that exhaustive evaluations for every person who presents with a chief complaint of low back pain be performed on a routine basis. Instead, a structured—yet individualized—approach should be taken with each patient. It is important for clinicians to recognize which patients are appropriate for referral for electrodiagnostic evaluation and how this information may guide or influence diagnostic or treatment options. The primary indications for electrodiagnostic testing include subjective symptoms of numbness, weakness, sensory disturbance, or pain or objective physical findings of disordered sensation, weakness, atrophy, abnormal reflexes, dural tension signs, or abnormal visible muscle contractions, such as fasciculations or myokymia. Axial back pain alone, without any associated signs or symptoms that suggest radiculopathy or other peripheral neuropathic processes, is not in and of itself a strong indication for electrodiagnostic evaluation. Abnormal imaging studies that identify structural pathology that may affect neurophysiologic function also may provide a reasonable indication for electrodiagnostic testing, particularly if an individual does not respond to treatment focused on the structural pathology.

Frequently, a patient's history and physical examination findings correlate well, and the treating physician is comfortable proceeding with treatment without the information provided by imaging studies or electrodiagnostic testing. When a patient responds to the treatment plan, further diagnostic evaluation is not necessary. Many patients with low back pain and related symptoms do not present with a classic constellation of history and corresponding physical examination findings, however, or do not respond to initial treatment measures as anticipated. In these situations, further diagnostic evaluation that includes imaging studies or electrodiagnostic testing may be indicated. Identifying the specific pain generators is important in developing an optimally effective treatment plan. In patients with signs or symptoms of suspected nerve root injury, electrodiagnostic testing can help to confirm or establish a diagnosis that was otherwise unclear and can offer insight on severity and prognosis when nerve root injury exists. Once a diagnosis of suspected lumbosacral radiculopathy is confirmed, specific and targeted treatment options can be implemented. A patient with radiating leg pain and sensory disturbance might benefit most from a selective nerve root injection and specific therapy interventions if an isolated single nerve root abnormality is identified. The patient also might be best served by surgical nerve root decompression if severe or more widespread nerve root axonal damage is demonstrated.

When significant nerve root pathology is confirmed and there is strong correlation with imaging studies, the decision for surgical intervention becomes much clearer. Profound electrophysiologic abnormalities may not only strengthen the decision to proceed with surgery but also suggest that the postoperative course may be prolonged with a more guarded prognosis, even with surgery. On the other hand, even when a patient's signs or symptoms point to a diagnosis of lumbosacral radiculopathy, electrodiagnostic testing may reveal normal nerve root function or unexpected abnormalities, such as a more peripheral neuropathic process (eg, plexopathy, mononeuropathy, or polyneuropathy). Such information may lead to an alteration in the patient's treatment plan, including the potential to prevent patients from undergoing unnecessary surgery or invasive procedures, or redirect treatment efforts to more potentially effective interventions. Normal electrodiagnostic findings can assist in reducing or eliminating the worry or concern a patient may have about possible nerve damage and allow the treating physician to be confident in offering reassurance that an individual's symptoms do not come from actual nerve damage. Low back pain or leg pain is often referred from injury to nonneural structures, in which instance electrodiagnostic testing is likely to be normal and treatment options modified accordingly. For example, a course of oral or epidural steroids and physical therapy that might be provided based on an assumed diagnosis of radiculopathy may be unwarranted or less effective than other measures if the primary pain generators are facet or soft tissue pathology, in which case the electrodiagnostic studies would be normal.

Electrodiagnostic studies can establish the severity and extent of nerve damage and the chronicity of neurologic insult and ultimately provide insight into prognosis and potential for recovery. Although the severity of an injury does not always correlate well with a patient's subjective complaints of pain, the assessment of CMAP amplitudes, degree of abnormal spontaneous activity, degree of motor unit loss, and recruitment patterns collectively correlate well with severity and prognosis related to nerve function. A significantly longer and less complete recovery is to be expected when there is more than one level of nerve root involvement or when there is evidence of significant axonal degeneration, compared with a less severe injury that involves primarily conduction block, which is associated with a more favorable prognosis.

Chronicity of injury can be determined through electrodiagnostic studies, because MUAPs of long duration and increased amplitudes indicate a more chronic process. MUAPs of normal size in the presence of increased insertional activity without abnormal spontaneous activity indicate that the lesion may have occurred within the past several days. The presence of abnormal spontaneous activity with normal MUAPs implies an injury of approximately 3 weeks or longer. Some clinicians even advocate avoiding vigorous muscle strengthening during this early period of acute denervation.

Summary

Establishing a specific diagnosis is important in the effective management of individuals who present with a complaint of low back pain. Electrodiagnostic studies are an integral part of the diagnostic evaluation when the history or physical examination suggests that neural structures may contribute as symptom generators. Lumbosacral radiculopathies, plexopathies, and peripheral nerve injuries are of primary concern when evaluating individuals with low back pain, and electrodiagnostic studies assist in identifying and quantifying neurophysiologic injuries and abnormalities using techniques as previously identified and described. A thorough, thoughtful, and individualized electrodiagnostic study performed by qualified physicians as an extension of a detailed history and physical examination can be an important and useful component in the proper evaluation of individuals with low back pain.

References

[1] Cole A, Herring S, editors. The low back pain handbook: a practical guide for the primary care clinician. Philadelphia: Hanley & Belfus; 1997.
[2] DeLisa J, editor. Rehabilitation medicine principles and practice. Philadelphia: JB Lippincott; 1988.
[3] Dumitru D. Electrodiagnostic medicine. Philadelphia: Hanley & Belfus; 1995.
[4] Malanga G, editor. SPINE: state of the art reviews. Cervical flexion-extension/whiplash injuries. Philadelphia: Hanley & Belfus; 1998.
[5] American Association of Electrodiagnostic Medicine. Guidelines in electrodiagnostic medicine: muscle and nerve. Rochester (MN): American Association of Electrodiagnostic Medicine; 1999.
[6] Lambert EH. Neurophysiological techniques useful in the study of neuromuscular disorders. In: Adams RD, Eaton LM, Shy G, editors. Neuromuscular disorders. Baltimore (MD): Williams and Wilkins; 1960. p. 247–73.
[7] Martinez AC, Perez Conde M, DelCampo F, et al. Ratio between the amplitude of sensory evoked potentials at the wrist in both hands of left-handed subjects. J Neurol Neurosurg Psychiatry 1980;43:182–94.
[8] Kimura J. Electrodiagnosis in diseases of nerve and muscle: principles and practice. 2nd edition. Philadelphia: FA Davis Company; 1989.
[9] Kikuchi S, Sato K, Honno S, et al. Anatomic and radiographic study of dorsal root ganglia. Spine 1994;19:6–11.
[10] Upton RM, McComas AJ. The double crush syndrome in nerve entrapment syndromes. Lancet 1984;9:19–22.
[11] Kimura J. F-wave determination in nerve conduction studies. In: Desmedt JE, editor. Motor control mechanisms in health and disease. New York: Raven Press; 1983. p. 961–75.
[12] Fisher MAF. Response latency determination. Muscle Nerve 1982;5:730–4.
[13] Panayiotopoulos CP, Scarpalezos S, Nastas PE. F wave studies on the deep peroneal nerve. J Neurol Sci 1977;31:319–29.

[14] Aminoff MJ, Goodin DS, Parry GJ. Electrophysiologic evaluation of lumbosacral radiculopathies: electromyography, late responses, and somatosensory evoked potentials. Neurology 1985;34:1514–8.
[15] Young RR, Shahani BT. Clinical value and limitations of F-wave determination. Muscle Nerve 1978;1:248–9.
[16] Levin KH, Maggiano JH, Wilbourn AJ. Cervical radiculopathies: comparison of surgical and EMG localization of single root lesions. Neurology 1996;45:1022–5.
[17] Eisen A. Electrodiagnosis of radiculopathies. Neurol Clin 1985;3:495–510.
[18] Jankus WR, Robinson LR, Little JW. Normal limits of side-to-side H reflex amplitude variability. Arch Phys Med Rehabil 1994;75:3–7.
[19] Nishida T, Kompoliti A, Janssen K, et al. H reflex I S-1 radiculopathy: latency versus amplitude controversy revisited. Muscle Nerve 1996;19:915–7.
[20] Schuchmann J. H-reflex latency in radiculopathy. Arch Phys Med Rehabil 1978;59: 185–7.
[21] Levin KH. Electrodiagnostic approach to the patient with suspected radiculopathy. Neurol Clin N Am 2002;20:397–421.
[22] Wilbourn AJ. The value and limitations of electromyographic examination in the diagnosis of lumbosacral radiculopathy. In: Hardy RW, editor. Lumbar disc disease. New York: Raven Press; 1982. p. 65–109.
[23] Aminoff MJ. Electromyography in clinical practice. 3rd edition. New York: Churchill-Livingstone; 1998.
[24] Kuroglu R, Oh SJ, Thompson B. Clinical and electromyographic correlations of lumbosacral radiculopathy. Muscle Nerve 1994;17:250–1.
[25] Kimura J. Electrodiagnosis in diseases of nerve and muscle: principles and practice. 2nd edition. Philadelphia: FA Davis Company; 1989.
[26] Weichers DO. Mechanically provoked insertional activity before and after nerve section in rats. Arch Phys Med Rehabil 1977;58:402–5.
[27] Weichers DO, Stow R, Johnson EW. Electromyographic insertional activity mechanically provoked in the biceps brachii. Arch Phys Med Rehabil 1977;58:573–8.
[28] Goodgold J, Eberstein A. Electrodiagnosis of neuromuscular diseases. 3rd edition. Baltimore: Williams & Wilkins; 1983.
[29] Elmqvist D, Johns TR, Thesleff S. A study of some electrophysiological properties of human intercostal muscle. J Physiol 1960;154:602–7.
[30] Elmqvuist D, Hoffman WW, Kugelberg J, et al. An electrophysiological investigation of neuromuscular transmission in myasthenia gravis. J Physiol 1964;174:417–34.
[31] Elmqvist D, Quastel DMJ. A quantitative study of endplate potentials in isolated human muscle. J Physiol 1965;178:505–29.
[32] Buchthal F, Rosenfalck P. Spontaneous electrical activity of human muscle. Electroencephalogr Clin Neurophysiol 1966;20:321–36.
[33] Buchthal F. Fibrillation: clinical electrophysiology. In: Culp WJ, Ochoa J, editors. Abnormal nerves and muscle generators. New York: Oxford University Press; 1982. p. 632–62.
[34] Thesleff S. Physiological effects of denervation of muscle. Ann N Y Acad Sci 1974;228: 89–103.
[35] Emeryk B, Hausmanowa-Petrusewicz I, Nowak T. Spontaneous volleys of bizarre high frequency potentials in neuromuscular diseases. Electromyogr Clin Neurophysiol 1974;14: 339–54.
[36] Brumlik J, Dreschler B, Vannin TM. The myotonic discharge in various neurological syndrome: neurophysiologic analysis. Electromyography 1970;10:369–83.
[37] Brown WF. The physiological and technical basis of electromyography. Boston: Butterworth; 1984.
[38] Litchy WJ. A practical demonstration of EMG activity. In: Standard needle electromyography of muscles. Rochester (MN): American Association of Electrodiagnostic Medicine; 1988. p. 23–33.

[39] Preston DC, Shapiro BE. Needle electromyography fundamentals, normal and abnormal patterns. Neurol Clin N Am 2002;20:361–96.

[40] Daube JA, Kelly JJ, Martin RA. Facial myokymia with polyradiculoneuropathy. Neurology 1979;29:662–9.

[41] Stalberb EV, Trontelj JV. Abnormal discharges generated within the motor unit as observed with single-fiber electromyography. In: Culp WJ, Ochoa J, editors. Abnormal nerves and muscles as impulse generators. New York: Oxford University Press; 1982. p. 445–74.

[42] Albers JW, Allen AA, Bastron JD, et al. Limb myokymia. Muscle Nerve 1981;4:494–504.

[43] Clamann HP. Activity of single motor units during isometric tension. Neurology 1970;20: 254–60.

[44] Petajan JH. Clinical electromyographic studies of diseases of the motor unit. Electroencephalogr Clin Neurophysiol 1974;36:395–401.

[45] Warmolts JR, Engel WK. Open biopsy electromyography: correction of motor unit behavior with histochemical muscle fiber type in human limb muscle. Arch Neurol 1972;27:512–7.

[46] Clairmont AC, Johnson EW. Evaluation of the patient with possible radiculopathy. In: Johnson EW, Pease WS, editors. Practical electromyography. 3rd edition. Baltimore: William & Wilkins; 1997. p. 115–30.

[47] Wilbourn A, Aminoff M. The electrodiagnostic examination in patients with radiculopathies. Rochester (MN): American Association of Electrodiagnostic Medicine; 1998.

[48] Petajan J. Motor unit recruitment. Rochester (MN): American Association of Electrodiagnostic Medicine; 1991.

[49] Dillingham TR, Lauder TD, Andary M, et al. Identification of cervical radiculopathies: optimizing the electromyographic screen. Am J Phys Med Rehabil 2001;80(2):84–91.

[50] Cherington M. Long thoracic nerve conduction studies. Dis Nerv Syst 1972;33:49–51.

[51] Davis FA. impairment of repetitive impulse conduction in experimentally demyelinated and pressure injured nerves. J Neurol Neurosurg Psychiatry 1972;35:537–44.

[52] Aminoff MJ, Goodin DS, Barbaro NM, et al. Dermatomal somatosensory evoked potentials in unilateral lumbosacral radiculopathy. Ann Neurol 1985;17:171–6.

[53] Aminoff MJ. Use of somatosensory evoked potentials to evaluate the peripheral nervous system. J Clin Neurophysiol 1987;4:135–44.

[54] American Electroencephalographic Society. Recommended standards for short-latency somatosensory evoked potentials. J Clin Neurophysiol 1984;1:41–53.

[55] American Electroencephalographic Society. Recommended standards for the clinical practice of evoked potentials. J Clin Neurophysiol 1984;1:6–14.

[56] Aminoff MJ, Goodin DS. Dermatomal somatosensory evoked potentials in lumbosacral root compression [letter]. J Neurol Neurosurg Psychiatry 1988;51:740–1.

[57] Aminoff NJ. Evoked potential studies in neurological diagnosis and management. Ann Neurol 1990;28:706–10.

[58] Eisen A, Elleker G. Sensory nerve stimulation and evoked cerebral potentials. Neurology 1980;30:1097–105.

[59] Eisen A, Hoirch M, Moll A. Evaluation of radiculopathies by segmental stimulation and somatosensory evoked potentials. Can J Neurol Sci 1983;10:178–82.

[60] Perlik S, Fisher MA, Patel DV, et al. On the usefulness of somatosensory evoked responses for the evaluation of lower back pain. Arch Neurol 1986;43:907–13.

[61] Rodriquez AA, Kanis L, Rodriques AA, et al. Somatosensory evoked potentials from dermatomal stimulation as an indicator of L5 and S1 radiculopathy. Arch Phys Med Rehabil 1987;68:366–8.

[62] Scarff TB, Allman DE, Toleikis JR, et al. Dermatomal somatosensory evoked potentials in the diagnosis of lumbar root entrapment. Surg Forum 1981;332:488–91.

[63] Walk D, Fisher MA, Doundoulakis SH, et al. Somatosensory evoked responses in the evaluation of lumbosacral radiculopathy. Neurology 1991;43:1197–202.

[64] Dumitru D, Dreyfuss P. Dermatomal/segmental somatosensory evoked potential evaluation of L5S1 unilateral/unilevel radiculopathies. Muscle Nerve 1996;19:442–9.

[65] Seyal M, Sandhu LS, Mack YP. Spinal segmental somatosensory evoked potentials in lumbosacral radiculopathies. Neurology 1989;39:801–5.

[66] Zhu PY, Starr A. Neuroselective CPT evaluation in syringomyelia. Presented at the Meeting of the North American Spine Society. Washington, DC, 1995.

[67] Luis Kopacz DJ. Quantitative assessment of differential sensory nerve block after lidocaine spinal anesthesia. Anesthesia 1995;83:60–3.

[68] American Associations of Electrodiagnostic Medicine. Technology review: the neurometer current perception threshold (CPT): equipment and computer committee. Muscle Nerve 1991;22:523–31.

[69] Mironer YE, Somerville JJ. The current perception threshold evaluation in radiculopathy: efficacy in diagnosis and assessment of the treatment results. Pain Digest 1998;8:37–8.

[70] Tay B, Wallace M, Irving G. Quantitative assessment of differential sensory blockade after lumbar epidural lidocaine. J Anesth Analg 1997;84:1075.

[71] Liu S, Kopacz D, Carpenter R. Quantitative assessment of differential sensory nerve block after lidocaine spinal anesthesia. Anesthesiology 1995;82:60–3.

[72] Sakura S, Sumi M, Yamada Y, et al. Quantitative and selective assessment of sensory block during lumbar epidural anesthesia with 1% or 2% lidocaine. Br J Anesthesia 1998;81: 718–22.

[73] American Association of Electrodiagnostic Medicine. Guidelines in electrodiagnostic medicine. Muscle Nerve 1999;8(Suppl):239–41.

[74] Pullman SL, Goodin DS, Marquinez AI. Clinical utility of surface EMG: report of the therapeutics and technology assessment subcommittee of the American Academy of Neurology. Neurology 2000;55:171–7.

ELSEVIER
SAUNDERS

Clin Occup Environ Med
5 (3) 615–632

CLINICS IN
OCCUPATIONAL AND
ENVIRONMENTAL
MEDICINE

The Role of Exercise in the Prevention and Management of Acute Low Back Pain

Sheila A. Dugan, MD

Rush Medical College, 1725 West Harrison, Suite 970, Chicago, IL 60612, USA

Background

Patients commonly complain of low back pain (LBP). Studies completed over the last several decades demonstrated that 60% to 90% of individuals suffer with LBP at some point in their life and 5% of the population suffers annually [1–3]. LBP is the leading cause of disability in persons younger than age 45 years and the third leading cause of disability in persons aged 45 years and older [4]. In a review of patients seen by primary care providers, orthopedists and chiropractors, most individuals reported functional recovery at 6 months, although approximately one third continued to have low-grade disability and ongoing symptoms [5]. A study of industrial workers found that 62% of patients had one or more relapses in 1 year and up to 40% still had LBP at 6 months [6].

The transition from acute pain to chronic pain and onward to disability is burdensome emotionally and financially to individual sufferers, loved ones, employers, and the health care system. Up to 40% of acute LBP cases can become chronic and lead to disability in some cases [1,7,8]. Treatments that reduce the risk of chronic pain by successful management of acute LBP are highly desirable. Prevention of acute LBP is even more desirable. Exercise has been part of the armamentarium of treating and preventing acute LBP, especially as a means of avoiding disability. This article critically reviews studies of the role of exercise in the management and prevention of LBP. One also must take into account some variability in the definition of acute LBP, which ranges from <7 days to <6 weeks in various studies.

This article relies heavily on the previous review of this topic by Casazza and colleagues [9]. Many of the studies of exercise and LBP are flawed by

E-mail address: Sheila_Dugan@Rush.edu

1526-0046/06/$ - see front matter © 2006 Elsevier Inc. All rights reserved.
doi:10.1016/j.coem.2006.03.003   *occmed.theclinics.com*

inappropriate design, subject heterogeneity, or limited outcome measurements. Acute LBP also is a symptom associated with a wide variety of conditions, of which a subset have significant morbidity compared with others, such as radiculopathy with neurologic impairment compared with lumbar strain. Many studies do not adequately describe the clinical presentation and assume homogeneity of individuals with nonspecific LBP. The identification of defined LBP subgroups has been a focus of studies published since the previous review. The Cochrane Back Review Group has referred to the identification of subgroups and predictors of chronicity as the Holy Grail of LBP [10]. Exercise treatments require funding and patient availability. The use of rehabilitation services has come under scrutiny by health care delivery systems and employers who are faced with limited financial resources. In the setting of restricted reimbursements and evidence-based medical and rehabilitation practices, critical review of the literature is important. As Casazza and colleagues noted, however, the absence of proof because of methodologic flaws in the literature is not equivalent to proof of the lack of effectiveness of exercise in acute LBP.

Clinical guidelines for acute low back pain

The Agency for Health Care Policy and Research (AHCPR) established guidelines in 1994 for clinicians treating acute LBP [11]. Their review of the literature resulted in recommendations that have not been well accepted by most spine treating specialists [9]. The AHCPR general guidelines advocate remaining active and returning early to normal activity as a means of faster recovery and less disability, in keeping with other LBP clinical guidelines in Europe [12,13]. One should note that exercise therapy is not equivalent to recommendations for staying active; however, the AHCPR recommendations are reviewed as a starting point for the review of the role exercise in treating and preventing acute LBP.

Bed rest for acute low back pain

The underlying principle of bed rest to reduce lumbar intervertebral disc pressure in LBP sufferers is grounded in Nachemson's human studies, which demonstrated differential interdiscal pressure based on positioning [14]. The AHCPR guidelines summarized the use of bed rest for acute LBP with these four major recommendations [11]: (1) Gradual return to normal activities is more effective than prolonged bed rest. (2) Prolonged bed rest (longer than 4 days) is not recommended. (3) Most persons who have LBP do not require bed rest. (4) Bed rest may be an option for patients with initial symptoms of severe leg pain. There are many well-recognized deleterious effects of bed rest, however, including

1. Loss of maximal aerobic capacity [15–18]
2. Elevation of resting heart rate [15–18]

3. Altered fibrinolysis/coagulation [19]
4. Reduced oxidative enzyme levels in skeletal muscle [20,21]
5. Reduced plasticity of connective tissue [22]
6. Reduced bone mineralization [15,22]
7. Reduced cross-sectional area and strength of muscle [23–25]
8. Psychological effects, such as adoption of the sick role [22]

Deyo and colleagues [26] studied bed rest in LBP and compared the consequences of limited (2 days) bed rest versus generous (7 days) bed rest. They concluded that 2 days of bed rest was as efficacious as 7 days. The study participants were heterogeneous in regards to the type of pain (acute and chronic) and level of education. Information about neurologic signs and symptoms or previous episodes of LBP was not provided. The study did not include an activity as tolerated control group. The group that had 2 days of bed rest was better educated. Compliance with bed rest also was limited, more so in the group that had 7 days of bed rest. In a prospective, randomized trial of patients with LBP with and without radiating leg pain, Gilbert and colleagues [17] studied patients who had 4 days of bed rest compared with patients who had no bed rest. The authors noted a 42% longer time to return to normal activity for the bed rest groups and no difference in respect to recovery at 6 weeks, 12 weeks, and 1 year. Two days of bed rest was compared with mobilizing exercises in a prospective, randomized, controlled trial by Malmivaara and colleagues [27], including a control group that had activity as tolerated. The study subjects suffered with acute LBP or recently exacerbated chronic LBP. The bed rest group had significantly greater absence from work at 3 and 12 weeks; however, the bed rest group was significantly less satisfied with work and had more pain radiating below the knee, which may account for some of the difference in work outcomes.

The bed rest literature cited by the AHCPR is limited in many of the ways noted previously, including poor subject description and heterogeneity of subjects in regards to length of time and number of episodes of LBP, previous surgery, or radicular signs and symptoms [17,26,28–30]. The guidelines do not support the use of prolonged bed rest in patients with nonradicular acute LBP. The literature is inadequate to determine efficacy of bed rest in the setting of lumbosacral radiculopathy. Bed rest may be counterproductive to early functional restoration, an approach aimed at promoting tissue healing and strengthening. Multifidus muscle recovery was studied by Hides and colleagues [31] after acute, first episode LBP. The control group, treated with 2 to 3 days of bed rest and oral medications, had decreased multifidus cross-sectional muscle area at the 10-week follow-up visit.

Exercise in the setting of acute low back pain

Exercise is included in the management of painful conditions for the known physiologic benefits of improved cardiovascular fitness, increased

strength and flexibility, and increased conditioning. One or all of these parameters may be compromised in patients who have LBP. Other benefits of
exercise for some individuals who have LBP include improved sleep, mood,
and pain tolerance [32,33]. Biomechanical studies have linked spinal motion
with disc nutrition and elimination of local waste products [34]. Presentations and findings on manual assessment of patients who have LBP drive
manual treatments toward exercises that remediate strength and flexibility
deficits. LBP exercise programs have been developed with consideration
of a combination of biomechanical and clinical factors. The AHCPR guidelines recommend that exercise should be increased gradually over time [11].

More studies over the last decade have used LBP population subgroups
defined by individual clinical signs on mechanical assessment, some of which
required particular positioning to define a patient's directional preference
[35–39]. The directional preference is an immediate, lasting improvement
in pain from performing repeated lumbar flexion, extension, or sideglide/ro-
tation tests [35]. It is identified when particular postures or repeated end
range motions decrease or abolish lumbar pain or cause referred pain to re-
treat progressively in a proximal direction. This method of subgrouping patients who have LBP and using patient-specific exercise programs derives
from clinical practice patterns of using directional preference to guide treatments aimed at controlling and eliminating pain.

Exercise versus usual care in acute nonspecific low back pain

Exercise has been studied compared with usual medical management of
acute LBP. Multiple meta-analyses and reviews for clinical guidelines of exercise and LBP are available in the literature [10,12,29,30,40,41]. One must
consider critically the aims of the review. These analyses include various
combinations of trials depending on their aims. A recent meta-analysis assessed the effectiveness of exercise therapy for reducing pain and disability
in adults with acute, subacute, and chronic nonspecific LBP compared
with no treatment and other conservative treatments by reviewing randomized, controlled trials [40]. They deemed only 11 trials of acute LBP (<6
weeks' duration) feasible for their analysis, defining high-quality studies as
those that included appropriate randomization, adequate concealment of
treatment allocation, adequacy of follow-up, and outcome assessor blinding.
They defined exercise therapy as a series of specific movements with the aim
of training or developing the body by a routine practice or as physical training to promote good physical health [12]. The trials showed positive, negative, and neutral outcomes of exercise therapy. Meta-analysis showed no
advantage of exercise therapy over no treatment or other conservative treatments for pain and functional outcomes over the short- or long-term follow-up.
The literature on exercise and LBP is comprised of individual studies with
conflicting outcomes, however.

Malmivaara and colleagues [27] prospectively compared mobilizing exercises, activity as tolerated, and 2 days of bed rest in 186 patients with acute or recently exacerbated chronic LBP. They found mobilizing home exercises given to patients in an occupational setting to be less effective than usual care. Patients with radiating pain to the level of the knee were included, but neurologic deficit resulted in exclusion. At 3- and 12-week follow-up, the control group fared better with respect to pain duration and intensity, lumbar flexion, ability to work, and number of days absent from work. Patients randomized to the exercise therapy group received one visit to physical therapy and then performed an independent home exercise program, including back extension and lateral bending, with no reference to how this affected their pain. There were twice as many subjects with chronic LBP in the exercise group than the control group.

Other randomized and prospective studies by Coxhead and colleagues [42], Gilbert and colleagues [17], Faas and colleagues [28], and Evans and colleagues [43] also failed to demonstrate a benefit of exercise over placebo treatment in acute LBP. Methodologic flaws make these results more difficult to interpret and apply. Coxhead and colleagues [42] studied patients with sciatica and randomly divided patients into 16 groups of varying treatment regimens, including traction, exercise, manipulation, and corset use, and compared these groups to a control group. They did not document duration or intensity of exercise or the particulars of the exercise intervention, which was described as including all ranges of motion and all muscle groups. Three fourths of all subjects improved regardless of treatment. Gilbert and colleagues [17] found no difference in recovery at 6 and 12 weeks between an exercise and education group and a control group of 187 patients in a primary care setting. In this study, subjects performed adapted Kendall flexion exercises regardless of their presenting symptoms. The exercise group had a higher percentage of workers' compensation cases. They were noted to discontinue oral medications sooner than controls. Faas and colleagues [28] studied 473 patients in a primary care setting comparing flexion-based exercises for all individuals randomized to exercise therapy. They found no benefit with the exercise therapy delivered individually compared with care from a general practitioner or sham treatment.

Chok and colleagues [44] demonstrated a benefit to exercise therapy in a study of 62 patients referred for specialty LBP care. An extensor endurance program delivered by a physical therapist improved short-term functioning better than no treatment. Flaws were noted in the study, including questionable allocation concealment. The outcome assessor was not blinded to the treatment group.

A multicenter randomized, controlled trial of 230 subjects, who were subgrouped by directional preference, compared contrasting exercise prescriptions [35]. The study enrollment included approximately 13% of patients who had acute pain (<7 days), 30% who had subacute pain (<7 weeks), and the remainder who had chronic pain (>7 weeks) who presented for physical therapy. Each subject received a mechanical diagnosis, which noted directional preference, and was then randomized to one of three groups: (1) exercise matched to the directional preference, (2) exercise opposite the directional preference, or (3) exercise considered to be evidenced based (multidirectional, midrange lumbar exercises, and stretches for the hip and thigh muscles). Two thirds of 312 patients were found to have a directional preference (an immediate, lasting improvement in pain from performing repeated lumbar flexion, extension, or sideglide/rotation tests), whereas one third did not, which resulted in 230 patients for randomization. The subjects were seen for at least three visits (maximum six visits) with a credentialed McKenzie Institute–trained therapist over a 2-week period. Patients were included with LBP and radicular pain; however, subjects with more than two neurologic signs were excluded. Seventy percent of patients had had previous incidents of LBP. Although all three treatment groups improved in all outcome measures, there were statistically significant improvements in every outcome in the group in which exercises matched the subjects' directional preferences. Patients in the matched exercise group had significantly greater satisfaction with care. One limitation of the study was the potential bias introduced by McKenzie Institute–trained therapists administering the opposite and evidenced-based treatments, counter to their training in mechanical diagnosis and treatment matched to directional preference. Because all subjects were enrolled when they were seeking care, the authors were not able to compare the exercise interventions to a no-treatment group.

As noted in the review by Casazza and colleagues [9], trials of LBP exercise programs may need to be diagnosis driven. Patient presentation and examination findings may serve as a proxy for diagnosis [10,41]. Treatment efficacy has been demonstrated in trials using patient-specific LBP subgroups; however, methodologic flaws also limit this body of literature [45–49]. It is unreasonable to expect to observe specific benefits from an exercise program if no specific diagnosis or subgroup identification was made before initiation of the treatment arm of the study. Fortunately, the need for more uniform identification of subjects and outcomes and uniform reporting of clinical trials drives future LBP research [50,51].

Aerobic training and cardiovascular conditioning

Clinical practitioners advise patients that aerobic fitness confers some protective effect from developing LBP or causing LBP to worsen. Aerobic conditioning is easily lost if one's back injury results in more than 1 week of reduced activity level. It is less clear how the known benefits of aerobic exercise (reducing heart rate, blood pressure, and ventilatory drive for any standard intensity level of work) impact stress encountered by the spine. Exercise training of 8 to 12 weeks' duration usually results in a 10% to 20% increase in VO_{2max}, with submaximal exercise parameter and subjective endurance improvements observed beforehand [18,52].

The AHCPR recommends low stress aerobic exercise to prevent debilitation caused by inactivity during the first month of LBP symptoms and thereafter to help return patients to their highest level of functioning [11]. Patients who have acute LBP are encouraged to start low impact aerobic exercise during the first 2 weeks of symptoms. Aerobic training has been studied primarily in regards to prevention of LBP or in relation to chronic LBP. Few studies in the LBP literature use direct or indirect metabolic measurements of fitness to characterize patients at study onset or to quantify response to training. McQuade and colleagues [53] retrospectively studied the association between LPB and cardiovascular fitness and found a negative correlation between LBP and fitness level. In a cross-sectional study, Brennan and colleagues [54] demonstrated reduced fitness levels in patients with disc herniation compared with age-matched controls. Because of study design, neither study allowed for causal determination.

Observational studies of fire fighters by Cady and colleagues [55] sparked interest in aerobic fitness and injury prevention, particularly related to health care costs. Subjects who were less fit had more episodes of LBP and were more costly to care for. The less fit subjects were older, however, which confounded the results. It is not clear what percentage of fire fighters studied had previous back injuries. Cady and colleagues did follow a group of fire fighters prospectively for 10 years and noted that the individuals who continued to be less fit had higher medical costs [56]. Fire fighters with improved fitness level had lower medical costs; however, no data were given on the number of medical claims for LBP. Studies by Battie and colleagues [57] and Dehlin and colleagues [58] failed to demonstrate a beneficial effect of cardiovascular fitness on LBP. Battie and colleagues [57] prospectively studied industrial back pain complaints related to baseline fitness level and cardiovascular risk factors. There were no longitudinal data on fitness level or aerobic training. The subjects also were not matched for previous LBP or lumbar surgery history. In a nonrandomized trial, Dehlin and colleagues [58] studied nursing aides with LBP and did not show a positive effect of improved cardiovascular fitness level on duration of recurrent back pain episodes.

Kellet and colleagues [59] looked prospectively at cardiovascular exercise in subjects with and without prior episodes of LBP randomized to exercise or no exercise. At an 18-month follow-up, no significant improvement in aerobic capacity was achieved, but subjects in the exercise group reported fewer sick days and less back pain. The exercise intervention included 1 hour of supervised and 1 hour of unsupervised aerobic training per week without assessment of adequate training, such as heart rate monitoring. Linton and colleagues [60] showed that nurses with previous history of LBP had fewer self-reported symptoms of pain, fatigue, and difficulties with activities of daily living after a 5-week program that included 4 hours of aerobic exercise and 4 hours of back education. In a prospective study of postmicrodiscectomy patients, aerobic training with walking was prescribed to the exercise group compared with a matched postoperative group [61].

Exercise metabolic measurement testing demonstrated significantly greater gains in aerobic fitness in the exercise group without any increase in LBP.

A literature review by Lahad and colleagues [62] concluded that aerobic exercise may be protective against low back injury in the workplace, with outcomes of fewer days of back pain and fewer days of lost work, at least in follow-up of 18 months. A 10-year prospective observational study by Leino [63] noted that increased leisure exercise correlated with decreased LBP symptoms in men; because of study design, however, causality could not be determined.

Regarding the relationship between cardiovascular fitness and the development or recurrence of LBP, one can summarize that (1) it is unclear if LBP reduces fitness or if reduced fitness promotes LBP, (2) patients who have LBP are capable of improving their aerobic fitness, (3) more fit individuals have less LBP, and (4) aerobic exercise as part of a rehabilitation treatment program seems to be a reasonable approach.

Strength training

To review the literature on strength training and LBP, one must first define strength (the maximum force produced from a single effort), power (work over a specific time), and endurance (the ability to sustain work at a given percent of maximum). Strength gains are brought about by overloading muscles and are specific to the muscle and joint angle. Early changes in strength are related to neuromuscular retraining and changes in motor unit recruitment, with muscle hypertrophy occurring later [64,65]. The AHCPR guidelines state that gradual conditioning exercises for the trunk muscles, especially back extensors, may be helpful for acute LBP that persists; however, strength training may aggravate acute LBP during the first 2 weeks [11]. The AHCPR guidelines state that back-specific exercise machines provide no apparent benefit over traditional exercise for patients with acute LBP. The time required for measurable strength improvements prohibits, in part, the study of strength training for acute LBP, lending itself more so to LBP prevention or chronic LBP management. The strength training literature is also fraught with imprecise characterizations of subjects related to their presenting symptoms or presumed diagnosis. An additional problem with reviewing strength trials relates to the usefulness of isokinetic testing in predicting LBP in the industrial population.

Donchin and colleagues [66] performed a prospective, randomized, controlled study of hospital employees with more than three annual episodes of LBP. Subjects in the exercise group (lumbar flexion and pelvic tilt training) had fewer months of back pain and had increased abdominal strength for the next 12 months compared with a back school group and a control group. They did not demonstrate increase in isometric back strength or endurance, which likely reflects the specificity of strength training. Gundewall and colleagues [67] studied nurses and nursing aides with and without previous

LBP. The group given six exercise treatments per month of trunk strengthening and endurance demonstrated increased back strength, less pain, and less absenteeism.

Trunk extension endurance testing was predictive for the development of LBP in previously asymptomatic men but not women in a population-based study by Biering-Sorenson [1]. Troup and colleagues [68] studied British workers in a nonrandomized trial and were not able to demonstrate a positive predictive value of trunk endurance and LBP incidence. Plowman [69] analyzed retrospective studies and concluded that a link between trunk strength and LBP was plausible. Limiting factors noted by the author included difficulty with maximal strength measurement in individuals with pain and the impact of apparent deconditioning in individuals with longstanding pain.

Regarding clinically relevant strength testing, an extensive review concluded that there was inadequate evidence to support isokinetic testing for pre-employment, clinical, or medicolegal purposes [70]. Reimer and colleagues [71] suggested that isokinetic testing may be a useful tool as part of a fitness test battery after reviewing retrospective data that low back injuries declined by 32% and 41% over the next 2 years after screening out workers who could not perform 15 of 17 minimum standard tests. McGill and colleagues [72] found an association between having a history of LBP and predicting individuals who would develop LBP in the future and the test of torso isometric flexor and extensor muscle endurance.

Study design that does not attempt to subgroup patients based on diagnosis or presentation has led to mismatching of patients and interventions. The mismatch results in the conclusion that neither flexion nor extension exercises are particularly useful in the treatment of LBP [28,29,43]. For example, randomization without screening of pathology or individual posture preference or directional preference may lead to dilution of potential treatment effects, because individuals would be randomized to treatment that would provoke their symptoms [73–75]. In a prospective, randomized study by Dettori and colleagues [76], soldiers with acute LBP exercised for 8 weeks in the flexion exercise and posture group or the extension exercises and posture group or did not exercise in the control group. At 1 week, both exercise groups fared better than the control group in regards to disability score, straight leg raise testing, and return to work. On the follow-up survey administered 6 to 12 weeks after study entry, however, there was no significant difference between groups for recurrent LBP. The authors concluded that flexion or extension exercises were only slightly better than no exercise. They stated that there was no difference between using flexion- or extension-based exercise therapy.

One can look to the body of literature in which patient-specific exercises are studied to find examples of strength training studies that differentiate between flexion- and extension-based programs [77,78]. In a prospective, randomized, noncontrolled study, Stankovic and Johnell [79] compared the McKenzie method of treatment to mini back school in 100 patients who had acute and subacute LBP. Both groups received one session of instruction. The McKenzie group received a 20-minute session that reviewed extension exercises, postural corrections, and ergonomics. The mini back school included one 45-minute session with nonspecific exercise recommendations. In the McKenzie group, all participants returned to work in 6 weeks compared with the mini back school group, which required 11 weeks for the entire cohort to return to work. At 1 year, the McKenzie group had fewer LBP recurrences. Delitto and colleagues [45] studied individuals who had LBP and sciatica who improved with two extension movements and worsened with at least one flexion movement. They were randomized to extension plus sacroiliac mobilization or a flexion exercise program. The extension group improved more rapidly. Erhard and colleagues [46] performed a follow-up study on 24 individuals to determine the differential benefit of sacroiliac mobilization versus exercise in subjects with acute and subacute LBP. The mobilization group improved more rapidly than the exercise group; however, the exercise group had higher Oswestry scores at baseline.

Strength training and LPB studies generally include a heterogeneous patient population described by LBP symptoms, with and without referral to the lower limb. Neurologic signs or symptoms are included as descriptors in some studies. Saal and Saal's retrospective cohort study [80] of patients with herniated lumbar discs noted that 90% of patients obtained good to excellent results with an aggressive lumbar stabilization program and 92% returned to work. Of the six patients who required surgery, four had spinal stenosis.

Nadler and colleagues [81] studied the influence of the kinetic chain in LBP and its prevention. In a prospective study of college athletes, they found that previous lower extremity injuries correlated positively with incidence of acute LBP episodes during the ensuing year. One theory to explain the phenomenon of increased LBP in athletes with lower extremity injury is an alteration or inhibition of the proximal hip musculature, rather than muscle inflexibility or leg length discrepancy, neither of which was significantly correlated with LBP. Nadler and colleagues [82] demonstrated a significant asymmetry in hip extensor strength in female athletes with reported LBP but not in male athletes. They studied exercise interventions to prevent LBP and found no significant difference in incidence of LBP after incorporating a core strengthening program [83]. In female athletes the incidence of LBP increased, with the authors conjecturing that core strengthening programs may require gender-specific modification. They also noted that the small number of athletes with LBP (7/162 male athletes and 7/74 female athletes) makes any conclusions difficult. This series of studies identifies an area of further research regarding strength training and the prevention of LBP in athletes and may provide some important insights into LBP prevention in work-related LBP.

Regarding the relationship between strength training and the prevention or treatment of LBP, the literature cannot be used to establish guidelines.

There is a need for more carefully designed studies with well-described patient populations and exercise interventions. Operational definitions of strength differ across studies, which makes interpretation of results difficult. LBP sufferers, even in the face of disc herniation, are candidates for exercise training. There seems to be at least a mild relationship between trunk muscle strength and LBP. Specific exercises should be implemented in pain-free subjects who are followed longitudinally for development of LBP to study exercise and prevention of acute LBP.

Flexibility training

The overall goal of stretching or flexibility training is to increase the available range of motion and decrease the feeling of joint stiffness. Stretching may improve comfort during activities of daily living. There may be less biomechanical stress on joints with greater flexibility. It generally takes 1 to 2 months to change range of motion with flexibility training. The AHCPR guidelines do not support stretching of the back muscles in the treatment of acute LBP [11]. The literature on the role of flexibility in acute LBP has more limitations than those previously reviewed in regards to aerobic and strength training.

Operational definitions of flexibility and measurements vary greatly from study to study. Intertester and intratester reliability is poor. The sit-and-reach test has been used to represent low back flexibility [84,85]. This test, or the similar fingertip-to-floor test, is thought to estimate trunk flexibility or mobility [1,85]. Several authors have questioned whether the sit-and-reach test is related to low back status [84,86]. Although the test seems to be valid and reliable, it involves whole body motion, which may be influenced by many anthropometric and flexibility issues of the upper spine and shoulder girdle. Grenier and colleagues [87] examined the relationship between the sit-and-reach test, lumbar flexibility, and previous history of LBP in 72 blue collar workers. Of the 72 workers, 28 had no history of LBP, 26 had an injury that resulted in LBP and lost work, and 18 had a history of LBP but no work loss. They found that the sit-and-reach test scores did not correlate with previous history of LBP; however, lumbar sagittal flexion scores did correlate with previous history of LBP.

In a cross-sectional study, Pope and colleagues [88] noted that men with current or previous LBP had diminished extension and rotation of the spine compared with men without LBP. Lumbar flexion was similar in both groups. Bilateral lateral bending and rotation were summed for a total score, which would dilute the impact of any side-to-side differences. Cady and colleagues [55] measured flexibility in fire fighters, again noting that individuals with poorer flexibility cost seven times more in regards to work-related low back injuries than the most flexible fire fighters. As noted in the cardiovascular outcomes, the fire fighters with greater flexibility were younger and stronger and had greater work capacity. Battie and colleagues

[57] prospectively studied flexibility and LBP in 3000 aircraft manufacturing workers over 3 years using the modified Schober test, sit-and-reach test, and lateral bending test to document trunk flexibility. They were unable to demonstrate a significant difference in flexibility between persons with and without LBP. Pain severity, function, sick time, and cost were not analyzed.

Biering-Sorenson reported that men with better mobility on modified Schober testing and no prior history of LBP were more likely to develop LBP over the next year, whereas for women the opposite was true [1]. In a study of athletes and LBP by Kujala and colleagues [89], male athletes with low maximal lumbar flexion, as measured by a modification of a flexi-curve technique, were more likely to have LBP 3 years later compared with men with higher maximal lumbar flexion. In female athletes, low maximal extension and decreased lumbar range of motion were associated with greater likelihood of LBP 3 years later. This study illustrated how direction of activity may be important in the development of back pain, because the female athletes performed more extension-based sports, whereas the men performed more flexion-based sports.

Regarding the relationship between flexibility and the prevention or treatment of LBP, the literature cannot be used to establish guidelines. The variability in study design and measurements limits the clinical usefulness of this literature. Although stretching exercises may be included in usual physical therapy care for LBP, no stretching intervention studies show their efficacy in treating or preventing LBP.

Summary and future directions

There are several fruitful examples of innovative research on the role of exercise in treating and preventing acute LBP. The study by Long and colleagues [35] showed how previously validated subgroups of LBP subjects had a significantly different response to exercises that either matched or were opposite to the subjects' directional preference. Response to manual assessment was one means of accurately describing and classifying patients who presented with LBP. This subgrouping was useful in directing exercise therapy likely to succeed in reducing pain and improving function. Nadler and colleagues [83] have laid groundwork in defining the impact of the kinetic chain on preventing LBP and started to look critically at the role of core strengthening in athletic populations. Grenier and colleagues [87] raised and answered questions about validity and utility in regards to lumbar strength and flexibility testing, because they used cadaveric studies and computer modeling of electromyographically derived data aimed at more precisely defining the role of particular lumbar muscles in supporting the spine.

As noted by Cassaza and colleagues, exercise and therapy regimens can be beneficial and cost-effective when they are constructed to address specific conditions associated with accurate clinical diagnosis. Precisely prescribed rehabilitation programs tailored toward specific anatomic, biomechanical, and

Box 1. The role of bed rest and exercise in patients who have acute or subacute low back pain

1. There is no proven benefit of prolonged bed rest (ie, >4 days) in acute LBP without radiculopathy.
2. The literature does not provide adequate information to establish guidelines for the amount of rest required in the face of proven acute disc injury with or without radicular symptoms.
3. There is no conclusive proof that aerobic exercise prevents development of LBP. Based on the literature, however, aerobic fitness may be mildly protective against low back injury and LBP.
4. There is no conclusive evidence that aerobic exercise hastens recovery from an episode of acute LBP.
5. Acute LBP results in reduction of physical activity, which leads to reduction of aerobic fitness. This problem is accentuated if LBP is recurrent. It may have significant consequences with regard to physical working capacity and cardiovascular risk. On this basis alone, it is recommended that aerobic exercises be incorporated into the spine rehabilitation program as early as possible.
6. Future studies that examine the role of aerobic conditioning exercises/aerobic fitness in the prevention and treatment of LBP should use direct quantification of oxygen consumption via respiratory gas analysis rather than predictive nomograms or population-based norms. Longitudinal studies that include asymptomatic cohort groups must be performed to determine if the presence of back pain is associated with greater deterioration of aerobic fitness over time.
7. Because most of any individual's daily activities are not performed at maximum levels, future studies that examine the role of aerobic exercise should incorporate submaximal parameters, such as submaximal heart rate response and rating of perceived exertion at standard workloads, or relative percentages of maximal aerobic capacity.
8. Findings of reduced strength, endurance, and flexibility are common in patients who have LBP. These findings may be consequences of acute deconditioning and a potential causative factor for dysfunction in the future.
9. Isokinetic strength testing does not seem to be helpful in the assessment of risk of development of LBP. Isokinetic

devices may prove to be useful in the quantification of work capacity.

10. Operational definitions of strength, power, and endurance are inconsistent across studies, which makes generalized statements about the efficacy of strength training or strength testing difficult. There seems to be at least a mild relationship between trunk muscle strength and LBP.

11. The literature supports neither the notion that flexibility training confers protection against the development of LBP nor the notion that it is essential in the treatment of acute LBP. There seems to be at least a mild relationship between decreased flexibility in the direction of repeated spinal motion and LBP, however.

12. The causes of LBP are multifactorial, even when a pain generator is identified. Treatment of LBP by randomizing patients to only one method of treatment is unrealistic. It is an error to equate exercise with rehabilitation. The patient always must be taken into account.

Adapted from Young JL, Herring SA, Press JM. Bed rest and exercise as clinic management tools for acute low back pain. In: Gonzalez E, editor. The nonsurgical management of acute low back pain. New York: Demos Vermande; 1997. p. 209–10; with permission.

functional deficits are needed to optimize function after low back injury. Clinicians can work collaboratively with researchers to define more precisely the neuromuscular patterns involved in lumbar spine mobility and stability to modify and upgrade their approach to individual patients rather than follow predetermined algorithmic flow charts. A multifaceted approach seems to be more effective [8,80,90,91]. The literature reviewed provides a framework for decision making. Box 1 summarizes the role of bed rest and exercise in patients with acute or subacute LBP. One is warned against the notion that absence of proof because of methodologically flawed studies is equivalent to proof of absence of the beneficial effect of exercise for acute LBP. Because of the multifactorial nature of LBP, more innovative research is required to define adequately the role of exercise in treating and preventing LBP.

References

[1] Biering-Sorenson F. Physical measurements as risk indicators for low back trouble over a one year period. Spine 1984;9:106–19.
[2] Frymoyer JW, Pope MH, Clements JH, et al. Risk factors in low back pain: an epidemiological study. J Bone Joint Surg Am 1983;65A:213–8.

[3] Svensson H, Vedin A, Wihelmsson C, et al. Low back pain in relation to other diseases and cardiovascular risk factors. Spine 1983;8:277–85.

[4] Pope MH, Andersson GBJ, Frymoyer JW, et al, editors. Occupational low back pain: assessment, treatment and prevention. St. Louis: Mosby; 1991.

[5] Carey TS, Garrett J, Jackson A, et al. The outcomes and costs of care for acute low back pain among patients seen by primary care practitioners, chiropractors, and orthopedic surgeons. N Engl J Med 1995;333:913–7.

[6] Bergquist-Ullman M, Larsson U. Acute low back pain in industry: a controlled prospective study with special reference to therapy and confounding factors. Acta Orthop Scand Suppl 1977;170:1–117.

[7] Frymoyer JW. Back pain and sciatica. N Engl J Med 1988;318:291–300.

[8] Herring SA, Weinstein SM. Assessment and nonsurgical management of athletic low back injury. In: Nicholas JA, Hershman EB, editors. The lower extremity and spine in sports medicine. 2nd edition. St. Louis: Mosby-Year Book; 1995. p. 1171–97.

[9] Casazza BA, Young JL, Herring SA. The role of exercise in the prevention and management of acute low back pain. Occup Med State Art Rev 1998;13:47–60.

[10] Bouter L, Pennick V, Bombardier C. Cochrane back review group. Spine 2003;28: 1215–8.

[11] Bigos S, Bowyer O, Braen O, et al. Acute low back problems in adults: clinical practice guidelines. Quick reference guide no. 14. Rockville (MD): Agency for Health Care Policy and Research; 1994.

[12] Abenheim L, Rossignol M, Valat JP, et al. The role of activity in the therapeutic management of back pain: report of the International Paris Task Force on Back Pain. Spine 2000; 25(Suppl):1–33.

[13] Royal College of General Practitioners. Clinical guidelines for the management of acute low back pain. London: Royal College of General Practitioners; 1999.

[14] Nachemson AL. The lumbar spine: an orthopedic challenge. Spine 1976;1:59.

[15] Astrand PO, Rodahl K. Textbook of work physiology. 3rd edition. New York: McGraw-Hill; 1986.

[16] Coyle EF, Hemmert MK, Coggan E. Effects of detraining on cardiovascular responses to exercise: role of blood volume. J Appl Physiol 1985;60:95–9.

[17] Gilbert JR, Taylor DW, Hildebrand A, et al. Clinical trials of common treatments for low back pain in family practice. BMJ 1985;291:789–94.

[18] Saltin B, Blomqvist B, Mitchell JH, et al. Response to submaximal and maximal exercise after bed rest and training. Circulation 1968;38(Suppl 5):1–78.

[19] Bowman K, Hellsten G, Bruce A, et al. Endurance physical activity, diet and fibrinolysis. Atherosclerosis 1994;196:65–74.

[20] Henriksson J, Reitman JS. Time course of changes in human skeletal muscle succinic dehydrogenase and cytochrome oxidase activities and maximal oxygen uptake with physical activity and inactivity. Acta Physiol Scand 1977;99:91–7.

[21] Klaussen K, Andersen LB, Pelle I. Adaptive changes in work capacity, skeletal muscle capillarization and enzyme levels during training and detraining. Acta Physiol Scand 1981;113:9–16.

[22] Halar EM, Bell K. Contracture and other effects of immobility. In: DeLisa JA, editor. Rehabilitation medicine. Philadelphia: JB Lippincott; 1988. p. 448–62.

[23] Booth FW, Gollnick PD. Effects of disuse on the structure and function of skeletal muscle. Med Sci Sports Exerc 1983;15:415–20.

[24] Eichelberger L, Roma M, Moulder PV. Effects of immobilization on the histochemical characterization of skeletal muscle. J Appl Physiol 1958;12:42–7.

[25] Muller EA. Influence of training and inactivity on muscle strength. Arch Phys Med Rehabil 1970;51:449–62.

[26] Deyo RA, Diehl AK, Rosenthal M. How many days of bed rest for acute low back pain: a randomized trial. N Engl J Med 1986;315:1064–70.

[27] Malmivaara A, Hakkinen U, Aro T, et al. The treatment of acute low back pain: bed rest, exercises, or ordinary activity? N Engl J Med 1995;332:351–5.

[28] Faas A, Chavannes AW, van Eijk JTM, et al. A randomized placebo-controlled trial of exercise therapy in patients with acute low back pain. Spine 1993;18:1388–95.

[29] Koes BW, Bouter LM, Beckerman H, et al. Physiotherapy exercises and low back pain: a blinded review. BMJ 1991;302:1572–6.

[30] Koes BW, Bouter LM, van der Heijden GJMG. Methodological quality of randomized clinical trials on treatment efficacy in low back pain. Spine 1995;20:228–35.

[31] Hides JA, Richardson CA, Jull GA. Multifidus muscle recovery is not automatic after resolution of acute, first-episode low back pain. Spine 1996;21:2763–9.

[32] O'Connor PJ, Youngstedt SD. Influence of exercise on human sleep. Exerc Sport Sci Rev 1995;23:105–34.

[33] Rejeski WJ, Brawley LR, Shumaker SA. Physical activity and health related quality of life. Exerc Sport Sci Rev 1996;24:71–108.

[34] Holm S, Nachemson A. Variations in nutrition of the canine intervertebral disc induced by motion. Spine 1983;8:867–74.

[35] Long A, Donelson R, Fung T. A randomized control trial of exercise for low back pain. Spine 2004;29:2593–602.

[36] McKenzie R, May S. Mechanical diagnosis and therapy. 2nd edition. Waikane, New Zealand: Spinal Publications New Zealand Limited; 2003.

[37] Donelson R, Grant W, Kamps C, et al. Pain response to end-range spinal motion in the frontal plane: a multi-centered, prospective trial. Heidelberg, Germany: International Society for the Study of the Lumbar Spine; 1991.

[38] Donelson R, Grant W, Kamps C, et al. Pain response to repeated end-range sagittal spinal motion: a prospective, randomized, multi-centered trial. Spine 1991;16:206–12.

[39] Williams M, Hawley J, McKenzie R, et al. A comparison of the effects of two sitting postures on back and referred pain. Spine 1991;16:1185–91.

[40] Hayden JA, van Tulder MW, Malmivaara AV, et al. Meta-analysis: exercise therapy for nonspecific low back pain. Ann Intern Med 2005;142:765–75.

[41] Borkan J, Koes B, Reis S, et al. A report from the second international forum for primary care research on low back pain: reexamining priorities. Spine 1998;23:1992–6.

[42] Coxhead CE, Meade TW, Inskip H, et al. Multicentre trial of physiotherapy in the management of sciatic symptoms. Lancet 1981;229:1065–8.

[43] Evans C, Gilbert JR, Taylor W, et al. A randomized controlled trial of flexion exercises, education and bed rest for patients with acute low back pain. Physiother Can 1987;33:96–101.

[44] Chok B, Lee R, Latimer J, et al. Endurance training of the trunk extensor muscles in people with subacute low back pain. Phys Ther 1999;79:1032–42.

[45] Delitto A, Cibulka MT, Erhard RE, et al. Evidence for use of an extension-mobilization category in acute low back pain syndrome: a prospective validation pilot study. Phys Ther 1993;73:216–22.

[46] Erhard RE, Delitto A, Cibulka MT. Relative effectiveness of an extension program and a combined program of manipulation and flexion and extension exercises in patients with acute low back pain syndrome. Phys Ther 1994;74:1093–100.

[47] Fritz J, George S. The use of a classification approach to identify subgroups of patients with acute low back pain. Spine 2000;25:106–14.

[48] Kopp JR, Alexander AH, Turocy RH, et al. The use of lumbar extension in the evaluation and treatment of patients with acute herniated nucleus pulposus: a preliminary report. Clin Orthop 1986;202:211–8.

[49] Spratt K, Lehrmann T, Weinstein J, et al. A new approach to the low back physical examination: behavioral assessment of mechanical signs. Spine 1990;15:96–102.

[50] Deyo RA, Battie M, Beurskens AJ, et al. Outcome measures for low back pain research: a proposal for standardized use. Spine 1998;23:2003–13.

[51] Begg C, Cho M, Eastwood S, et al. Improving the quality of reporting randomized controlled trials: the CONSORT statement. JAMA 1996;276:367–9.

[52] Grimby G, Saltin B. Physiological effects of physical training. Scand J Rehabil Med 1971;3: 6–14.

[53] McQuade KJ, Turner JA, Buchner DM. Physical fitness and chronic low back pain. Clin Orthop 1988;233:198–204.

[54] Brennan GP, Ruhling RO, Hood RS, et al. Physical characteristics of patient with herniated intervertebral lumbar discs. Spine 1987;12:699–702.

[55] Cady LD, Bischoff DP, O'Connell ER, et al. Strength and fitness and subsequent back injury in fire fighters. J Occup Med 1979;21:269–72.

[56] Cady LD, Thomas PC, Karwasky RJ. Program for increasing health and physical fitness of fire fighters. J Occup Med 1985;27:110–4.

[57] Battie MC, Bigos SJ, Fisher LD, et al. A prospective study of the role of cardiovascular risk factors and fitness in industrial back pain complaints. Spine 1989;14:141–7.

[58] Dehlin O, Berg S, Hedenrud B, et al. Effects of physical training and ergonomic counseling on the psychological perception of work and the subjective assessment of low back insufficiency. Scand J Rehabil Med 1981;13:1–9.

[59] Kellett KM, Keller DA, Nordhom LA. Effects of an exercise program on sick leave due to low back pain. Phys Ther 1991;4:283–93.

[60] Linton SJ, Bradley LA, Jensen I, et al. The secondary prevention of low back pain. Pain 1989; 36:197–207.

[61] Brennen GP, Schultz BB, Hood RS, et al. The effects of aerobic exercise after lumbar microdiscectomy. Spine 1994;19:735–9.

[62] Lahad A, Malter AD, Berg AO, et al. The effectiveness of four interventions for the prevention of low back pain. JAMA 1994;272:1286–90.

[63] Leino PI. Does leisure time physical activity prevent low back disorders? Spine 1993;18: 863–71.

[64] Basford JR. Weightlifting, weight training and injuries. Orthopedics 1985;8:1051–6.

[65] Sale DG. Neural adaptation to resistance training. Med Sci Sports Exerc 1988;20: S135–45.

[66] Donchin M, Woolf O, Kaplan L, et al. Secondary prevention of low back pain: a clinical trial. Spine 1990;15:1317–20.

[67] Gundewall B, Liljeqvist M, Hansson T. Primary prevention of back symptoms and absence from work. Spine 1993;18:587–94.

[68] Troup JDG, Foreman TK, Baxter CE, et al. The perception of back pain and the role of physiological tests of lifting capacity. Spine 1987;12:645–57.

[69] Plowman SA. Physical activity, physical fitness and low back pain. Exerc Sport Sci Rev 1992; 20:221–42.

[70] Newton M, Waddell G. Trunk strength testing with iso-machines. Part I: Review of a decade of scientific evidence. Spine 1993;18:801–11.

[71] Reimer DS, Halbrook BD, Dreyfuss PH, et al. A novel approach to preemployment worker fitness evaluations in a material-handling industry. Spine 1994;19:2026–32.

[72] McGill SM, Childs A, Liebenson C. Endurance times for low back stabilization exercises: clinical targets for testing and training from a normal database. Arch Phys Med Rehabil 1999;80:941–5.

[73] Bunch RW. Letter. Spine 1996;21:1119.

[74] McGavin JC, Low-McGavin T. Letter. Spine 1996;21:1120.

[75] Sommer HM. Letter. Spine 1996;21:1121.

[76] Dettori JR, Bullock SH, Sutlive TG, et al. The effects of spinal flexion and extension exercises and their associated postures in patients with acute low back pain. Spine 1995;20: 2303–12.

[77] Battie M, Cherkin D, Dunn R, et al. Managing low back pain: attitudes and treatment preferences of physical therapists. Phys Ther 1994;4:219–26.

[78] Foster N, Thompson K, Baxter D, et al. Management of nonspecific low back pain by physiotherapists in Britain and Ireland. Spine 1999;24:1332–42.

[79] Stankovic R, Johnell O. Conservative management of acute low-back pain: a prospective randomized trial. McKenzie method of treatment versus patient education in "mini back school." Spine 1990;15:120–3.

[80] Saal JA, Saal JS. Nonoperative treatment of herniated lumbar intervertebral disc with radiculopathy. Spine 1989;14:431–7.

[81] Nadler SF, Wu KD, Galski T, et al. Low back pain in college athletes: a prospective study correlating lower extremity overuse injuries or acquired ligamentous laxity with low back pain. Spine 1998;23:828–33.

[82] Nadler SF, Malanga GA, Feinberg JH, et al. Relationship between hip muscle imbalance and occurrence of low back pain in collegiate athletes: a prospective study. Am J Phys Med Rehabil 2001;80(8):572–7.

[83] Nadler SF, Malanga GA, Bartoli LA, et al. Hip muscle imbalance and low back pain in athletes: influence of core strengthening. Med Sci Sports Exerc 2002;34:9–16.

[84] Jackson A, Morrow JR, Brill PA, et al. Relation of the sit-up and sit and reach tests to low back pain in adults. J Orthop Sports Ther 1998;27:22–6.

[85] Minkler S, Patterson P. The validity of the modified sit and reach test in college age students. Res Q Exerc Sport 1994;65:189–92.

[86] Hui SSC, Yuen PY. Validity of the modified back saver sit and reach test: a comparison with other protocols. Med Sci Sports Exerc 2000;32:1655 9.

[87] Grenier SG, Russell C, McGill SM. Relationship between lumbar flexibility, sit-and-reach test, and a previous history of low back discomfort in industrial workers. Can J Appl Physiol 2003;28:165–7.

[88] Pope MH, Bevins T, Wilder G, et al. The relationship between anthropomorphic, postural, muscular, and mobility characteristics of males age 18–55. Spine 1985;10:644–8.

[89] Kujala UM, Taimela S, Oksanen A, et al. Lumbar mobility and low back pain during adolescence: a longitudinal follow-up study in athletes and controls. Am J Sports Med 1997;25:363–8.

[90] Wiesel SW, Boden SD, Feffer HL. A quality-based protocol for management of musculoskeletal injuries. Clin Orthop 1994;301:164–76.

[91] Young JL, Press JM, Cole AJ. Physical therapy options for lumbar spine pain. In: Cole AJ, Herring SA, editors. The low back pain handbook. Philadelphia: Hanley and Belfus; 1996. p. 125–40.

ELSEVIER
SAUNDERS

Clin Occup Environ Med
5 (3) 633–642

CLINICS IN
OCCUPATIONAL AND
ENVIRONMENTAL
MEDICINE

Spinal Stabilization Exercises for the Injured Worker

Kim Janeck, PT[a], Barbara Reuven, PT[a],*,
Christopher T. Romano, MS, PT[b]

[a]The Center for Physical Therapy and Sports Rehabilitation, Atlantic Health,
Morristown, NJ 07960, USA
[b]The Kessler Institute for Rehabilitation, 1199 Pleasant Valley Way,
West Orange, NJ 07052, USA

Spinal stabilization exercises (SSE) have become an integral component in the treatment of the injured worker, and they have been useful in improving the function and return-to-work rate in this population [1,2]. Stability of the spine is necessary for normal human functioning. A stable spine allows for the movement of body parts, carrying of loads, and protection of the spinal cord and nerve roots [3]. The spinal stability mechanism is thought to be an integration of active, passive, and neural feedback systems. Damage to any of these systems, such as by injury or disease, may result in spinal instability, which has been identified as a major source of low back pain and is defined as a greater than normal amount of vertebral movement [3]. SSEs involve the cocontraction of muscles to restore stability to the spine and protect it from biomechanical stresses and further injuries [2,4,5]. These biomechanical stresses include tension, compression, torsion, and shear, which occur as a result of occupational activities involving spinal flexion, extension, and rotation. As a result of these stresses, an individual may be susceptible to further injury. SSEs focus on improving the dynamic stability of the spine. This chapter demonstrates how these exercises can be a valuable tool in helping the injured worker return to work and in preventing reinjury.

This article was originally published in Occupational Medicine: State of the Art Reviews 1998;13(1):199–207.

* Corresponding author. The Center for Physical Therapy and Sports Rehabilitation, 310 Madison Avenue, Madison, NJ 07960.

E-mail address: barbara.reuven@ahsys.org (B. Reuven).

Passive stabilizers of the spine

Spinal injuries can affect workers of any occupation. They can occur as a result of the occupational stresses placed on the passive stabilizers of the spine. The passive stabilizers are noncontractile tissues that resist the end ranges of spinal movement [3]. Injury to any of these structures can result in additional injuries to the remaining passive stabilizers. It is theorized that injuries to this system may produce unstable spinal segments [3].

The passive stabilizers of the spine include the vertebrae, intervertebral discs, apophyseal joint capsules, and ligaments. These structures provide stability in two ways. The first is by limiting the amount of spinal motion, which is achieved by the mechanical restriction of the ligaments, joint capsules, discs, and apophyseal joint configuration. For example, forward flexion is limited by the supraspinatus ligament. The second mechanism of stability occurs via the neural system. Sensory receptors located in the passive stabilizers provide information to the central nervous system about the intervertebral joint position and movement [3]. This information is necessary to protect the passive stabilizers from excessive loading and allows the active system to make muscular adjustments to improve spinal stability.

Occupational stresses can injure the apophyseal joint capsules, ligaments, and discs. These stresses produce tension, compression, torsion, and shear forces that may result in stretching or tearing of the collagen fibers that make up the passive stabilizers. For example, a secretary is at risk for mechanical stress to the spine as a result of the compressive and shearing forces produced as a result of prolonged sitting. Studies have shown torsional forces to cause articular cartilage destruction in the facets of the apophyseal joints [6,7]. Additional studies demonstrate injury to the posterior lateral fibers of the anulus with tension, shear, and torsion [8–10].

Occupational stresses can be sustained or repetitive. The secretary who is sitting is subjected to sustained compressive and shearing loads. The truck driver who is lifting and loading boxes is subjected to repeated compressive, shearing, and torsional loads. These forces result in stretching and, ultimately, tearing of the collagen fibers. These injuries are explained by the stress-strain curve [11,12]. Under loading, collagen fibers exhibit a characteristic pattern of elongation that produces the stress-strain curve (Fig. 1). This curve reflects the elastic properties of collagen tissue and demonstrates the amount of loading a passive stabilizer can sustain before an injury occurs. There are two ways that an injury can occur. The first mechanism of injury occurs with high loads. When a high load is applied in a sustained or repeated manner, injuries occur as a result of failure of the collagen fibers. The second mechanism of injury occurs with sustained low loads. It is theorized that sustained low loading results in permanent stretching of the collagen fibers [11]. Both mechanisms of injury result in a passive stabilizer that allows a greater excursion of vertebral movement. This increased mobility is believed to produce unstable spinal segments [3]. A worker

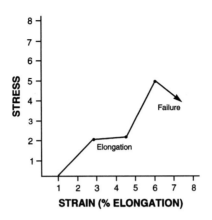

Fig. 1. Stress-strain curve. Collagen fibers elongate during loading. Two mechanisms of injury—high loads and sustained low loads—can lead to failure of collagen fibers.

who has an unstable spinal segment is at risk for further injury and more dependent on the active stabilizers to provide spinal stability.

Dynamic stabilizers of the spine

The active system provides spinal stability through the synergistic actions of muscles that corset the spine with the goal of maintaining the spine in mid-range and limiting excessive movement [7]. The muscles work in force couples to counter-balance the external forces in the sagittal, coronal, and transverse planes. When the spine is maintained in mid-range, as compared with end-range flexion, extension, or rotation, there is less stress on the passive stabilizers and a decreased risk for injury [6,7,10,13,14]. Therefore, it is important for the worker to stabilize the spine in mid-range.

When flexion forces are experienced, the body must produce countering extension forces to maintain a stable spine. Flexion forces are resisted through the muscular actions of the back extensors and muscles producing tension via the thoracolumbar fascia. The back extensors consist of the multifidus and the lumbar portions of the erector spinae muscles. These muscles are capable of producing back extension through their direct attachment to the spine. The thoracolumbar fascia provides extension moments via two mechanisms. The first is the tension placed on the thoracolumbar fascia by the synergistic contraction of the internal oblique abdominis, transverse abdominis, gluteus maximus, and latissimus dorsi. This tension results in an extension moment, which resists flexion of the lumbar spine [11,15,16]. The second mechanism involves a retinacular effect of the thoracolumbar fascia. It is proposed that the thoracolumbar fascia resists the expansion of the back muscles surrounding the spine, which increases the strength and effectiveness of the muscles as stabilizers. In modular form, Hukins et al demonstrated that the retinacular effect of the thoracolumbar fascia can increase the strength of the back muscles by 30% [17].

Not only does the worker have to resist flexion forces, but he has to stabilize against extension forces. To avoid these end-range extension forces, the body produces flexion forces through the coupling action of the rectus abdominis, internal oblique abdominis, external oblique abdominis, and the gluteus maximus, semi-membranosus, semitendinosus, and biceps femoris muscles. These muscles synergistically pull on the pelvis, causing a posterior pelvic tilt that secondarily flexes the spine [18,19]. Maintaining the spine in this slightly flexed position will limit the end-range extension forces and protect the passive stabilizers of the spine.

Rotation of the spine is predominantly produced by the ipsilateral internal oblique abdominis and the contralateral external oblique abdominis. When rotation occurs, there is usually an accompanied action of flexion secondary to the fiber orientation of the oblique muscles [11]. Torsional forces can be damaging to the passive stabilizers. Stabilizing the spine against these forces is accomplished by the eccentric contractions of the opposite oblique muscles and the extensor mechanisms, which can limit the effects of the flexion.

The neural feedback system is a link between the active and passive stabilizing systems. Panjabi states that the passive system, while the lumbar spine is in mid-range, is insufficient in providing stability [3]. These noncontractile tissues need to be near end-range or put on stretch to provide stability. However, the sensory receptors in these structures provide essential feedback on the position and movements of the spine. In a similar fashion, the muscle spindles and Golgi tendon organs in the active stabilizers provide feedback that allows the muscles to coordinate their actions for appropriate spinal stability. For example, when a worker starts to pick up a heavy box the spine usually experiences a flexor moment followed by an extensor moment, when the box is at waist level or higher. Throughout the lift there is a tendency for rotation to occur. The receptors in the passive and active system will continuously send messages to the muscles that control the extension, flexion, and rotation stabilizing mechanisms via the central nervous system. This continuous loop finetunes the active stabilizers so that the spine will be stable throughout all phases of the lift. Damage to any part of the loop will put additional stress on the remaining structures, which increases the chance of injury and challenges the dynamic stability of the spine.

Once an understanding of how the passive, active, and neural systems are involved in the control of spinal stability is achieved, it must be determined if an injured worker has any deficiencies in these systems. Various studies demonstrate that individuals with low back pain have impaired active systems [14,20–25]. The causes of these impairments are debatable.

Roy et al used surface electromyography (EMG) to study the multifidus and erector spinae muscles and suggested that there is abnormal muscle functioning in people with work-related back injuries [25]. The authors raise the possibility that the alterations could be due to deconditioning or muscular inhibition resulting from pain or the fear of reinjury. The authors concluded that isometrically training these muscles can be beneficial in decreasing their ability to fatigue.

It has been hypothesized that the stability of the spine could be decreased as a result of motor control problems. Cresswell et al performed EMG on various trunk muscles in normals while they experienced unexpected and expected loading in standing [20]. The authors found that the transverse abdominis was always activated first. Hodges et al compared EMG recordings of the transverse abdominis between normals and people with low back pain while performing upper extremity velocity-dependent tasks [23]. These authors also found the transverse abdominis to be the first muscle activated in normals. However, the people with low back pain had a delayed onset pattern of activation, suggesting motor control problems, which may decrease the dynamic stability of the spine.

O'Sullivan et al compared abdominal contractions between a physically active control group and a physically active chronic low back pain group [24]. The chronic low back pain group had spinal instability and pain secondary to spondylolysis and spondylolisthesis. The chronic low back pain group had an inability to selectively activate the internal oblique abdominis without significant activation of the rectus abdominis. The authors suggested that neuromuscular dysfunction could alter the dynamic stability of the spine.

Using real-time ultrasound images, Hides et al were able to detect ipsilateral multifidus wasting at one vertebral level on the symptomatic side of subjects experiencing their first episode of low back pain [22]. In another study by Hides et al, the authors found that the multifidus was again asymmetrical in size and and determined that the multifidus does not spontaneously recover after the first episode of low back pain [21]. The authors demonstrated that the multifidus requires specific exercising to regain its symmetry. Rantanen et al found that 5 years after disc herniation surgery the multifidus was deficient in type II muscle fibers [14]. This atrophy could subject the intervertebral joints to increased loads and compromise the stability. The authors suggested that with adequate exercise these findings could be reversed.

Spinal stabilization is a complex process involving the passive, active, and neural feedback system. Damage to any one of these systems can jeopardize spinal stability and put a worker at further risk for injury. There is also significant evidence that people with back injuries have an impaired active system. Therefore, rehabilitation of the person with a back injury should include exercises that train the active system with the goal of increasing dynamic spinal stability.

Spinal stabilization exercises

Theoretically, SSEs may be used in the treatment of acute, subacute, and chronic low back injuries. The goal in all stages of rehabilitation is to decrease the biomechanical stresses placed upon the spine, for the promotion of healing (acutely) and prevention of further degeneration and injury (subacute and chronic). When the patient is considered to have an active disc derangement, the authors favor the use of the McKenzie approach before initiating SSE. This rationale is based on the findings that muscular cocontractions, which occur during stabilization exercises, have been found to increase intradiscal pressure and cause additional stress to the anular fibers [26,27].

SSE can be divided into three stages [1,2], which progress from the least stressful exercises to the most stressful. In stage one, the patient identifies the spinal position that is most comfortable and begins to exercise using minimal muscular effort. In stage two, or dynamic stabilization, an individual maintains a mid-range spinal position, which requires more muscular effort, while performing upper extremity (UE) and lower extremity (LE) exercises. During stage three, or transitional stabilization, a person is trained to stabilize his spine against the forces that are encountered while performing functional or occupational activities. A spinal stabilization program may be commenced at any stage depending on the physical abilities of the individual [1].

Stage one

In the first stage of an SSE program, the therapist assists the patient in obtaining a pain-free or comfortable position of the spine, which is called the *functional position* [1] or *neutral position* [2]. After injury, many patients have lost kinesthetic awareness and muscular strength and are unable to actively move their spine out of painful positions. The therapist must position the patient's spine in the desired position. This is termed *passive positioning* (Fig. 2) [1,2,5]. As a patient's kinesthetic awareness and strength improve, he may begin to actively preposition his spine using his muscles (Fig. 3).

Stage two

Stage two, or dynamic spinal stabilization, is introduced as the patient's physical condition improves [1,2,5]. In this stage, a mid-range spinal position is maintained, which is more difficult to maintain because the patient is required to make continuous neuromuscular adjustment. During stage two, a neurodevelopmental progression is used that begins with low-level or less stressful positions (supine, prone, and side lying) and then advances to high-level positions (Fig. 4). In each developmental position, muscles are cocontracted to maintain the mid-range position of the spine while UE and LE movements are used to challenge these stabilizers. During these exercises the patient works on improving neuromuscular endurance, kinesthetic awareness, and strength. Improvement is demonstrated by his ability to maintain these postures for prolonged periods against increasing forces.

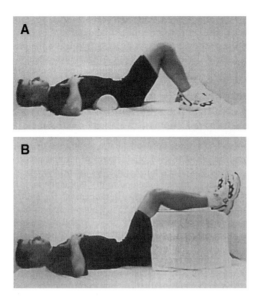

Fig. 2. Passive positioning to obtain functional (neutral) posture. To avoid lumbar flexion and maintain lordosis, a lumbar roll is placed under the spine in the supine position (*A*). To avoid lumbar lordosis, the lower extremity is placed on a chair and the hips are maintained at 90° flexion (*B*).

Stage three

In the third stage, transitional stabilization, the focus is having the patient perform his activities of daily living and occupational activities with proper spinal stabilization [1,2,26]. This stage is most relevant to the successful rehabilitation of the injured worker. It has been demonstrated that introducing the injured worker back into the environment early in the recovery period reduces fears of reinjury and improves the probability of return to work [28,29]. Job-specific exercises have been shown to be more effective than general muscle strengthening. This principle is called specific adaptation to imposed demand (SAID) [18]. Based on this concept, all muscles must be trained in the specific movement patterns that are required to

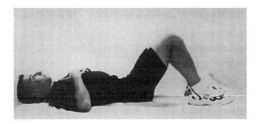

Fig. 3. Active positioning of functional (neutral) posture. With strengthening, the patient can actively contract the gluteal and abdominal muscles to maintain lumbar flexion.

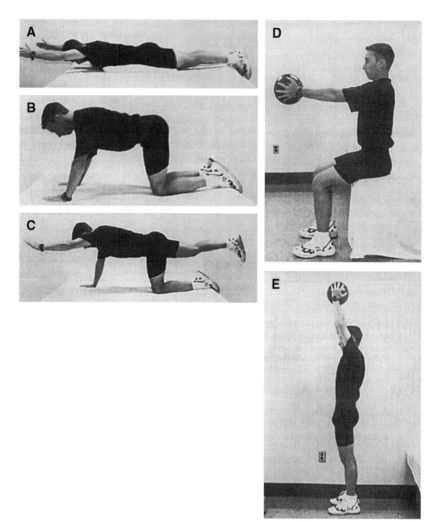

Fig. 4. Dynamic spinal stabilization. (*A*) Shoulder flexion/extension is performed while contracting the abdominal muscles and spinal extensor muscles. Difficulty is increased with hand weights. (*B,C*) In a quadruped position, the patient can start lifting one extremity and progress to two extremities. (*D,E*) A ball can be lifted to challenge muscles maintaining the mid-range position of the spine in seated and standing positions.

perform the activity. Industrial rehabilitation uses the SAID principle through job simulation, which involves the patient performing his specific occupational duties in a controlled environment.

An example of a patient in industrial rehabilitation may be a driver/delivery worker who experiences a diversity of physical demands. This type of occupation involves medium to heavy work and includes the following occupational demands: (1) lifting boxes weighing up to 70 pounds from the floor to overhead, (2) carrying boxes weighing up to 70 pounds various distances on all surfaces and elevations, (3) pushing/pulling a hand truck with a load of boxes on all surfaces and elevations, and (4) driving a truck using a clutch and standard stick shift. The therapist should emphasize proper spinal stabilization while the worker practices his occupational activities.

Summary

Returning the injured worker to his previous occupation can be a difficult and complex rehabilitation process. The goal of SSE is to facilitate the active system for improved dynamic spinal stability. Improving dynamic spinal stability can decrease the forces placed on the intervertebral joints, which minimizes the chance of reinjury. When used in conjunction with industrial rehabilitation, SSEs offer the optimal environment for an injured worker to practice his occupational demands while using appropriate spinal stabilization.

References

[1] Morgan D. Concepts in functional training and postural stabilization for the low back injured. Top Acute Care Trauma Rehabil 1988;2:8–17.
[2] Saal JA, Saal JS. Later stage management of lumbar spine problems. Phys Med Rehabil Clin N Am 1991;2:205–20.
[3] Panjabi M. The stabilizing system of the spine. Part I: Function, dysfunction, adaptation and enhancement. J Spinal Disord 1992;5:383–9.
[4] McKenzie RJ. The lumbar spine, mechanical diagnosis and therapy. Upper Hutt (New Zealand): Spinal Publications; 1981.
[5] Norris CM. Spinal stabilisation: 5. An exercise programme to enhance lumbar stabilisation. Physiotherapy 1995;81:138–46.
[6] Adams MA, Huhon WC. The relevance of torsion to the mechanical derangement of the lumbar spine. Spine 1981;6:241–8.
[7] Saal JA. Dynamic muscular stabilization in the nonoperative treatment of lumbar pain syndrome. Orthop Rev 1990;16:75–122.
[8] Adl-Shrrazi A. Strain in fibers of a lumbar disc analysis of the role of lifting in producing disc prolapse. Spine 1989;14:96–103.
[9] Gordon SJ, Yang KH, Mayer PJ, et al. Mechanism of disc rupture: A preliminary report. Spine 1991;16:450–6.
[10] Hickey SD, Hukins DWL. Relation between the structure of the annulus fibrosus and the function and failure of the intervertebral disc. Spine 1980;5:106–16.
[11] Bogduk N, Twomey LT. Clinical anatomy of the lumbar spine. New York: Churchill Livingstone; 1991.
[12] Oakes BW. Physiology responses to injury: Ligament, tendon, and bone. In: Zuluaga M, editor. Sports physiotherapy applied science and practice. New York: Churchill Livingstonel; 1995. p. 43–59.
[13] Liu YK, Goel VK, DeJong A, et al. Torsional fatigue of the lumbar intervertebral joints. Spine 1985;10:894–900.
[14] Rantanen J, Hurme M, Falck B, et al. The lumbar multifidus muscle five years after surgery for a lumbar intervertebral disc herniation. Spine 1993;18:568–74.

[15] Bogduk N, Macintosh JE. The applied anatomy of the thoracolumbar fascia. Spine 1984;9: 164–70.
[16] Vleeming A, Pool-Goudzwaard AL, Stoeckart R, et al. The posterior layer of the thoraco-lumbar fascia. Spine 1995;20:753–8.
[17] Hukins DWL. Disc structure and function. In: Ghosh P, editor. The biology of the interver-tebral disc. Boca Rotan (FL): CRC Press; 1988. p. 1–37.
[18] Hamil J, Knutzen KM. Biomechanical basis of human movement. Baltimore (MD): Williams & Wilkins; 1995.
[19] Kendall FP, McCreary EK, Provance PG. Muscles testing and function with posture and pain. Philadelphia: Williams & Wilkins; 1993.
[20] Cresswell AG, Oddsson L, Thorstensson A. The influence of sudden perturbations on trunk muscle activity and intra-abdominal pressure while standing. Exp Brain Res 1994;98:336–41.
[21] Hides JA, Richardson CA, Jull GA. Multifidus muscle recovery is not automatic after resolution of acute, first-episode low back pain. Spine 1996;21:2763–9.
[22] Hides JA, Stokes MJ, Saide M, et al. Evidence of lumbar multifidus muscle wasting ipsilat-eral to symptoms in patients with acute/subacute low back pain. Spine 1994;19:165–72.
[23] Hodges PW, Richardson CA. Inefficient muscular stabilization of the lumbar spine associated with low back pain. Spine 1996;21:2640–50.
[24] O'Sullivan P, Twomey L, Allison G, et al. Altered patterns of abdominal muscle activation in patients with chronic low back pain. Aust J Physiother 1997;43:91–8.
[25] Roy SH, DeLuca CJ, Emley M, Buijs RJC. Spectral electromyographic assessment of back muscles in patients with low back pain undergoing rehabilitation. Spine 1995;20:38–48.
[26] May P. Movement awareness and stabilization training. In: Basmajian JV, Nyberg R, edi-tors. Rational manual therapies. Baltimore (MD): Williams & Wilkins; 1993. p. 347–58.
[27] Nachemson A, Morris JM. In vivo measurements of intradiscal pressure. J Bone Joint Surg Am 1964;46:1077–92.
[28] Kelsey JL, White AA III. Epidemiology and improvement of low back pain. Spine 1980;5: 133–4.
[29] Lepore BA, Olson CN, Tomer GM. The dollars and sense of occupational back injury prevention training. Clin Manage 1982;4:210–3.

ELSEVIER SAUNDERS

Clin Occup Environ Med
5 (3) 643–653

CLINICS IN
OCCUPATIONAL AND
ENVIRONMENTAL
MEDICINE

Use of Medications in the Treatment of Acute Low Back Pain

Gerard A. Malanga, MD[a,b,c],*, Robin L. Dennis, MD[d]

[a]Department of Rehabilitation Medicine, Overlook Hospital, 99 Beauvoir Avenue,
Summit, NJ 07901, USA
[b]Department of Sports Medicine, Mountainside Hospital, Bay and Highland Avenues,
Montclair, NJ 07092, USA
[c]Department of Physical Medicine and Rehabilitation, University of Medicine and Dentistry
of New Jersey, 30 Bergen Street, Newark, NJ 07101, USA
[d]Spine Center, Resurgens Orthopaedics, 5671 Peachtree Dunwoody Road,
Suite 700, Atlanta, GA 30342, USA

The prescription of medications continues to be one of the mainstays of treatment for acute low back pain episodes. The goals of pharmacologic treatment for acute low back are reduction of pain and return of normal function [1]. Often, nociception is a result of secondary inflammation and muscle spasm after the acute injury of a structure of the spine, which may include muscle, tendon, ligament, disc, or bone. An understanding of the appropriate use of medications to address the underlying pain generator and the current evidence for using these medications is essential for any physician who sees and treats patients with acute low back pain.

Acetaminophen

Acetaminophen is a para-aminophen derivative with analgesic and antipyretic effects equal to those of aspirin, but it has weak anti-inflammatory effects (ie, it is a reversible but weak inhibitor of cyclo-oxygenase and does not inhibit the activation of neutrophils, as do nonsteroidal anti-inflammatory drugs [NSAIDs]). Its therapeutic effects seem to be secondary to an inhibition of prostaglandin biosynthesis, with a resultant increase in the pain threshold and modulation of the hypothalamic heat-regulating center [2].

* Corresponding author. Department of Rehabilitation Medicine, Overlook Hospital, 99 Beauvoir Avenue, Summit, NJ 07901.
E-mail address: gmalanga@pol.net (G.A. Malanga).

1526-0046/06/$ - see front matter © 2006 Elsevier Inc. All rights reserved.
doi:10.1016/j.coem.2006.03.002   *occmed.theclinics.com*

Past studies have shown acetaminophen to be superior to placebo in the treatment of osteoarthritis pain, and because of its efficacy, it has been recommended as a first-line agent in treatment of osteoarthritis. In 1991, Bradley and colleagues [3] compared the analgesic properties of acetaminophen to ibuprofen for pain associated with osteoarthritis of the knee. Acetaminophen was found to be as efficacious as low-dose analgesic and high-dose anti-inflammatory regimens of ibuprofen in providing pain relief and improved function.

Acetaminophen is relatively inexpensive and available without prescription. The accepted oral dose of acetaminophen is 325 to 1000 mg every 4 to 6 hours, with a total 24-hour intake not to exceed 4000 mg. (Tablets are available in 160-, 325-, 500-, and 650-mg doses.) Peak plasma levels and analgesic effects are usually seen 30 to 60 minutes after ingestion. The most serious adverse effect of acute overdose is hepatotoxicity, which may result from a single dose of 10 to 15g. More chronic abuse has been associated with nephrotoxocity. Minor effects include urticarial skin rashes.

Nonsteroidal anti-inflammatory drugs

The primary mechanism of action of NSAIDs is reversible inhibition of cyclo-oxygenase isoenzymes (COX-1 and COX-2), which block conversion of arachidonic acid into prostaglandins, which are active mediators of the inflammatory cascade and serve to sensitize peripheral nociceptors. (Note: aspirin is a salicylic NSAID that irreversibly inhibits cyclo-oxygenase.) Reduced local prostaglandin concentration could explain the combined anti-inflammatory and analgesic properties of NSAIDs. Nonsteroidal medicines are also believed to inhibit neutrophil function and interfere with phospholipase C activity, which increases intracellular Ca^{++} and can lead to production of arachidonic acid metabolites.

There are several subclasses of NSAIDs: salicylates (eg, aspirin, diflunisal, salsalate), phenylacetics (eg, diclofenac), indoleacetic acids (eg, etodolac, indomethacin, sulindac, tolmetin), oxicams (eg, piroxicam, meloxicam), propionic acids (eg, ibuprofen, ketorolac, naprosyn, oxaprozin), and naphthylkanones (eg, nabumetone). Each subclass and a given drug within each subclass can demonstrate varying characteristics. For example, oxaprozin, a propionic acid, has a long half-life (42–50 h) compared with ketorolac (4–6 h), which is also a propionic acid. Ketorolac is remarkable for analgesic potency comparable to the opioids; however, significant renal toxicity limits its use to 5 days maximum. Sulindac, an indoleacetic acid, does not decrease renal function, however, and may be relatively renal sparing.

The selective COX-2 inhibitor nonsteroidal agents (eg, rofecoxib, celecoxib, valdecoxib) are discussed in a separate section. In 2003, Schattenkirchner and Milachowski [4] examined the efficacy and tolerability of aceclofenac compared with diclofenac in a double-blind, randomized, controlled trial of persons with acute low back pain. Two hundred twenty-seven patients treated with current recommended doses over 10 days demonstrated similar analgesic efficacy of aceclofenac versus diclofenac but demonstrated superiority in pain relief, which was statistically—although not clinically—significant. Van Tulder and colleagues [5] completed a meta-analysis of 51 trials of NSAIDs for low back pain in 2000 patients using the Cochrane Controlled Trials register, which showed evidence that NSAIDs were superior to placebo in short-term relief of acute low back pain. No specific type of NSAID was found to be clearly more effective than any other. McCormack and Brune [6] reviewed 26 studies that investigated the role of NSAIDs in acute soft tissue injuries and found a significant difference between placebo and nine different NSAIDs.

In 2002, Dreiser and colleagues [7] completed a 7-day randomized, controlled, double-blind study to assess the effects of diclofenac, ibuprofen, and placebo for acute low back pain relief. They found diclofenac to be superior to placebo and ibuprofen for initial dosing. Ibuprofen was superior to placebo for initial dosing. Both active treatments were as well tolerated as placebo.

In 2000, in a prospective, randomized double-blind study for 10 days of drug treatment, Pohjolainen and colleagues [8] evaluated the efficacy and tolerability of nimesulide (100 mg twice daily), a COX-2 selective anti-inflammatory drug, versus ibuprofen (600 mg three times daily) in patients who had acute lumbosacral back pain. Results confirmed that nimesulide is an effective and well-tolerated agent for acute low back pain with a lower incidence of gastrointestinal side effects compared with ibuprofen.

The dosing and cost of each NSAID vary significantly by chemical family and agent. Because steady states of plasma concentration are not typically observed until dosing has continued for three to five half-lives, plateau concentrations and maximal therapeutic effects are not realized as quickly in agents with longer half-lives. Prescribing an initial loading dose followed by regular dosing achieves adequate plasma levels and adequate therapeutic effects.

The major adverse reactions caused by nonselective NSAID use are gastrointestinal and renal damage. They are nonselective inhibitors of COX-1 (thromboxane and prostaglandin synthesis; maintenance of gastrointestinal mucosa), which can lead to gastrointestinal dyspepsia, erosion, and hemorrhage, often without clinical symptoms. They also inhibit prostaglandin formation (involved in the autoregulation of renal blood flow and glomerular filtration), which can cause acute renal failure, nephrotic syndrome, and minimal change glomerulonephropathy, especially in individuals with preexisting renal insufficiency or persons in hypovolemic states.

In more recent studies, NSAIDs have been shown to inhibit or delay bone healing in nonhuman models. In 2002, Riew and colleagues [9] reviewed a time-dependent deleterious effect of indomethicin on fusion after spine arthrodesis of New Zealand white rabbits. The study showed the greatest inhibition during the early phases of fusion (2–4 weeks postoperatively). Also in 2002, Goodman and colleagues [10] compared a 4-week course of a nonselective COX-1 and COX-2 inhibitor (naprosyn), a selective

COX-2 inhibitor (rofecoxib), and a placebo as inhibitors on in vivo bone ingrowth and tissue differentiation of eight New Zealand white rabbits 6 weeks after harvest chambers were implanted in their unilateral tibiae. Naprosyn and rofecoxib decreased the number of CD51+ osteoclast-like cells harvested compared with placebo, and rofecoxib decreased osteoblasts compared with controls, which suggested that bone formation is suppressed by oral administration of an NSAID that contains a COX-2 inhibitor. Although current human studies are ongoing, these findings have changed postoperative protocols by some orthopedic surgeons to preclude use of NSAIDs for 6 to 8 weeks to prevent possibility of a nonfusion.

NSAIDs are a reasonable choice as a first-line agent for the control of low back pain. Researchers recommended using them for less than 4 weeks to reduce risk of toxicity.

Choice is empiric and is guided by prior patient experience, cost, dosing schedule, and specific side-effect profile. Because patient response to NSAIDs varies, it is advisable to consider an NSAID of a different class before choosing another analgesic [11].

COX-2 selective nonsteroidal anti-inflammatory drugs

Rofecoxib (Vioxx), celecoxib, and valdecoxib are the main three NSAID selective COX-2 inhibitors. These medications were developed to create a more selective inhibition of the inducible COX isoform (COX-2), which is expressed at sites of inflammation, while sparing inhibition of the constitutive COX-1 isoform, which produces prostaglandins that are gastrointestinal protective.

The Vioxx Gastrointestinal Outcomes Research (VIGOR) trial was a double-blind, randomized, controlled trial of 8076 patients that compared rofecoxib to naproxen for anti-inflammatory efficacy with reduced gastrointestinal complications [12]. The study noted a fivefold higher incidence of myocardial infarction in the Vioxx group compared with naproxen, and this difference was initially attributed to a cardioprotective effect of naproxen rather than a cardiotoxic effect of Vioxx. Results of the Adenomatous Polyp Prevention on Vioxx (APPROVe) study (unpublished data) showed an increased cardiovascular risk (myocardial infarction) in patients who took Vioxx for more than 18 months. Merck Pharmaceuticals withdrew Vioxx from the market on September 30, 2004 [13].

From 1998 to 2000, Silverstein and colleagues [14] conducted the Celecoxib Long-term Arthritis Safety Study (CLASS) to compare gastrointestinal toxicity of celecoxib versus conventional NSAIDs. Results showed that celecoxib was associated with a lower incidence of symptomatic ulcers and ulcer complications, renal toxicity, and hepatotoxicity. Aspirin use for cardiovascular prophylaxis was permitted in the CLASS trial but not in the VIGOR trial. The CLASS trial reported no differences in the incidence of cardiovascular events between NSAIDs and celecoxib, regardless of aspirin use.

The proposed mechanism by which selective COX-2 inhibitors increase the risks of cardiovascular incidents lies in the natural balance between prothrombotic and antithrombotic prostaglandins. The COX-1 isoform results in production of prostaglandins that not only maintain gastric mucosa but are also found in platelets, and it mediates thromboxane A2 production, a platelet activator and aggregator. The inducible COX-2 isoform leads to prostaglandin PGI2 production, which is an inhibitor of platelet aggregation and a vasodilator. If selective COX-2s "inhibit the inhibitor" of platelet aggregation while allowing the unopposed platelet activator activity, an increase in prothrombotic mediators is inevitable.

In 2001, Mamdani and colleagues [15] concluded a retrospective cohort study in Ontario, Canada to compare the rates of acute myocardial infarction among 70,000 elderly patients (>66 years) given celecoxib, refecoxib, naproxen, or nonselective NSAIDs and a control group. They found no significant increase in the short-term (<1 year) risk of acute myocardial infarction among COX-2 users compared with non–COX-2 users. They also found no short-term reduced risk of acute myocardial infarction with naproxen.

The cardiovascular effects of COX-2 inhibitors used for osteoarthritis and musculoskeletal pain in patients without coronary artery disease was studied by Mukherjee and colleagues in 2001 [16], when they conducted a meta-analysis of the VIGOR and CLASS studies and studies 085 and 090. These last two studies were smaller (approximately 1000 subjects each), double-blind, randomized, controlled trials that compared rofecoxib, nabumetone, and placebo after 6 weeks of treatment for knee osteoarthritis. They found increased risk of cardiovascular events with rofecoxib in the VIGOR trial (rofecoxib, 50 mg/d) and no increased risk in studies 085 and 090 (rofecoxib, 12.5 mg/d) or the CLASS trial. Low-dose aspirin for cardioprotection was permitted in studies 085 and 090 and the CLASS trial. Selective COX-2 nonsteroidal drugs were effective in reducing musculoskeletal pain and gastrointestinal toxicity, but their increased risk of thrombotic cardiovascular events precluded their safe use. Celecoxib is the sole remaining selective COX-2 available for prescription use. Dosing varies from 100 to 200 mg twice daily, and an acute "pain pack" dose is also available. The dose is 400 mg initially followed by 200 mg 4 to 6 hours later, which may be repeated one time.

Muscle relaxants

Limiting muscle spasm and improving range of motion prepares patients who are experiencing back pain for therapeutic exercise as part of their rehabilitation. Muscle relaxants are often prescribed in the treatment of acute low back pain in an attempt to improve the initial limitations in range of motion from muscle spasm and interrupt the pain-spasm-pain cycle.

The muscle relaxing properties of these medications arise from inhibition of central polysynaptic neuronal events rather than direct activity on the motor unit (possible central nervous system depression by acting on the brainstem to reduce skeletal muscle hyperactivity). The 1994 Agency for Health Care Policy and Research guidelines for low back pain noted that muscle relaxants are an option in acute low back pain treatment—probably more effective than placebo and as effective as NSAIDs—but no additional benefit is gained with their combination with NSAIDs over NSAIDs alone. This information has evolved over the past 10 years to be more supportive of the combination of an NSAID with a muscle relaxant [17,18].

In 2003, Borenstein and Korn [19] studied the efficacy of a low-dose cyclobenzaprine in acute skeletal muscle spasm compared with placebo in two randomized controlled trials using 2.5-, 5-, and 10-mg doses three times daily. These studies demonstrated that the 5- and 10-mg doses gave significantly higher pain relief versus placebo and were equally effective, with a 5-mg dose associated with a significantly lower incidence of sedation.

In 1989, Basmajian [20] originally studied the efficacy of cyclobenzaprine alone and combined with an NSAID. He demonstrated superior pain relief and range of motion for the combination during the first 7 to 10 days after the initial insult. In 2002, Bernstein and colleagues [18] performed a secondary data analysis of a 1633 participant cohort with low back pain and their use of muscle relaxants. They found that muscle relaxants were not associated with a more rapid functional recovery. In 2001, Browning and colleagues [17] completed a meta-analysis of the cyclobenzaprine literature, which found consistent evidence of a moderate effect on pain, range of motion, and activities of daily living compared with placebo.

What follows is a list of commonly prescribed muscle relaxants:

Cyclobenzaprine, 5- or 10-mg tabs, dosing 10 mg three times daily, maximum 60 mg/d

Metaxalone, 400-mg tabs, dosing 800 mg orally three or four times daily

Methocarbamol, 500- and 750-mg tabs, dosing 1500 mg orally four times daily × 48 to 72 hours, then 1000 mg orally four times daily (or 1500 mg three times daily) maintenance

Carisoprodol, 350-mg tabs, dosing 350 mg three or four times daily (note: this drug has abuse potential and should be used only after failure of other muscle relaxants)

Tizanidine, diazepam, and baclofen are also muscle relaxants but have greater indication in the chronic management of spasticity, such as that seen after spinal cord injury. The most commonly reported adverse effect of most muscle relaxants is sedation. This side effect has been reduced in cyclobenzaprine, which currently has a 5-mg tablet taken on a three-times-daily basis. Metaxalone has been noted to have little to no sedation, but its efficacy has not been well supported in independent medical literature.

Opioids

Opioid medications act by binding to mu-opioid receptors and producing analgesia. These receptors are located peripherally on sensory nerves and immune cells and centrally in the spinal cord and brainstem. Opioids are an analgesic option for severe, nonmalignant, acute low back pain only when used on a time-limited course. They offer more potent analgesia than acetaminophen or NSAIDs and provoke no end-organ toxicity.

Orally administered opioids reach peak plasma concentration 60 to 90 minutes after ingestion. Half-lives of oxycodone, hydrocodone, morphine, and codeine are approximately 3 to 4 hours. Steady-state is reached in four to five half-lives, or approximately 24 hours. The potency of the opioid agonists is generally compared with that of morphine. Adverse side effects associated with chronic opioid use include constipation, nausea, and somnolence.

In 2001, Grilo and colleagues [21] reviewed 67 patients who suffered from nonmalignant low back pain with sciatica to determine if an opioid rotation (including oral morphine, hydromorphone, buprenorphine, and transdermal fentanyl) could be useful for establishing a more advantageous analgesic/side-effect relationship in rheumatologic pain, with results showing improvement in the visual analogue scales. This study did not compare opioids to placebo for efficacy; however, it did demonstrate the variability and perhaps tolerance of a given opioid and the effectiveness of trying another drug in the class if the first one fails. In a study with 200 patients who presented with acute low back strain, Weisel and colleagues [22] compared analgesic efficacy of acetaminophen with codeine and aspirin with oxycodone. A significantly greater level of pain reduction was noted for patients who received acetaminophen or aspirin with oxycodone over the non–opioid-containing preparations, especially within the first 3 days of treatment.

Although it is not chemically related to opiates, tramadol hydrochloride is a centrally acting analgesic that binds to mu receptors and has demonstrated its ability to provide superior analgesia to combined acetaminophen-propoxyphene in patients experiencing severe postoperative pain. Its mechanism of action is not completely understood but is believed to be at least partly secondary to its inhibition of the reuptake of serotonin and norepinephrine. In 2001, Reig [23] reviewed literature that illustrated the efficacy of tramadol alone or in conjunction with an NSAID in the management of low back pain, osteoarthritis, and breakthrough pain. He concluded that tramadol is more appropriate than NSAIDs for patients who suffer from gastrointestinal and renal problems and that tramadol caused fewer opioid-type adverse effects (eg, nausea, drowsiness, vomiting, dry mouth, constipation).

Successful opioid prescription involves achieving a tolerable balance between analgesia and the side effects associated with opioid use. Regular, rather than as-needed dosing, should be prescribed and their use limited to a short course to control pain. Tolerance to adverse effects, such as somnolence, nausea, and impaired thought processes, occurs within days to weeks of initial opioid administration. Constipation is a more persistent side effect that can be managed with concomitant stool softeners and laxatives. Opioids should be used with caution in patients with chronic obstructive pulmonary disease, emphysema, severe obesity, or cor pulmonale because of their respiratory depressant effects and blunting of the respiratory response to carbon dioxide. Despite the stigma and fears of addiction associated with their use, when properly used by a knowledgeable physician, opioid analgesics can treat otherwise intractable pain successfully.

Corticosteroids

Oral steroids have been found effective in the treatment of inflammatory conditions by interfering with the inflammation cascade by inhibiting phospholipase A2 actions and preventing the leukotriene and prostaglandin-mediated inflammatory response. They interact with receptor proteins in target tissues to regulate gene expression and, ultimately, protein synthesis by the target tissue, which accounts for their delayed effect. In the late 1970s, phospholipase A2, a potent inflammatory mediator, was found to be released by intervertebral discs after injury, possibly causing a chemical radiculitis, which might explain radicular pain in the absence of a more mechanical stressor.

Studies designed to investigate the use of oral steroids in the setting of acute low back pain remain limited. Haimovic and Beresford [24] compared oral dexamethasone with placebo in the treatment of lumbosacral radicular pain. Although patients treated with a dexamethasone taper had diminished pain compared with placebo, the use of additional analgesics, the small subject number, and loss of several patients to follow-up presented confounders that limited the study's use. Because of these obstacles (and the lack of current oral steroid/acute low back pain studies), the Agency for Health Care Policy and Research guideline has not recommended oral steroids for the treatment of acute low back pain. Despite the guideline, in the setting of acute low back pain with radiculopathy, oral corticosteroids are typically prescribed in a dosepak (methylprednisolone) taper of 21 4-mg tabs over 7 days, although this dose is probably insufficient. The author's preference is to prescribe oral prednisone beginning with 60 mg daily and tapering off within 6 days. The half-life of methylprednisolone is 18 to 36 hours. They are contraindicated in individuals with systemic fungal infections; precaution is required for patients who have diabetes (transient hyperglycemia). Complications are seen with chronic use (including immunosuppression, aseptic necrosis, gastric upset, impaired wound healing, osteoporosis, suppression of hypothalamic-pituitary-adrenal axis). The effectiveness of oral steroids in persons who have acute low back pain remains unproven; further research in this area is needed.

Other medications

Although colchicine is a powerful anti-inflammatory agent, it is not recommended by the Agency for Health Care Policy and Research guidelines for the treatment of acute low back pain. Current literature that involves colchicine trials for treatment of chronic low back pain versus placebo shows mixed responses and tolerance for colchicine's adverse effects (diarrhea and vomiting).

Although several classes of antidepressants have been used successfully in the treatment of various pain syndromes, the literature most strongly supports the analgesic efficacy of the tricyclic antidepressants. Migraine headaches, neuropathic pain associated with diabetic neuropathy, and postherpetic neuralgia have been found to respond favorably to antidepressant administration. Tricyclics also have been found to alleviate pain associated with musculoskeletal conditions, such as fibromyalgia, rheumatoid arthritis, and osteoarthritis. These more chronic pain conditions require lower doses than those prescribed for effective antidepressive effects. Most antidepressants require a minimum of 4 weeks to begin efficacy for their antidepressive effects, but it is unknown if this same time period is required to demonstrate pain relief.

Etanercept is a tumor necrosis factor-α inhibitor normally used for treatment of rheumatoid arthritis, with the usual dosage being 25 mg administered subcutaneously twice a week. A 2003 pilot study in Switzerland by Genevay and colleagues [25] studied the efficacy of etanercept in the treatment of 20 patients who were hospitalized for acute and severe sciatica. Ten consecutive patients received three subcutaneous injections (25 mg, every 3 days) in addition to standard analgesia, compared with ten control subjects with severe sciatica who received intravenous methylprednisolone. Compared with the steroid group, pain and disability ratings were significantly better in the etanercept group, which suggested that inhibition of tumor necrosis factor-α is a beneficial treatment option for sciatica. The presence of concomitant standard analgesia and the small study numbers confound the results, however. Further research is necessary before this treatment can be recommended.

Kanayama and colleagues [26] studied the efficacy of sarpogrelate hydroxychloride, a serotonin (5-HT) receptor blocker, in patients with symptomatic lumbar disc herniation. Serotonin is a chemical mediator associated with nerve root inflammation and sciatic symptoms in lumbar disc herniation. Kanayama and colleagues examined 44 patients who had symptomatic lumbar disc herniations and were given sarpogrelate hydroxychloride, 300 mg, orally every day for 14 days. They demonstrated that 64% of patients who had uncontained disc herniations had good pain relief, compared with none of the patients who had contained disc herniations.

Willow bark extract (salicin) is an herbal medicine widely used in Europe for treatment of low back pain. In 1999, Chrubasik and colleagues [27] evaluated its effectiveness in patients with an acute exacerbation of chronic low back pain compared with placebo in a 4-week blind trial. High- and low-dose salicin were compared with placebo. The principal outcome measures were the proportion of patients who were pain free at least 5 days at final week of study and the amount of tramadol rescue doses required. More patients in the high- and low-dose salicin groups versus placebo group were pain free at the end of the study. In 2000, Chrubasik and colleagues [28] compared salicin to rofecoxib (COX-2) in patients with acute exacerbation of low back pain. Doses used were chosen according to existing recommendations. They found no significant difference in effectiveness between the two groups, although salicin treatments were 40% less expensive than rofecoxib.

Summary

An understanding of the indications, risks, and benefits is necessary to prescribe properly the various medications that can be beneficial to patients who require treatment for acute low back pain. The scientific evidence supports the use of a nonselective NSAID combined with a muscle relaxant for most episodes of acute lumbar strain. These medications, in conjunction with nonpharmacologic modalities (eg, ice, heat, exercise), can help control pain, normalize function, and facilitate rehabilitation and recovery. There is variable evidence for the use of other medications, and their use must be reviewed and discussed by physicians and their patients to decide which therapeutic is most appropriate.

References

[1] McGuirk B, et al. Safety, efficacy, and cost effectiveness of evidence-based guidelines for the management of acute low back pain in primary care. Spine 2001;26(23):2615–22.
[2] Agency for Health Care Policy and Research. Low back guideline panel. Publication #14. Washington, DC: Agency for Health Care Policy and Research; 1994.
[3] Bradley, et al. Comparison of an antiinflammatory dose of ibuprofen, an analgesic dose of Ibuprofen, and acetaminophen in the treatment of patients with osteoarthritis of the knee. N Engl J Med 1991;325:87–91.
[4] Schattenkirchner M, Milachowski KA. A double-blind, multicentre, randomised clinical trial comparing the efficacy and tolerability of aceclofenac with diclofenac resinate in patients with acute low back pain. Clin Rheumatol 2003;22(2):127–35.
[5] Van Tulder MW, et al. Nonsteroidal anti-inflammatory drugs for low back pain: a systematic review within the framework of the Cochrane Collaboration Back Review Group. Spine 2000;25(19):2501–13.
[6] McCormack K, Brune K. Toward defining the analgesic role of nonsteroidal anti-inflammatory drugs in the management of acute soft tissue injuries. Clin J Sports Med 1993;3(2).
[7] Dreiser RL, et al. Relief of acute low back pain with diclofenac-K 12.5mg tablets: a flexible dose, ibuprofen 200mg and placebo-controlled clinical trial. International Journal of Clinical Pharmacologic Therapy 2003;41(9):375–85.

[8] Pohjolainen T, et al. Treatment of acute low back pain with the COX-2-selective anti-inflammatory drug nimesulide. Spine 2000;25(12):1579–85.

[9] Riew KD, et al. Time-dependent inhibitory effects of indomethacin on spinal fusion. J Bone Joint Surg Am 2003;85A(4):632–4.

[10] Goodman S, et al. COX-2 selective NSAID decreases bone ingrowth in vivo. J Orthop Res 2002;20(6):1164–9.

[11] Malanga G, Dennis R. Treatment of acute low back pain: use of medications. Journal of Musculoskeletal Medicine 2005;22(2).

[12] Bombardier C, et al. Comparison of upper gastrointestinal toxicity of rofecoxib and naproxen in patients with rheumatoid arthritis. N Engl J Med 2000;343:1520–8.

[13] Juni P, et al. Risk of cardiovascular events and rofecoxib: cumulative meta-analysis. Lancet 2004;364:2021–9.

[14] Silverstein F, et al. Gastrointestinal toxicity with celecoxib vs nonsteroidal anti-inflammatory drugs for osteoarthritis and rheumatoid arthritis: the CLASS Study. A randomized controlled trial. JAMA 2000;284(10):1247–55.

[15] Mamdani M, Rochon P, Juurlink DN, et al. Effect of selective cyclooxygenase 2 inhibitors and naproxen on short-term risk of acute myocardial infarction in the elderly. Arch Intern Med 2003;163(4):481–6.

[16] Mukherjee D, Nissen SE, Topol EJ. Risk of cardiovasular events associated with selective COX-2 inhibitors. JAMA 2001;286(8):954–9.

[17] Browning R, et al. Cyclobenzaprine and back pain: a meta-analysis. Arch Intern Med 2001; 161:1613–20.

[18] Bernstein E. The use of muscle relaxant medications in acute low back pain. Spine 2004; 29(12):1346–51.

[19] Borenstein DG, Korn S. Efficacy of a low-dose regimen of cyclobenzaprine hydrochloride in acute skeletal muscle spasm: results of two placebo-controlled trials. Clin Ther 2003;25(4): 1056–73.

[20] Basmajian JV. Acute back pain and spasm: a controlled multicenter trial of combined analgesic and antispasm agents. Spine 1989;14:438–9.

[21] Grilo RM, et al. Opioid rotation in the treatment of joint pain: a review of 67 cases. Joint Bone Spine 2002;69(5):491–4.

[22] Weisel SW, Cuckler JM, DeLuca F, et al. Acute low back pain: an objective analysis of conservative therapy. Spine 1980;4:324–30.

[23] Reig E. Tramadol in musculoskeletal pain: a survey. Clin Rheumatol 2002;21(Suppl 1): S9–11.

[24] Haimovic IC, Beresford HR. Dexamethasone is not superior to placebo for treating lumbosacral radicular pain. Neurology 1986;36:1593–4.

[25] Genevay S, et al. Efficacy of etanercept in the treatment of acute and severe sciatica: a pilot study. Ann Rheumatol Dis 2004;63(9):1120–3.

[26] Kanayama M, et al. Efficacy of serotonin receptor blocker for symptomatic lumbar disc herniation. Clin Orthop Relat Res 2002;411:159–65.

[27] Chrubasik S, et al. Treatment of low back pain exacerbations with willow bark extract: a randomized double-blind study. Am J Med 2000;109:9–14.

[28] Chrubasik S, et al. Treatment of low back pain with an herbal or synthetic anti-rheumatic: a randomized controlled study. Willow bark extract for low back pain. Rheumatology (Oxford) 2001;40(12):1388–93.

ELSEVIER
SAUNDERS

Clin Occup Environ Med
5 (3) 655–702

CLINICS IN
OCCUPATIONAL AND
ENVIRONMENTAL
MEDICINE

Lumbar Spine Injection
and Interventional Procedures
in the Management of Low Back Pain

Frank J.E. Falco, MD[a,b,*], Lee Irwin, MD[a],
Jie Zhu, MD[a]

[a]Mid Atlantic Spine and Pain Specialists, P.A., 139 East Chestnut Hill Road,
Newark, DE 19713, USA
[b]Physical Medicine and Rehabilitation Department, Temple University Medical School,
3420 North Broad Street, Philadelphia, PA 19140, USA

Low back pain has had and continues to have a substantial medical and financial impact in the United States. The incidence of low back pain is 5%, with a 60% to 90% lifetime prevalence [1,2]. Low back pain is the most common cause of disability in persons younger than age 45 and ranks second to cardiovascular disease in disability for persons older than age 45 [3]. The cost of low back pain in the United States has been estimated at billions of dollars annually in medical expenses, lost income, lost productivity, insurance costs, compensation payments, and legal fees [4–6].

Sedentary and physical laborers develop low back pain, with no significant gender predilection [7–9]. There is an increased risk for back injury as strength demands increase beyond the capabilities of the worker, as seen with manual labor occupations (eg, construction, warehouse, and textile workers) and in the nursing profession [10]. Individuals who drive heavy machinery or vehicles have a two- to fourfold greater incidence of low back pain compared with other workers because of the associated vibrational stresses [11–13]. Low back pain is responsible for 20% of all workers' compensation claims and accounts for 25% of all disabling work-related injuries, resulting in the loss of 30 days per 100 workers each year, which amounts to 38.5 million workdays annually in the United States [11,14,15].

Making the correct diagnosis is critical to treating low back pain effectively. The history and physical examination findings commonly fail to

* Corresponding author. Mid Atlantic Spine and Pain Specialists, P.A., 139 East Chestnut Hill Road, Newark, DE 19713.
   E-mail address: CSSM01@aol.com (F.J.E. Falco).

1526-0046/06/$ - see front matter © 2006 Elsevier Inc. All rights reserved.
doi:10.1016/j.coem.2006.04.001   *occmed.theclinics.com*

provide an accurate diagnosis [16–18]. Imaging studies can reveal anatomic abnormalities that might or might not have clinical significance and are unable to disclose soft tissue injuries [19–23]. Specific lumbar spine injections can identify the source of pain (the pain generator), which has a significant impact on making the diagnosis and identifying patients who would benefit from other types of treatment that can give long-term pain relief. These injections alone can provide prolonged pain relief that can maximize treatment and improve functional outcome. This article discusses the different types of lumbar spine injections used in the evaluation and management of low back pain and lumbar radiculopathy and several interventional procedures that can deliver lasting pain relief.

Lumbar epidural injections

Indications

Lumbar spine epidural injections have been used to treat various low back conditions, including generalized low back pain, radiculopathy, spinal stenosis, herniated lumbar discs, discogenic pain, and postlaminectomy syndrome. The first report of an epidural steroid injection was published in 1952 by Robecchi and Capra [24], who performed a periradicular S1 injection with hydrocortisone for a woman who suffered from back pain and sciatica. The next published report of an epidural injection was by Lièvre in 1953 [25]. In 1961, Goebert and colleagues [26] were the first to report the use of epidural steroids in the United States, in which 72% of 113 patients had good relief of radicular pain.

The diagnostic evaluation for radiculopathy includes radiographs to evaluate the disc space and vertebral body height and can reveal degenerative osseous and disc changes and foraminal narrowing. Electrodiagnostic studies can be helpful to differentiate radiculopathy from a peripheral neuropathy or compression mononeuropathy. MRI can provide an in-depth anatomic evaluation of the spinal canal, neuroforamen, spinal cord, thecal sac, nerve roots, and intervertebral discs. CT and myelography are helpful in evaluating osseous structures and spinal canal dimensions. Clinical correlation always must be used to interpret the results of diagnostic testing, however, particularly with anatomic studies, such as imaging techniques [19,27–30].

Technique

Lumbar epidural injections can be performed with any of three different techniques. Interlaminar, caudal, and foraminal epidural approaches all provide access to the epidural space. The epidural injections are performed primarily to treat lumbar radiculopathy. Interlaminar and foraminal epidural injections place the corticosteroid and anesthetic agents in the vicinity or at the site of pathology. Foraminal epidural injections also can provide diagnostic information in regard to confirming the presence of radicular pain and the root level. Caudal epidural injections are less specific and typically are used for therapeutic purposes when treating lower lumbar or sacral radiculopathies.

Interlaminar epidural injections are performed under fluoroscopic guidance with a patient in the prone position by passing an epidural needle between the lamina using a median (between the spinous processes) or paramedian (oblique to the spinous processes) approach. An epidural needle is advanced through the skin until contact with the lamina and then is "walked off" onto the ligamentum flavum and slowly advanced into the epidural space using a loss-of-resistance technique (Fig. 1A). A 2- to 3-mL volume of nonionic contrast is slowly injected under fluoroscopy after negative aspiration to produce an epidurogram (Fig. 1B) to confirm appropriate needle placement. A 1-mL test dose of lidocaine is injected, after which the anesthetic and corticosteroid solution is slowly injected into the epidural space.

The patient is positioned in the prone position for a lumbar foraminal epidural steroid injection, and the C-arm or the patient is positioned obliquely until the tip of the ipsilateral subjacent superior articular process divides the pedicle in half. The safe triangle technique, which has been described commonly for performing a lumbar foraminal epidural steroid injection (Fig. 2), might not be so safe because the needle tip is placed in the anterior portion of the foramen superior to the exiting nerve root (Fig. 3). This procedure potentially risks an arterial injury to the radicular artery and subsequent spinal cord infarction. Alternative methods position the needle tip in either the posterior/inferior (Fig. 4) or posterior portion of the foramen. These needle placements are chosen to reduce potentially the risk or arterial injury by avoiding the radicular or Adamkiewicz artery that is most commonly located along the superoanterior portion of the nerve.

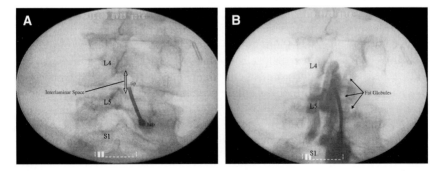

Fig. 1. Interlaminar lumbar epidural injection. (*A*) The epidural needle is "walked off" the lamina into the L4/5 interlaminar space. (*B*) Contrast injection produces a lumbar epidurogram that demonstrates a fluffy, cloud-like, cobblestone pattern. hub, epidural needle hub; tip, epidural needle tip; L4, L4 vertebra; L5, L5 vertebra; S1, S1 vertebra.

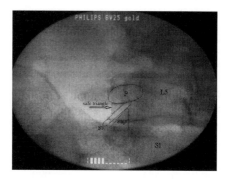

Fig. 2. Safe triangle. This is a triangle created by the lateral edge of the vertebral body (laterally), pedicle (superiorly), and nerve root (medially) that provides a safe area for needle tip placement to avoid contact with the exiting nerve root when performing lumbar transforaminal epidural injections. P, pedicle; sap, superior articular process; NR, nerve root; L5, L5 vertebra; S1, S1 vertebra.

The patient is placed in a prone position for an S1 foraminal epidural steroid injection. The S1 foramen is located with fluoroscopy caudad to the S1 pedicle. Repositioning the C-arm in a slightly cephalad or lateral position can allow for better visualization of the foramen. A spinal needle is advanced toward the superolateral aspect of the S1 foramen until contact with the sacrum and then is advanced into the foramen (Fig. 5).

The needle depth for all transforaminal epidurals is checked with a fluoroscopic anteroposterior and lateral view, which ensures that the needle tip does not extend any farther medially than the midpoint of the pedicles. This precaution, along with the use of blunt tip needles, is taken to avoid penetration of the nerve root dural cuff and the epidural vasculature. Care must be taken to avoid puncturing the dural sleeve, which can lead to an

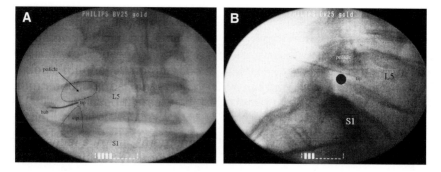

Fig. 3. Lumbar transforaminal epidural, safe triangle technique. (*A*) Needle placement oblique view. (*B*) Needle placement lateral view. hub, spine needle hub; tip, spine needle tip; sap, superior articular process; solid circle, approximate nerve root position in the foramen; L5, L5 vertebra; S1, S1 vertebra.

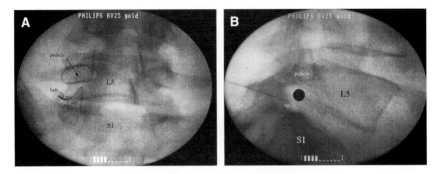

Fig. 4. Lumbar transforaminal epidural, posterior inferior technique. (*A*) Needle placement oblique view. (*B*) Needle placement lateral view. hub, spine needle hub; tip, spine needle tip; sap, superior articular process; solid circle, approximate nerve root position in the foramen; L5, L5 vertebra; S1, S1 vertebra.

inadvertent intrathecal injection. A radiculogram is produced by contrast injection to confirm that the needle tip is in proper position (Fig. 6) and ensure that there was no puncture of the dural sac. Injection tubing is then attached to the needle and to a syringe with contrast. Injection tubing is used mainly to avoid needle tip movement. At least 0.5 mL of nonionic contrast is injected under fluoroscopy to outline the nerve root and spread into the epidural space. The needle tip is repositioned if there is a venous, arterial, or intrathecal injection. Otherwise, syringes are exchanged for the anesthetic and steroid mixture. The needle tip position is confirmed by injecting the remaining contrast within the tubing. The solution is injected slowly after a negative 1 mL test dose.

Caudal epidurals, a unique third alternative for performing a lumbar epidural injection, are performed ideally under fluoroscopy. The patient is placed in the prone position and the sacral hiatus and sacral cornu are

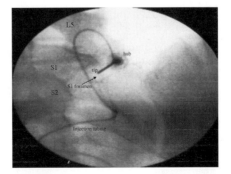

Fig. 5. Sacral transforaminal epidural needle placement. Anterior posterior view of spinal needle within the S1 foramen with injection tubing attached to the needle hub. hub, spine needle hub; tip, spine needle tip; L5, L5 vertebra; S1, S1 vertebra; S2, S2 vertebra.

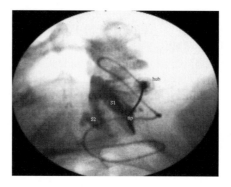

Fig. 6. Sacral transforaminal epidural contrast injection. Anterior posterior view of spinal needle within the S1 foramen with injection tubing attached to the needle hub and contrast outlining S1 and S2 nerve roots. hub, spine needle hub; tip, spine needle tip; S1, S1 nerve root; S2, S2 nerve root.

identified by palpation and with fluoroscopy. A spinal needle penetrates the skin at a 45° angle between the sacral cornu and is advanced until it contacts the sacrum. The needle is slightly withdrawn and advanced at a shallow 10° angle through the sacrococcygeal ligament into the epidural space. The needle position is confirmed with biplanar fluoroscopy, with the needle tip kept inferior to the S2 foramen to avoid thecal sac puncture. Contrast is injected after negative aspiration under fluoroscopy into the epidural space (Fig. 7) to produce a sacral epidurogram that identifies proper needle tip placement and to ensure that the needle tip has not entered a vascular structure or the thecal sac. Anesthesia and corticosteroid are then injected into the epidural space.

Caudal epidurals are primarily helpful in treating L5 or S1 radiculopathies. Injections are less likely to be effective in treating radiculopathies at higher levels because the injectant travels a farther distance. Caudal

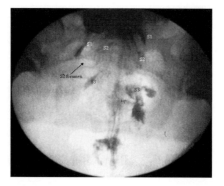

Fig. 7. Caudal epidural. tip, spine needle tip; S1, S1 nerve root; S2, S2 nerve root; S3, S3 nerve root.

epidurals are particularly advantageous when treating lumbosacral radiculopathies in patients who have had lower lumbar spine surgery, in which there is often epidural scarring or obliteration of the epidural space at the surgical site. The caudal epidural route avoids the high risk of dural puncture and any potential complications associated with an interlaminar approach that is attempted at or close to the operative site.

Complications

There are rare complications associated with epidural steroid injections. There have been reports of epidural hematoma, septicemia, bacterial meningitis, epidural abscess, arachnoiditis, Cushing's syndrome, chemical meningitis, epidural lipomatosis, dural-cutaneous fistula, retinal hemorrhage, and one case of death from an epidural abscess [31–39]. Dural puncture with subsequent spinal headache has a low reported incidence with caudal and lumbar epidural injections [40,41]. Although not frequent, a more common complication is a vasovagal episode that typically occurs during the injection. Hyperglycemia can occur in patients who have diabetes.

A subarachnoid or intravascular anesthetic injection can lead to periorbital numbness, disorientation, lightheadedness, nystagmus, tinnitus, complete sensory or motor block, muscle twitching, respiratory depression, and seizures. The risk of complications from intrathecal and intravascular injections of local anesthesia is proportionate to the injected volume.

Complications of transforaminal epidural steroid injections include infection, allergic reaction, and bleeding. Reports have demonstrated negative aspiration of blood to be inaccurate in predicting intravascular injection, and contrast injection is recommended to identify vascular uptake [41]. Although rare, transforaminal lumbar epidurals can lead to spinal cord infarction and hemiplegia [42]. Injury to the radicular artery, particularly the artery of Adamkiewicz (lower thoracic and upper lumbar levels), or other collateral arteries within the foramen are believed to occur as a result of spasm, puncture, thrombosis, or embolization by corticosteroid particulate matter [42–44]. This complication might be reduced or eliminated by inserting needles into the posterior portion of the foramen, avoiding injections in the presence of significant foraminal stenosis, using blunt tip needles [43,45], using injection tubing, injecting contrast under live fluoroscopy, administering a lidocaine test dose, and injecting with nonparticulate corticosteroids.

Patients are instructed to stop aspirin or nonsteroidal anti-inflammatory medications several days before an epidural injection to reduce the risk of bleeding [46]. Patients who take warfarin are instructed to stop the medication in accordance with their primary care physician and have bleeding parameters evaluated before an injection [47]. Epidurals should be avoided in patients with a platelet count less than 100,000/μL or abnormal bleeding parameters, such as a prolonged international normalized ratio. Other contraindications to performing lumbar epidural injections include bleeding disorders, infection, and spinal stenosis.

Efficacy

Lumbar epidural steroid injections are effective in the treatment of radiculopathy. Other than the exception of a few uncontrolled reports, most studies have demonstrated some degree of benefit from epidural injections [48]. The efficacy of lumbar epidural steroid injections is detailed in the Australian National Health and Medical Research Council Advisory Committee report, which supports the therapeutic use of caudal and transforaminal epidural steroid injections [49]. A published meta-analysis study in 1990 of the few available controlled studies showed to a statistically significant degree that lumbar epidurals are efficacious for treating radiculopathy [48]. A few of the controlled studies evaluated the long-term benefits of lumbar epidural steroid injections.

Manchikanti and colleagues [50] reviewed combined randomized, double-blinded, and nonrandomized trials for all three approaches to lumbar epidural steroid injections. The evidence for caudal epidurals is strong for short-term relief and moderate for long-term relief. The findings for interlaminar epidurals are moderate for short-term relief and limited for long-term relief of symptoms. The results for transforaminal epidural steroid injections are strong for short- and long-term relief.

Zygapophyseal joint injections

Indications

Goldthwaite [51] first considered the facet joint as a source of low back pain in 1911. He believed that the lumbar facet joint was responsible for low back pain, lumbar spine instability, and leg pain. Putti [52] supported the concept of facet joint generated low back and leg pain in 1927. Ghormley [53] coined the term "facet syndrome" in 1933, which is still used currently to describe this condition. The prevalence of symptomatic lumbar facet joints has been reported as 8% to 45% in chronic low back pain [18,54,55].

Mooney and Robertson [56] evaluated the lumbar facet joint in a group of individuals with and without low back pain with provocative hypertonic saline facet joint injections. The subjects described the pain produced from the injections as deep, dull, and vague. The location of the pain produced by stimulating the facet joints with the intra-articular injections was recorded, and pain referral maps were constructed for both groups (Fig. 8). The information derived from these maps has been helpful in the assessment of patient pain drawings [57,58]. The pain drawing is often used in clinical practice to help a physician evaluate lumbar disorders.

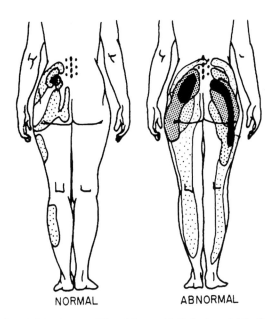

NORMAL   ABNORMAL

Fig. 8. Lumbar facet joint pain map. (*From* Mooney V, Robertson J. The facet syndrome. Clin Orthop 1976;115:149–56; with permission.)

Facet syndrome has been described as nonspecific low back pain with a deep and achy quality. Facet joint dysfunction can result from osteoarthritis or trauma. The syndrome is considered in a patient with low back pain that radiates into the buttock and posterior thigh. Patients might complain of symptoms that increase with twisting the back or bending backward. Physical examination typically reveals local lumbar paravertebral muscle tenderness to palpation. Radicular findings are commonly absent. The pain often can be increased with hyperextension and rotation of the lumbar spine consistent with historical complaints as described previously. Although these findings might be somewhat helpful in evaluating for lumbar facet syndrome, no history or physical examination findings are unique to this condition [59–62].

Technique

Facet joint injections not only are a potential therapeutic modality but also provide information regarding the source of the pain and ultimately a diagnosis. Facet joint blocks are performed in one of two ways: either the medial branch nerves that provide innervation to the joint can be injected with medication or the intra-articular facet joint can be injected. These blocks are performed with fluoroscopy to pinpoint and confirm needle placement before the injection.

Medial branch nerve injections are performed for diagnostic purposes. The injections are performed with anesthesia to determine whether the suspected facet joint or joints are responsible for the symptoms. The cephalad and subjacent medial branch nerves must be blocked to anesthetize or "block" a lumbar facet joint (Fig. 9). The procedure for lumbar medial branch block is performed by obtaining oblique views of the specific lumbar vertebra to visualize the "Scotty dog." The injection site for L1-4 medial branch is the "eye" of the "Scotty dog" over which the nerve travels (Fig. 10). Contrast is injected after negative aspiration to assess needle placement (Fig. 11). A volume of 0.3 to 0.5 mL of local anesthesia is injected with the needle bevel in an inferomedial orientation to prevent flow to the nearby nerve roots [63]. The injection for the L5 dorsal ramus involves placing the C-arm in a 10° to 15° ipsilateral oblique position. The spinal needle is

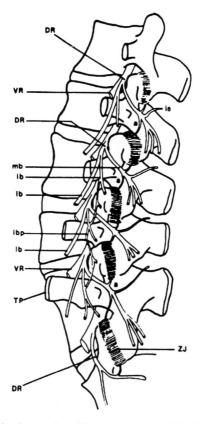

Fig. 9. Lumbar facet joint innervation. VR, ventral ramus; DR, dorsal ramus; mb, medial branch; ib, intermediate branch; ibp, intermediate branch plexus; is, interspinous branch; a, articular branch; ZJ, zygapophyseal (facet) joint. (*From* Bogduk N, Twomey LT, editors. Clinical anatomy of the lumbar spine. 2nd edition. New York: Churchill-Livingstone; 1991. p. 113; with permission.)

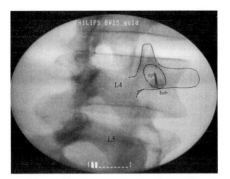

Fig. 10. Lumbar medial branch nerve injection. An oblique view of spinal needle placement for a right L3 medial branch nerve block. hub, spine needle hub; tip, spine needle tip; L4, L4 vertebra; L5, L5 vertebra.

positioned inferior to the superior aspect of the junction of the superior articular process with the sacral ala. The needle bevel should be directed medially to prevent flow into the S1 posterior sacral or the L5 intervertebral foramen. The L5 dorsal ramus is injected with 0.3 to 0.5 mL of local anesthesia after negative aspiration.

Injections are considered diagnostic for facet joint syndrome if there is significant relief of symptoms for the expected duration of the anesthetic effect. A higher diagnostic sensitivity and specificity from medial branch blocks can be accomplished if injections are performed on different occasions with anesthetic agents that possess different durations of action [62]. Patients with diagnostic pain relief from medial branch blocks are often

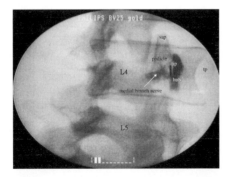

Fig. 11. Lumbar medical branch nerve injection. An oblique view of a right L3 medial branch nerve block. The first contrast injection demonstrated soft tissue accumulation. A second injection of contrast after repositioning the spinal needle outlined the medial branch nerve. This procedure was followed by an injection of local anesthesia and corticosteroid. hub, spine needle hub; tip, spine needle tip; sap, superior articular process; tp, transverse process; L4, L4 vertebra; L5, L5 vertebra.

considered for medial branch neurolysis, which has been reported to provide up to several years of symptom relief [64–67].

For percutaneous intra-articular lumbar facet joint injections, the patient or the fluoroscope is placed in a posterior oblique orientation until the joint cavity is first visualized. A spinal needle is advanced under fluoroscopy toward the midpoint of the facet joint cavity until contact with either articular process. The needle is directed toward either the articular joint itself or one of the capsular recesses. The needle tip is then "walked off" into the facet joint, with care taken not to pass through the joint and into the epidural space. After negative aspiration, contrast is injected to produce an arthrogram and confirm needle placement within the joint (Fig. 12). The typical lumbar facet joint has a volume of no more than 2 mL, and the physician should limit the amount of contrast used to allow for the subsequent injection of anesthesia and corticosteroid [68,69].

The medial branch nerve injection method is helpful in cases of severely degenerative facet joints, in which there can be extravasation of the injection material to bordering structures with intra-articular injections. The presence of extravasation can be determined during the injection of contrast. There might be a lack of effectiveness from the intra-articular injection in this situation. No diagnostic conclusion regarding the facet joint can be made regarding any clinical response in the presence of extravasation because the structure or structures anesthetized cannot be determined from the intra-articular injection.

Intra-articular zygapophyseal joint injections block the facet joint but not the other posterior elements, such as the facet joint capsule, multifidus muscle, interspinous muscle, or interspinous ligament. In addition to the facet joint, these structures are blocked with medial branch nerve injections. A nondiagnostic response to a facet joint injection does not rule out a posterior

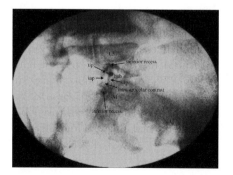

Fig. 12. Lumbar facet joint injection. An oblique view of an intra-articular contrast injection of the L5/S1 facet joint with some contrast extravasation beyond the superior recess. hub, spine needle hub; tip, spine needle tip; iap, inferior articular process; sap, superior articular process; L5, L5 vertebra; S1, S1 vertebra.

element injury, and a diagnostic response to medial branch injections does not necessarily implicate the facet joint as the specific pain generator.

Complications

Complications from facet joint injections are rare. Localized tenderness at the needle insertion site is not uncommon and typically lasts no more than a few days [70]. Spinal blockade has been recorded as a complication from facet joint injections [71]. Vasovagal episodes also can occur. Chemical meningitis has been reported as a result of puncture of the dural cuff [72]. Other complications include spinal cord trauma, intravascular injection, hematoma formation, and infection.

As with any spinal injection procedure, precautions are made regarding bleeding, such as stopping aspirin, nonsteroidal anti-inflammatory medications, and warfarin. Contraindications are similar to those for epidural injections, including bleeding disorders and infection.

Efficacy

Fluoroscopically guided facet injections are the only way to identify the facet joint as a pain generator [17]. Clinical suspicion by the examiner is the primary indication for diagnostic facet joint injections. Studies that demonstrated production of facet joint pain with capsular distension showed that lumbar medial branch blocks were 89% successful at relieving the provoked pain. Other outcome studies of facet joint nerve blocks have demonstrated short- and long-term relief [73,74]. False-positive rates have ranged from 22% to 47% in lumbar facet joint blocks [54,55,75,76]. The 8% false-negative rate in facet joint blocks has been caused by inadvertent intravascular uptake [63].

Lumbar facet joint blocks have been shown to be effective in providing diagnostic information as to whether the facet joint is responsible for low back symptoms [17,18,56,77,78]. The long-term therapeutic benefit from intra-articular facet joint injections has been controversial. Although many uncontrolled studies have reported a wide range of pain relief from lumbar facet blocks, only two controlled studies evaluated the long-term pain relief from fluoroscopically guided intra-articular facet joint injections.

The study by Carette and colleagues [79] investigated the long-term effectiveness of intra-articular methylprednisolone facet joint injections. Patients who had chronic low back pain underwent injection of the lower two lumbar facet joints with lidocaine. Individuals who had a 50% or more relief of back pain were equally and randomly divided into two groups. One group underwent lumbar facet joint injections with a methylprednisolone and saline mixture, whereas the other group received only saline. The two groups were followed for 6 months. The authors determined that there was no difference in pain relief between the two groups and concluded that intra-articular facet joint injections with methylprednisolone were not effective in treating chronic low back pain.

The study had several flaws. The authors established the presence of facet joint pain based on a single lidocaine injection as opposed to performing the injections with two different anesthetic agents on two different occasions. The double injection paradigm would have selected individuals with facet joint pain more accurately and excluded placebo responders [62]. Another error was the assumption that the saline was a true inert placebo. Other studies have shown that saline provides pain relief to a greater degree than would be expected from a placebo [80,81]. A review of the follow-up data during the study showed no significant difference between the groups at 1 and 3 months. At the 6-month follow-up, however, 46% of the steroid group and 15% of the saline group had good pain relief, a statistically significant difference ($P = 0.002$) between the two groups. The authors invalidated this finding, because only a portion of both groups that had pain relief at 1 month had actual pain relief at 6 months. The authors concluded that the methylprednisolone facet joint injections were no more effective than the saline injections.

The other controlled study, by Lilius and colleagues [82], evaluated different lumbar facet joint treatment groups. Patients were randomly distributed into one of three groups that received intra-articular cortisone/anesthesia, intra-articular saline, or pericapsular cortisone/anesthetic injections. Although there was substantial pain relief in all three groups at 3 months, there was no significant difference between the groups. There were also critical flaws with this study. The authors did not preselect subjects with diagnostic facet joint injections to identify properly the individuals with facet joint pain and exclude placebo responders. Another flaw was that the intra-articular facet joint injection volumes of up to 8 mL were excessive. Extravasation from the intra-articular facet joint injections would be expected with these large injection volumes, which would obscure any results from the intra-articular facet joint blocks, because nearby and potentially painful structures also would be affected by the injections.

Sacroiliac joint injections

Indications

The sacroiliac (SI) joint long has been implicated as a controversial source of low back and leg pain. The SI joint was regarded as the primary cause of sciatica at the turn of the century, and surgical fusion of the SI joint was commonly used to treat sciatica symptoms [83,84]. After the landmark publication of a lumbar disc herniation by Mixter and Barr [85] in 1934, the diagnosis of SI joint dysfunction became unpopular, and the lumbar intervertebral disc became the focus of low back and leg pain.

SI joint pain has been associated with metabolic, traumatic, degenerative, inflammatory, and infectious processes [86–90]. SI joint dysfunction has been described as a condition of joint hypomobility that might or might not lead to pain [16]. The diagnosis of SI joint dysfunction was once based primarily on clinical evaluation without a means to confirm whether it was responsible for any mechanical pain. No findings from imaging studies are specific for SI joint dysfunction [29,91–93]. Several structures near the SI joint potentially can lead to pain [18,55,94]. The inability to isolate and distinguish the SI joint as a pain generator has led to doubt in the past about it being a mechanical source of back and leg pain.

The concept of establishing the diagnosis of SI joint dysfunction by providing symptom relief from an anesthetic injection was reported as early as 1938 [95]. Many clinicians tried to perform intra-articular SI joint injections but were unable to puncture the joint, produce a joint arthrogram, or aspirate an uninfected joint [96,97]. Joint aspiration and injection of a non-infected joint were believed to be impossible. Recently, however, a technique was described that reliably allows for the injection of the SI joint [98]. The authors were able to produce joint arthrograms in normal volunteers and establish pain maps from SI joint provocation (Fig. 13). These maps were used in a subsequent study to identify patients with back pain

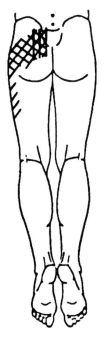

Fig. 13. SI joint pain map. (*From* Fortin JD, Dwyer AP, West S, et al. Sacroiliac joint: pain referral maps upon applying a new injection/arthrography technique. Part I: Asymptomatic volunteers. Spine 1994;19:1475–82; with permission.)

secondary to SI joint dysfunction who later underwent anesthetic injections that resulted in pain relief [99].

Although many questions remain about the SI joint regarding pain and its role in biomechanics, there is clear evidence that the SI joint does elicit pain. SI joint injections not only provide a means for establishing a diagnosis but are also a treatment option. The impact and role of SI joint injections on the management of SI joint dysfunction need further evaluation.

There is a 10% to 30% prevalence of SI joint dysfunction as the cause of low back pain [94,100]. SI joint dysfunction has been described to occur after a direct insult to the joint, such as falling on the buttocks or repetitive overuse activity, such as twisting and lifting [101]. Ipsilateral groin and posterior superior iliac spine pain are two complaints that have been shown to have a high correlation with SI joint dysfunction [94,101]. Other pain complaints are nonspecific, and the quality of pain has been described as deep, vague, and achy or stabbing [98,99]. The pain distribution associated with SI joint dysfunction is not unique but typically originates in the buttock area and can extend to the posterolateral thigh or distally into the leg [94,98]. Several maneuvers can be used on physical examination, including Patrick's, Gillet, seated flexion, and standing flexion tests, to evaluate for SI joint dysfunction, but there is little relationship between these tests and a symptomatic SI joint [16,93,103]. No specific findings on history, physical examination, or diagnostic studies are specific for SI joint pain.

Technique

Until recently, intra-articular SI joint injections were thought to be impossible. A posterior injection technique has been described that allows for reliable injection of the joint, however [98]. The injection is accomplished using fluoroscopic imaging with the patient lying in the prone position. Fluoroscopic imaging is essential, because only 22% of SI joint injections are performed successfully without fluoroscopic guidance [104]. The C-arm is rotated in an attempt to separate the anterior and posterior aspects of the joint to visualize the most inferior portion of the posterior joint. The C-arm rotation continues until direct visualization of the posterior limb is recognized by a lucent region in the inferior aspect of the joint, which represents overlap with the anterior limb. The medial aspect of the joint silhouette corresponds to the posterior limb, and the lateral aspect corresponds to the anterior limb. A spinal needle is advanced percutaneously using sterile technique 1 to 3 cm inferior to the joint. There is a characteristic feel to the needle as it penetrates the thick ligaments of the posterior joint. If there is resistance to advancement, the needle might need to be adjusted by rotating the bevel to conform to the bony contour of the joint. A small amount of contrast is then injected to produce a joint arthrogram to confirm needle placement (Fig. 14). A combination of corticosteroid and anesthesia is then instilled into the joint.

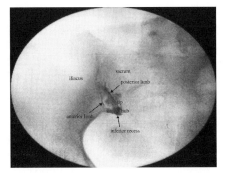

Fig. 14. SI joint injection. Contrast injection outlines the anterior and posterior limbs of the SI joint and the inferior recess. hub, spinal needle hub; tip, spinal needle tip.

Complications

The most common complications of SI joint dysfunction are caused by joint rupture or capsule extravasation. Posterior leakage of contrast into the dorsal sacral foramina, superior recess leakage onto the L5 epidural sheath, and ventral extravasation onto the lumbosacral plexus can affect the nearby neural structures [105]. Further complications include trauma to the sciatic nerve, infection, and adverse drug reactions. As with any injection procedure, there can be localized tenderness at the site of needle insertion, which typically lasts for only several days. Vasovagal episodes can occur during the injection. The same precautions regarding bleeding and infection apply with SI joint injections.

Efficacy

No well-controlled studies have evaluated the effectiveness of SI joint injections in treating SI joint dysfunction. Only recently was a reliable technique devised to perform intra-articular joint injections. SI joint injections are used diagnostically and therapeutically in clinical practice. Empirically, they have been helpful in reducing pain, which has resulted in better outcomes when combined with other forms of conservative care. There is a need for studies to evaluate the long-term effectiveness of SI joint injections on pain control and the impact of these injections on treatment regimens for SI joint dysfunction.

Lumbar discography

Indications

Disc injections were first performed by Schmorl [28] in 1929 to evaluate the structure of cadaveric intervertebral discs. In 1938, Steindler and Luck

[106] used in vivo disc injections of procaine to relieve low back pain. Hirsch [107] and Lindblom [108] introduced provocative discography in 1948 and noted that injections into ruptured discs exacerbated low back symptoms. The first disc injections in the United States were performed in 1951 by Wise and Weiford [109]. In 1952, Pierre Erlacher [73] established the correlation of the nucleogram to nuclear anatomy by investigating cadaver discs using contrast material and histologic stains. Cloward and Busaid [110] described the indications and technique for lumbar discography in 1952. Indications for lumbar discography include surgical planning of a lumbar fusion, identifying the presence or absence of a painful disc, testing the structural integrity of an adjacent disc to a known abnormality such as spondylolisthesis or fusion, and, in rare cases, evaluating a suspected lateral or recurrent disc herniation [111–117]. Over time, technologic advances, improved technique, and a better understanding of pain have contributed to the refinement of discography as a potentially valuable, albeit controversial, diagnostic test.

Internal disc disruption (IDD) is a term that was first used by H.V. Crock in 1970 to describe pathologic changes of the internal structure of the disc [118]. IDD is considered a chemically mediated abnormality that causes degradation of the nucleus and leads to annular deterioration without necessarily having an extradural disc defect [118]. Annular fiber deterioration can present as radial fissuring. Annular tears also are believed to result from axial rotation injuries. The risk for annular tearing with rotation increases if the lumbar spine is initially in a flexed position that places half of the annular fibers on stretch before the rotational movement [119–121]. Radial fissures into the innervated, outer disc margins might be painful because of mechanical or chemical irritation.

Plain film radiography, CT, or myelography cannot detect IDD because these studies are unable to detect abnormalities within the intervertebral disc. MRI study results can be normal or abnormal in the presence of IDD. T2-weighted MRI often demonstrates decreased nuclear signal intensity that reflects water loss from nuclear degradation [20,122–125]. The presence of high-intensity zones found within the posterior or posterolateral annulus typifies radial annular fissures associated with IDD (Fig. 15) [20,126,127]. Although MRI can demonstrate architectural abnormalities within the disc, it does not predict whether these changes are symptomatic [20]. Lumbar CT discography evaluates the disc architecture and pain. Many researchers believe that lumbar discography and postdiscography CT scanning are required to diagnose IDD [18,22,113].

The prevalence of discogenic pain in chronic low back pain was reported to be approximately 40% in one investigation [18]. Discogenic pain is typically described as a centralized and nonradicular pain produced during certain activities. Patients also can have diffuse, nondermatomal lower limb pain that is associated with low back pain that typically is not present in isolation [118]. Symptoms are typically increased with lifting and lumbar

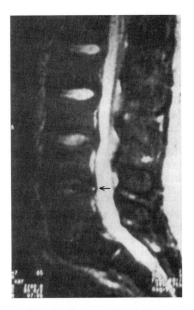

Fig. 15. High-intensity zone. A high-intensity zone (*arrow*) is present within the L4/5 posterior annulus, as seen on this T-2 weighted midsagittal view. The high-intensity zone is a bright (high-intensity) signal within the dark (low-intensity) signal of the central posterior annulus on this T-2 weighted image that is consistent for an annular tear.

flexion activities and with sitting. Physical examination is usually unremarkable except for restricted range of motion, pain on flexion, and tenderness with palpation of the lumbar spine. The neurologic evaluation is typically normal.

The North American Spine Society released its position statement on discography in 1988 and again in 1995, which summarized the indications for discography [128]. Indications include unremitting spinal pain for longer than 4 months, unresponsiveness to conservative treatment, and investigation with other modalities, such as CT, MRI, or myelography, that have failed to explain the source of pain. Contraindications include systemic infection, infection of the overlying skin, anticoagulation medications, and a bleeding diathesis. A contrast allergy is a relative contraindication that can be circumvented with either preventive premedication with antihistamines and corticosteroids or substituting gadolinium for nonionic contrast [129].

Technique

Three different discography techniques are described in the literature. The posterior (midline) and posterolateral (interlaminar) approaches are primarily of historical interest and involve dural penetration [73,108,130,131]. These techniques generally have been replaced by the lateral (extralaminar) approach, which does not require thecal sac penetration [132,133]. Patients selected for discography are interviewed for potential contraindications, such as current infection, unstable medical condition, and allergies. Screening laboratory studies, including erythrocyte sedimentation rate, complete blood count, chemistry profile, and urinalysis, are reviewed for abnormalities. Electrocardiogram and chest radiographs are obtained in patients with a history of smoking or cardiac or respiratory problems. Informed consent is obtained if no contraindications are noted with the preprocedural studies. The procedure is explained to patients, with special attention given to describing pain production, including pain quality, location, intensity, and similarity or dissimilarity.

The patient is transported into the radiology suite or procedure room equipped with resuscitative equipment. Light sedation is given to relieve any anxiety and promote tolerance to the procedure without compromising the patient's ability to participate. All discography procedures are performed under strict antiseptic technique. The procedure area is prepared and draped in a sterile fashion. The physician performs a disinfecting hand scrub and dons a gown, cap, and facemask. Intravenous antibiotics are administered as prophylaxis against disc infection [123,132,134,135]. Intradiscal antibiotics can be given as an alternative or in addition to the intravenous antibiotics for prevention of disc infection.

The patient is positioned in a modified lateral decubitus position when performing lumbar discography, with the symptomatic side down. The needles are placed into the discs from the asymptomatic side to avoid any confusion for the patient to distinguish needle-induced annular pain from a provocative pain response. For lumbar discography this position also facilitates optimal fluoroscopic imaging and mobilizes the bowel away from the needle path.

The patient or the fluoroscope is adjusted to provide a posterior oblique position, with the superior articular process dividing the intervertebral disc space in half (Fig. 16). The introducer needle tip is positioned just anterior to the superior articular process and superior to the subjacent endplate. The introducer needle is advanced to the outer annulus, with the surgeon being aware of any paresthesias from contact with the exiting nerve root at that level. The procedure needle is advanced through the introducer needle into the central third of the disc under biplanar fluoroscopic guidance. There is a characteristic firm, pliable tactile sensation as the needle enters the disc.

The iliac crests make it difficult to approach the L5/S1 disc with the straight single-needle approach used for the other lumbar levels. The previously described two-needle technique is often used with a curved 22- or 25-gauge, 6-inch procedure needle that is inserted through an 18- or 20-gauge introducer needle to enter into the L5/S1 disc [132].

Each disc is evaluated by injecting contrast, saline, or a combination of the two after all the needles are positioned in the discs. The injections are performed under lateral fluoroscopy, after which radiographs are obtained

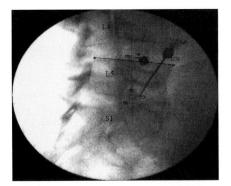

Fig. 16. Lumbar discogram. Oblique view for initial spinal needle position established by positioning the superior articular process tip (*vertical dashed line*) until it bisects the intervertebral disc (*solid horizontal line between asterisks*). HUB, introducer spine needle hub; TIP, introducer spine needle tip; hub, procedure spine needle hub; tip, procedure spine needle tip; sap, superior articular process; L4, L4 vertebra; L5, L5 vertebra; S1, S1 vertebra.

upon completion of the study. The nucleogram appearance is recorded after contrast injection based on several classification schemes (Fig. 17) [136,137]. The data recorded during the study include injection volume, discometry (end point), pain level, analgesia, pain quality, and nucleogram. The disc pressure (discometry) at the onset of pain during lumbar discography also can be measured and recorded with a pressure gauge in pounds per square inch (psi). Lumbar discs are defined as chemically sensitive (<15 psi), mechanically sensitive (15–50 psi), or intermediate (>50 psi) depending on the measured pressure above the opening pressure [138]. Lidocaine, 0.5% to 1%, is injected into the painful disc to determine if the

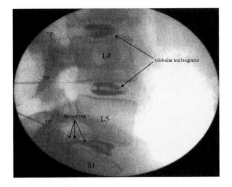

Fig. 17. Lumbar discogram. Lateral view of lumbar discogram demonstrates an L5/S1 posterior full-thickness annular tear with a normal nucleus. The outer annular fibers are intact, otherwise contrast would spread into the epidural space or surrounding soft tissue structures, an important finding when considering percutaneous intradiscal procedures. TIP, introducer spine needle tip; L4, L4 vertebra; L5, L5 vertebra; S1, S1 vertebra.

pain stems from the provocation injection or a neighboring painful disc. Data are recorded during the study (Fig. 18) about the injected volume, discometry (end point or recorded pressure), pain level, analgesia, pain quality, and nucleogram.

After the study the patient undergoes a CT scan of each injected level (Fig. 19) for further assessment of disc anatomy. Post-lumbar discography CT imaging provides further detailed information on the presence and degree of annular pathology and disc degeneration (Fig. 20). The extent of annular pathology on CT discography correlates with the likelihood of a concordantly painful disc [126,136,139]. The Dallas discogram classification for annular pathology and subsequent modifications to this system have shown a high correlation between grades 3, 4, and 5 tears (Fig. 21) with concordant low back pain [126,136,139]. The finding of a high-intensity zone on MRI in symptomatic patients is consistent for grade 3 and 4 tears [2,102]. This classification scheme assists in assessing patients with lumbar spine pain and selecting patients for surgical and intradiscal procedures [113,136,140,141].

Complications

Potential complications from discography include discitis, nerve root injury, bleeding, allergic reaction, subarachnoid puncture, soft tissue infection, and chemical meningitis [116,120,123,142–144]. Although discitis is a commonly reported complication, the incidence of discitis is relatively low, with a range of 0.05% to 4% [123,134,135,146]. The incidence of discitis can be reduced with meticulous aseptic technique, prophylactic antibiotics, styleted needles, and a two-needle technique [123,134,135].

Individuals who develop discitis after discography typically present with severe back pain 2 to 4 weeks after the procedure [144]. Back pain

Lumbar Discography Results

Patient: _____   Date: _____

Levels: _____   Physician: _____

Disc Level	Volume	End Point	Pressure	Pain Level	Lidocaine	Lidocaine Response	Pain Quality	Nucleogram
L2/3								
L3/4								
L4/5								
L5/S1								

Volume: Contrast volume injected into disc in millimeters or cubic centimeters.
End Point: Firm, Spongy, None.
Pressure: pounds per square inch, psi.
Pain Level: Pain intensity on verbal scale 1-10.
Lidocaine: Disc(s) injected with lidocaine.
Lidocaine Response: Pain level on disc re-injection after lidocaine disc injection.
Pain Quality: Pain description (achy, sharp, etc) and whether concordant or discordant.
Nucleogram: Normal, Degenerative, +/- Annular Pathology.

Fig. 18. Lumbar discography results worksheet.

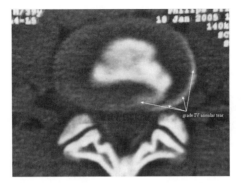

Fig. 19. Lumbar CT discogram. Postdiscography CT scan reveals a left posterolateral grade IV radial annular tear that extends into the left lateral outer annulus.

exacerbated by any motion and relieved by rest is characteristic of discitis. Patients might report fever and chills, but documented temperature elevations or elevated white blood cell counts are unusual [144]. A high level of suspicion is necessary to diagnose postdiscography discitis adequately. Bone scan, sedimentation rate, and MRI often produce normal results within the first 3 weeks of discitis [144]. Clinical presentation might warrant repeating these diagnostic tests if initial results are normal and there is continued clinical suspicion of discitis. MRI is considered the best means for early detection of discitis [145,146].

Excluding individuals with contrast dye allergies, using nonionic contrast, and using sterile technique can minimize adverse events from discography. A contrast allergy is a relative contraindication that can be circumvented either by using preventive premedication with antihistamines and corticosteroids or substituting gadolinium for nonionic contrast [128]. Prophylactic antibiotics might further decrease the risk of infection [123,135]. No significant risk of damaging discs from needle puncture has

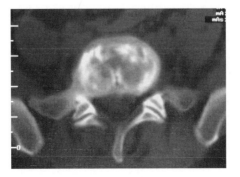

Fig. 20. Lumbar CT discogram. Postdiscography CT scan reveals a grade III degenerative L5/S1 disc.

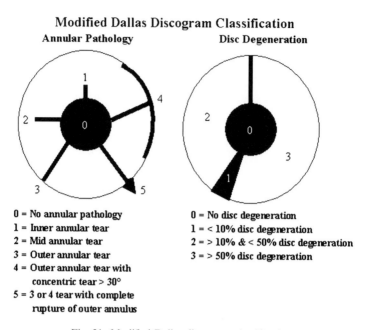

Modified Dallas Discogram Classification

Annular Pathology

0 = No annular pathology
1 = Inner annular tear
2 = Mid annular tear
3 = Outer annular tear
4 = Outer annular tear with
    concentric tear > 30°
5 = 3 or 4 tear with complete
    rupture of outer annulus

Disc Degeneration

0 = No disc degeneration
1 = < 10% disc degeneration
2 = > 10% & < 50% disc degeneration
3 = > 50% disc degeneration

Fig. 21. Modified Dallas discogram classification.

been reported in the literature. Disc herniation of a structurally intact disc after discography is rare [147].

Efficacy

Lumbar discography remains a controversial diagnostic technique [20,122,123,148–151]. Proponents believe discography uniquely demonstrates internal disc anatomy and identifies clinically symptomatic (ie, painful) discs [20,22,113,128,151]. A study published in 1968 by Holt [149] found a 37% false-positive rate and concluded that discography was an unreliable diagnostic tool. Holt's conclusions have been challenged seriously. Critics call attention to several design flaws, including suboptimal imaging equipment, irritating contrast material, inadequate needle placement, and not distinguishing if pain responses were concordant or disconcordant with the patient's typical pain pattern [112,151].

Walsh and colleagues [152] assessed discography in a normal and symptomatic population using modern equipment and technique to re-evaluate Holt's study. The study compared lumbar discography in seven patients with back pain to ten asymptomatic men aged 18 to 32 years. A positive discogram required an abnormal nucleogram and a concordant pain response. In the asymptomatic group, 5 of the 30 discs (17%) displayed structural abnormalities, but none of the discs was pain positive on provocation. In the symptomatic group, 13 of 20 discs (65%) had abnormal findings, and 8 discs

(40%) produced concordant pain. The significant finding of this study was the 0% false-positive rate for discography compared with the 37% false-positive rate reported by Holt. The authors concluded that with current technique and standardized protocol, discography is a highly reliable test. This study is limited by small sample size and a population bias of young men, however.

Although there has been a long, questionable history regarding the value of discography, it clearly has had an impact on the diagnosis of discogenic pain, surgical planning, and subsequent outcome for surgical fusions [113,138,153]. Discography has detected a 40% prevalence of discogenic pain in patients with 6 months of chronic low back pain and an unremarkable diagnostic evaluation, including imaging studies [18]. Results of MRI, CT, and myelography studies are commonly inconclusive regarding the presence or absence of discogenic pain [20,122,124]. Lumbar discography performed in asymptomatic volunteers has been demonstrated to be a reliable test [152]. More recently, the concept of zero false-positive discography has been challenged by some researchers on the grounds that abnormal psychometrics might result in misleading abnormal results [148]. On the contrary, others have not found any impact on discography results in persons with or without a somatoform disorder [150].

MRI and CT myelography adequately document most disc herniations. Lumbar CT discography is an appropriate diagnostic tool in the evaluation of suspected far lateral disc herniations [114,115,117,154,155]. Although MRI with gadolinium might be more accurate than CT discography in distinguishing recurrent disc herniations from postoperative scar, CT discography is more sensitive than myelography, CT, or CT myelography [114,115,117,154,155].

Discography performed on degenerative discs identified by MRI has been shown to produce similar and dissimilar pain patterns compared with a patient's typical pain [156–159]. The presence of degenerative disc changes does not necessarily correlate with clinical symptoms or a painful disc. There is evidence that the presence of outer annular ruptures is the best predictor of a painful degenerative disc rather than the degree of disc deterioration [126,139–141,156,157,158]. The presence of a high-intensity zone on MRI T2-weighted images might or might not correlate with pain on discography and requires further investigation [126,127,139,140].

Provocative testing for concordant pain is the most important aspect of discography and provides information regarding the clinical significance of the disc abnormality [20,22,113,128,151]. Although difficult to standardize, this portion of the evaluation distinguishes discography from other anatomic imaging techniques.

CT discography has been shown to be more sensitive and specific than CT, myelography, and CT myelography for IDD, herniated nucleus pulposus, recurrent disc herniation, and foraminal disc herniation [50,111,137,159,160]. CT discography interpretation is highly reproducible

for grading annular degeneration and disruption between different inter-
preters when using a common classification scheme [137]. Currently, MRI
does not seem to be as sensitive or specific as CT discography in determining
whether a disc is symptomatic [20,23,124]. Results of discography and CT
discography have been abnormal despite normal MRI scans, and they
have revealed asymptomatic discs in the presence of significantly abnormal
MRI studies [20,22,23,137,141,158].

Radiofrequency neurolysis techniques

The basic equipment needed to produce a radiofrequency (RF) tissue lesion from high-frequency waves includes a voltage generator, alternating
current, and active and reference electrodes. A patient's tissues serve as a re-
sistor within the circuit and provide impedance. The active electrode is an
insulated needle with an exposed tip, whereas the reference electrode is
a large surface adhesive pad. This configuration leads to the greatest current
concentration and heat being next to the tip, with diffusion of the current
and heat at the large reference electrode. The current causes vibration of
the electrons in the tissues in the vicinity of the RF probe, which results
in an increase in temperature. The greater the voltage and the tissue impedance, the higher the temperature that develops within the tissues.

The advantages of RF include controlled lesion size, accurate temperature monitoring, limited need for anesthesia, precise probe placement, low
incidence of morbidity or mortality, and rapid postprocedural recovery.
The lesion size depends on the probe diameter, length of the uninsulated
tip, temperature, time, and tissue vascularity. In general, the lesion size is
larger with a larger probe diameter, longer uninsulated tip, higher temperature, lower tissue vascularity, and longer lesioning time.

Pulsed RF uses 10- to 30-msec bursts of high-frequency alternating current. Lesions created by pulsed RF are low temperature (cold RF) and are
nondestructive lesions. When making an RF lesion, the tissue that sur-
rounds the tip of the electrode is exposed to an electromagnetic field.

Although the mechanism by which pulsed RF treatment works is not
known, there are several theories. One theory is that the electromagnetic
field might have a clinical neuromodulation effect that renders the nerve
less likely to transmit painful impulses. Another possibility is that it works
in a similar manner to transcutaneous electrical nerve stimulation, activating
spinal and supraspinal mechanisms, which can reduce pain perception.

Lumbar facet joint

Indications

Patients with functionally limited spinal facet joint pain that is resistant
to at least 3 months of conservative treatment are candidates for RF ablation (RFA) or neurolysis. This condition cannot be diagnosed definitively by

history, physical examination, or imaging studies. The current method for diagnosis is through facet joint injections or medial branch (facet joint) nerve blocks. The nerves that supply the facet joints from the cervical to the lumbar spine are the third occipital nerve, the medial branches of the dorsal rami, and the L5 dorsal ramus. Cervical and lumbar medial branch blocks have been shown to be target specific if anesthetic solutions are injected carefully at specific osseous target points, and contrast is necessary to ensure that inadvertent venous uptake does not occur. A dual injection paradigm of facet joint or medial branch nerve injections is recommended for a more accurate diagnosis of facet joint pain because of the false-positive rates associated with single lumbar and cervical facet joint or medial branch nerve blocks.

Technique

The patient is placed prone for RF lesioning of the lumbar facet joints. The RF probes are placed parallel to the nerves as opposed to the perpendicular approach used for medial branch nerve blocks. This approach allows for optimal denervation of the medial branch nerves. The probe is placed inferiorly and laterally to the targeted medial branch and advanced under fluoroscopy until contact at the junction of the superior articular process and the transverse process (Fig. 22A). An oblique "Scotty dog" view (Fig. 22B) is then obtained, and the needle should be seen to reside parallel to the target nerve in the osseous groove. The needle is advanced to the proximal junction of the superior articular process and transverse process for the L1-4 medial branch nerves (Fig. 22C) and the proximal junction of the S1 superior articular process and the sacral ala for the L5 dorsal ramus. A lateral view is obtained to ensure that the needle is placed no further anteriorly than the posterior aspect of the foramen (see Fig. 22C). The C-arm is finally repositioned in an anteroposterior projection to verify that the needles did not stray laterally while being advanced under oblique imaging. Electrical stimulation is performed as a safety precaution, and the area is anesthetized. This procedure is followed by an RFA lesion at 80° to 90°C for 30 seconds to 2 minutes.

Complications

Patients can feel increased soreness and local pain, especially in the first 3 to 5 days, but these symptoms usually disappear within 2 weeks. Other postoperative symptoms include itching, burning, and hypersensitivity, which usually subside in approximately 4 to 6 weeks. Gabapentin or tricyclic antidepressants can be helpful for this condition. Improper needle placement can lead to permanent limb weakness, permanent sensory deficit, or persistent neuritis. In the cervical spine, the proximity to the vertebral artery, combined with the vascular nature of this anatomic region, makes intravascular injection or vascular trauma a distinct possibility. The injection of small amounts of local anesthesia into the vertebral arteries can result in

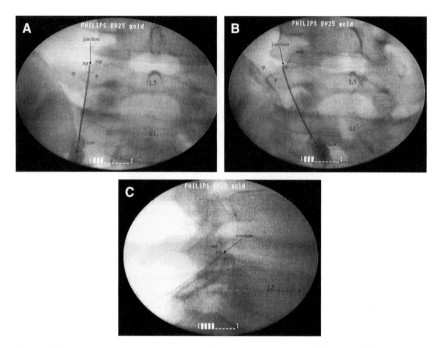

Fig. 22. RF neurolysis lumbar facet joint. RF probe in position for left C4 medial branch neurolysis. (*A*) Anteroposterior view. (*B*) Oblique view. (*C*) Lateral view. hub, RF probe hub; tip, RF probe tip; junction, junction of sap and tp; P, pedicle; tp, transverse process; sap, superior articular process; L5, L5 vertebra; S1, S1 vertebra.

seizures. In the thoracic spine, pneumothorax is a potential risk given the proximity of the pleural space. No long-term complications or serious adverse effects have been described with RF facet ablation procedures when motor stimulation was performed before lesioning to prevent inadvertent ventral ramus or nerve root injury. Needle electromyography of the multifidi muscles should be performed if the facet RFA fails to provide pain relief after several weeks. An electromyographic examination should show denervation potentials after this procedure, indicating that there was destruction of the medial branch nerves. If no denervation potentials are seen on electromyography and the patient is still symptomatic, the facet RFA can be repeated.

Efficacy

Dreyfuss and colleagues [64] reported the first prospective study to treat only patients with lumbar facet joint pain proven with dual diagnostic medial branch blocks. A 90% denervation rate was confirmed using multifidi electromyography 6 weeks after the procedure. At 1 year follow-up, nearly 90% of subjects had at least 60% pain relief, and 60% of subjects had at least 90% pain relief. Overall, one systematic review, two randomized trials, four prospective studies, and three retrospective evaluations of RF medial branch neurotomy have provided the best evidence to date for short-term relief and moderate evidence for long-term relief of chronic cervical and lumbar facet joint pain [50]. There have been no reports of long-term adverse side effects secondary to facet joint RF neurolysis, including any risk for creating a Charcot joint.

Sacroiliac joint

Indications

Candidates for SI joint RFA are patients who have been diagnosed with chronic SI joint pain resistant to at least 3 months of conservative treatment and who have experienced significant but transient relief after intra-articular SI joint corticosteroid injections.

Technique

One common technique for SI joint RFA is the bipolar technique, in which two RF probes are used to create a bipolar system. Under fluoroscopy, the first RF probe is inserted at the inferior joint margin. The second RF probe is placed more cephalad in the joint at a distance of less than 1 cm. RF lesions are created at 80°C. Another RF probe is then placed more cephalad in the SI joint at a distance of less than 1 cm from the second probe, and another lesion is created. Multiple subsequent lesions are created in a repetitive alternating "leapfrog" manner, going as high in the joint as possible. An alternative approach is to place a single RF probe and advance it cephalad along the posterior capsule creating overlapping lesions (Fig. 23). Another technique is to lesion at the origin of the multiple nerve branches that are believed to innervate the SI joint.

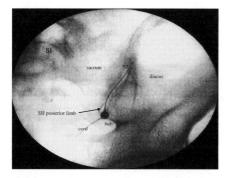

Fig. 23. RF neurolysis SI joint. Single RF probe overlapping technique. Note contrast in SI joint that confirms probe placement within posterior limb before RF neurolysis. hub, RF probe hub; tip, RF probe tip; cord, RF cord to generator; S1, S1 vertebra. (*From* Falco FJE, Kim D, Zhu J, et al. Interventional pain management procedures. In: Braddom RL, editor. Physical medicine and rehabilitation e-dition. 3rd edition. Philadelphia: WB Saunders; 2006; with permission.)

Complications

The major side effect of SI joint lesioning is postprocedural pain. Care must be taken to avoid placing the RF needle too laterally and traumatizing the sciatic nerve. There is a theoretical risk of dysesthesias if RF lesioning of the L5 dorsal ramus and lateral branches of the S1-3 dorsal rami is performed, because they provide sensory innervation to the skin of the buttock.

Efficacy

Formal peer-reviewed outcome studies for SI joint RFA are lacking. An uncontrolled study by Ferrante used a "leapfrog" technique along the posterior SI joint line [161]. He reported that about 36% of patients experienced a 50% decrease in the visual analog scale (VAS) pain scale for at least 6 months. Ferrante and colleagues [161] also noted that a significantly higher proportion of nonresponders had pain with lateral flexion to the affected side, implying that the presence of facet disease might have prevented these patients from experiencing at least 50% relief of their total back pain.

Dorsal root ganglia

Indications

Selection criteria include radicular pain for more than 6 months with no response to conservative treatment, no indication for surgical intervention, and a positive but short-lived response to a selective nerve root block or transforaminal epidural injection. Contraindications include infection, coagulopathy, platelet dysfunction, neck or back pain alone without any limb pain, deafferentation pain in the involved limb, and severe cardiopulmonary disease for procedures in the cervical and thoracic regions.

RF of the dorsal root ganglion (DRG) can be performed with the traditional or pulsed methods. Pulsed RF is being used more frequently to treat DRG than any other application, because the resulting temperature is below the threshold that causes irreversible nerve injury. The use of pulsed RF significantly reduces the risk of developing postprocedural neuritis.

Technique

The technique for probe placement in performing DRG RF neurolysis is the same whether using heat or cold (pulsed) RF. The probe is placed in the dorsal quadrant of the lumbar foramen. Sensory and motor stimulation is performed as a safety precaution and to improve the success rate of the procedure. The voltage at which the patient first perceives the stimulation in the appropriate dermatome is the sensory threshold. This threshold is usually 0.4 to 0.7 V when the tip of the needle is next to the DRG using a frequency of 50 Hz. The frequency is changed to 2 Hz for motor stimulation, and the voltage intensity must increase to at least twice the sensory threshold before motor activity in the myotomal distribution is typically seen. This is known as the disassociation of stimulation that occurs at a point over the DRG at which the sensory and motor nerves are still separate before crossing over into the ventral and dorsal rami. This is the probe placement site for DRG RFA when using conventional RF. The probe is typically placed next to the DRG for pulsed RF, obtaining a sensory threshold at 0.1 to 0.2 V. Lesions for traditional RF are created at 80° to 90°C for 1 to 2 minutes and from 2 to 4 minutes at 42°C for pulsed RFA.

Complications

Possible risks include nerve injury, vascular trauma, or entry into the subarachnoid space through the intervertebral foramen.

Efficacy

A limited case study report showed remarkable effectiveness of pulsed RF in patients with neuropathic pain syndromes that were poorly controlled with other oral and invasive treatments [162]. One study by Sluijter and colleagues [163] demonstrated that 56% of patients with radicular pain had a global perceived effect of more than 75% pain relief. In this same study, Sluijter and colleagues also showed that 8 of 15 patients were treated successfully at 6 months follow-up, and 3 of the 7 patients in the unsuccessful group reported that pain had improved on the side that was treated but they felt pain on the contralateral side afterwards.

Nucleoplasty

Indications

Nucleoplasty builds on the earlier percutaneous intradiscal treatment concepts of chemonucleolysis, nucleotomy, and RFA. The US Food and Drug Administration approved nucleoplasty for treatment of contained herniated discs in June 2001. Nucleoplasty is a non–heat-driven process that uses coblation and bipolar RF technology applied to a conductive medium, such as saline, to achieve tissue removal with minimal thermal damage to collateral tissues.

Like other decompressive procedures, nucleoplasty is designed to treat patients with limb pain caused by smaller disc protrusions. Inclusion criteria include chronic discogenic low back pain with radicular symptoms, contained disc herniation, adequate disc height of at least 50% of normal, and normal psychometric testing. Specific contraindications include severe disc space narrowing, large disc herniation, extruded or sequestered discs, spinal stenosis, spondylolisthesis, spinal fracture, and tumor. The usual general contraindications are the same as for any surgical procedure and include fever, infection, bleeding diathesis, and anticoagulant therapy.

Technique

The patient is positioned in a modified lateral decubitus position, and the lumbosacral area is prepared in the usual sterile manner. Intravenous antibiotics are given before the procedure with or without intradiscal antibiotics. Using a posterolateral approach under fluoroscopy, a 17-gauge, 6-inch Crawford needle (Fig. 24) is inserted through the skin into the center of the nucleus followed by the injection of nonionic contrast, which produces a nucleogram that outlines its borders (Fig. 25). A slightly curved wand with a bipolar coil at the distal tip (see Fig. 24) is advanced through the Crawford needle until the distal end of the tip touches the inside wall of the anterior annulus (anterior boundary of the nucleus) (Fig. 26A). The depth gauge is advanced down the shaft of the wand to the needle hub (Fig. 26B), which represents the depth of wand advancement through the Crawford needle for creating channels within the nucleus from coblation. The wand is withdrawn until the tip is inside the posterior wall of the annulus (Fig. 27A), which corresponds to the posterior boundary of the nucleus. A reference mark with a surgical pen is made on the wand at the needle hub (Fig. 27B). The proximal depth gauge and the distal reference mark on the wand represent the working length of the wand (see Fig. 27B) for creating channels within that specific nucleus. The dot indicator located on the wand handle (see Fig. 26B) is oriented to the 12 o'clock position, and the wand is advanced to the depth gauge using the coblation mode. The wand is withdrawn to the reference mark using the coagulation mode. Alternatively, the coblation mode can be used while advancing and withdrawing the wand in creating channels within the nucleus pulposus. The wand is advanced and withdrawn at an approximate rate of 0.5 cm/sec to create a single channel. This protocol is repeated to create six different channels by rotating the wand at 2 o'clock increments in either a clockwise or

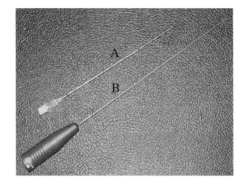

Fig. 24. Nucleoplasty instruments. (*A*) Crawford needle. (*B*) Bipolar wand nucleotome. (*From* Falco FJE, Kim D, Zhu J, et al. Interventional pain management procedures. In: Braddom RL, editor. Physical medicine and rehabilitation e-dition. 3rd edition. Philadelphia: WB Saunders; 2006; with permission.)

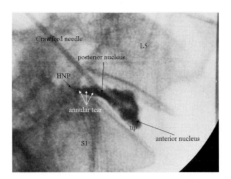

Fig. 25. Nucleoplasty. Contrast injected through the Crawford needle outlines the boundaries of the L5/S1 nucleus pulposus and reveals a posterior annular tear and disc herniation. tip, Crawford needle tip; L5, L5 vertebra; S1, S1 vertebra; HNP, disc herniation. (*From* Falco FJE, Kim D, Zhu J, et al. Interventional pain management procedures. In: Braddom RL, editor. Physical medicine and rehabilitation e-dition. 3rd edition. Philadelphia: WB Saunders; 2006; with permission.)

counter-clockwise direction. The result is removal of nuclear material by creating multiple intradiscal channels during coblation with the wand. These channels are sealed by way of coagulation after withdrawal of the wand. The products of the non–heat-driven process are elementary particles and low molecular weight gases, which are removed quickly from the surgical site through the Crawford needle. The reduction in nuclear tissue volume leads to a decrease in intradiscal pressure, which can result in pain reduction. The patient usually does not feel discomfort during the procedure because the coblation and coagulation take place within the nucleus pulposus that contains little sensory innervation. The

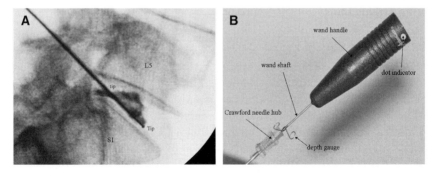

Fig. 26. Nucleoplasty. (*A*) Nucleoplasty wand tip at the anterior boundary of the nucleus pulposus. (*B*) Depth gauge (clamp-like device) positioned on the wand at the level of the Crawford needle hub represents the location of the wand tip at the anterior border of the nucleus pulposus. Tip, nucleoplasty wand tip; tip, Crawford needle tip; L5, L5 vertebra; S1, S1 vertebra. (*From* Falco FJE, Kim D, Zhu J, et al. Interventional pain management procedures. In: Braddom RL, editor. Physical medicine and rehabilitation e-dition. 3rd edition. Philadelphia: WB Saunders; 2006; with permission.)

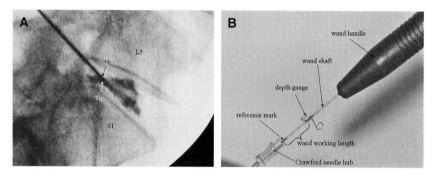

Fig. 27. Nuceloplasty. (*A*) Nucleoplasty wand tip at the posterior boundary of the nucleus pulposus. (*B*) Reference mark made by surgical pen distal to the depth gauge on the wand designates the position of the wand tip at the posterior border of the nucleus pulposus. Tip, nucleoplasty wand tip; tip, Crawford needle tip; L5, L5 vertebra; S1, S1 vertebra. (*From* Falco FJE, Kim D, Zhu J, et al. Interventional pain management procedures. In: Braddom RL, editor. Physical medicine and rehabilitation e-dition. 3rd edition. Philadelphia: WB Saunders; 2006; with permission.)

practitioner must be aware of any extreme pain or neurologic symptoms in the back or leg that can indicate damage to vital neural structures during the nucleoplasty procedure. If pain or symptoms occur, the physician should stop and reposition the Crawford needle or wand or abort the procedure to avoid potential damage.

Complications

There have been no reported significant complications after nucleoplasty. Possible complications include discitis, epidural abscess, pneumothorax, trauma to retroperitoneal structures, nerve root or spinal cord trauma, and cauda equina syndrome, however.

Efficacy

A recent study demonstrated that when coblation is performed at the central portion of the disc, there is minimal increased temperature in adjacent neurovascular structures [164]. The effectiveness of nucleoplasty recently was reported in two prospective trials. Singh and colleagues [165] followed 41 patients for 12 months and reported that 80% of patients indicated a statistically significant reduction in pain. They also reported improved sitting (2%), standing (59%), and walking (60%) ability. In a prospective cohort study of 48 patients, Sharps and Issac [166] reported a 79% decrease in pain scores at 12 months for 13 patients. Derby [167] reported that nucleoplasty gave an overall success rate of 79% and a success rate of 67% in previously operated patients. A cadaveric study demonstrated that nucleoplasty was highly effective at reducing intradiscal pressure in nondegenerated contained discs but had minimal effect in reducing intradiscal pressure in severely degenerative discs [168]. Nucleoplasty is probably not effective in treating severely degenerated discs because of the nuclear desiccation. Overall it seems that nucleoplasty is a promising treatment for contained disc herniation with or without radiculopathy, but clinical research in a larger patient population over a longer follow-up period is needed to validate its benefits. Nucleoplasty does not replace microdiscectomy or spinal fusion, but it can fill the gap between conservative treatments and open spinal procedures [169].

Intradiscal electrothermal therapy

Indications

Intradiscal electrothermal therapy (IDET) (annuloplasty) is a minimally invasive procedure for managing chronic discogenic low back pain in patients who have failed conservative treatment regimens and who otherwise are possible candidates for spinal fusion. The IDET procedure might relieve discogenic pain through numerous potential mechanisms, including thermal nociceptive fiber destruction, biochemical mediation of inflammation, cauterization of vascular ingrowth, induced healing of annular tears, and collagen modification. Whether collagen modification occurs is highly controversial, however, and the treated disc segment actually exhibits greater instability for a brief period of time after the procedure. Unlike other percutaneous intradiscal procedures, the objective of IDET is not to decrease intradiscal pressure.

Inclusion criteria include unremitting low back pain for at least 6 months, no significant response to conservative treatment (including injections), a negative straight leg raise test, an MRI unremarkable for a neural compressive lesion, less than 50% decrease in disc height, a small disc protrusion, absence of instability and stenosis, positive low pressure (<15 psi) discography, and no prior surgery [167,170,171]. Contraindications include severe radicular symptoms, previous disc surgery at the suspect level, severe loss of disc height more than 50%, imaging studies suggestive of nondiscogenic pathology, segmental instability on flexion and extension radiographs, inflammatory arthritides, extensive solid bone fusion, pregnancy, and psychological impairment.

Technique

The patient is positioned in a modified lateral decubitus position, and the lumbosacral area is prepared in the usual sterile manner. Intravenous antibiotics are given before the procedure with or without intradiscal antibiotics. A 17-gauge introducer spinal needle (Fig. 28) is inserted under fluoroscopic guidance into the center of the disc using a posterolateral approach. A navigable catheter (see Fig. 28) with a temperature-controlled

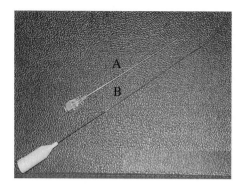

Fig. 28. IDET device. (*A*) Introducer needle. (*B*) IDET catheter. (*From* Falco FJE, Kim D, Zhu J, et al. Interventional pain management procedures. In: Braddom RL, editor. Physical medicine and rehabilitation e-dition. 3rd edition. Philadelphia: WB Saunders; 2006; with permission.)

thermal resistive coil is deployed through the needle and positioned intradiscally under two-plane fluoroscopic control. The catheter is navigated as far as possible adjacent to the inner posterior annulus. The catheter temperature is gradually increased according to a uniform protocol to 90°C during a period of 13 minutes and maintained at 90°C for an additional 4 minutes. The catheter should not be heated unless both radiopaque distal markers have exited the needle. The catheter also should be observed in various fluoroscopic views (Fig. 29) to ensure that no part of the heating element is in contact with the introducer needle, because heat could be transmitted along the needle. The catheter optimally should be placed so that the posterior half of the annulus is positioned between the distal makers. Patients often experience typical back pain and referred leg pain during the procedure. This pain must be differentiated from true radicular pain, especially if a patient

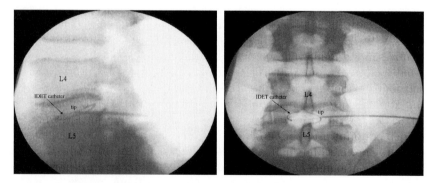

Fig. 29. IDET L4/5 annuloplasty. (*A*) Lateral view. (*B*) Anteroposterior view. tip, introducer needle tip; L4, L4 vertebra; L5, L5 vertebra. (*From* Falco FJE, Kim D, Zhu J, et al. Interventional pain management procedures. In: Braddom RL, editor. Physical medicine and rehabilitation e-dition. 3rd edition. Philadelphia: WB Saunders; 2006; with permission.)

experiences it early in the heating cycle. If this occurs, it usually indicates an attenuated posterolateral annulus or extradiscal positioning of the catheter that necessitates repositioning or removal of the catheter. After completing the procedure, the catheter is withdrawn carefully back through the needle to avoid any shearing of the catheter followed by removal of the introducer needle.

The recommended heating protocol begins at 65°C, and the catheter temperature is increased by one degree every 30 seconds until it reaches 90°C, which is sustained for a period of 4 minutes. If a patient cannot tolerate the recommended heating protocol, however, a lower temperature can be used to perform the procedure based on the belief that the amount of heat delivered over a period of time is more important than the final temperature. It is strongly suggested that the temperature reach at least 80°C, which should be maintained for 6 minutes at that particular temperature.

Complications

Potential complications include bleeding, catheter fracture within the disc, inadvertent puncture of the dura, headache, damage to the thecal sac and its contents, infection (including discitis), and traumatic disc herniation caused by the weakened state of the annulus during the first month after the procedure.

Efficacy

Initial published results for IDET showed positive response rates of 73% and 80%, respectively. Subsequent studies showed average decreases in VAS scores of 62% to 72% and decreases of 59% to 78% in SF-36 body pain [172,173]. In general, one third of the patients were significantly better, one third were slightly better, and one third were the same or worse. Spinal fusion subsequently was performed in less than 5% of patients treated with IDET, although some patients required spinal surgery 6 to 18 months after the procedure [174–176]. Pauza and colleagues [170] evaluated the efficacy of IDET for the treatment of chronic discogenic low back pain after 6 months in a randomized, double-blind, placebo-controlled trial. They reported a statistically significant improvement in bodily pain, VAS, overall disability and handicap based on the Oswestry scale, significant improvement in physical functioning on SF-36, and statistically significant improvement in the Beck Depression Inventory. Pauza and colleagues [171] later reported that although mean improvements were statistically significant in the group treated with the IDET procedure, only approximately 40% of the patients obtained more than 50% pain relief, whereas approximately 50% of the patients experienced no appreciable benefit. Kapural and colleagues [177] showed that IDET was effective in patients with multilevel degenerative disc disease even if all symptomatic discs were not initially treated, but the pain relief and improvement in pain disability index questionnaires were significantly better in IDET patients with only one or two symptomatic discs.

Epidural lysis of adhesions

Indications

Epidural fibrosis with or without adhesive arachnoiditis is a possible complication of spinal surgery. The fibrosis can be caused by manipulation of the supporting structures of the spine, bleeding into the epidural space after surgery, or leakage of disc material. Epidural fibrosis is related to inflammatory reactions that result in the entrapment of nerves within dense scar tissue. Arachnoiditis is most frequently seen in patients who have undergone multiple surgical procedures of the spine. Presumably, inflammation and compression of nerve roots by epidural scar or fibrosis (adhesions) are the mechanisms of persistent pain after back surgery, a ruptured or herniated disc, or a vertebral body fracture.

Percutaneous epidural lysis of adhesions (also referred to as epidural neuroplasty or epidural adhesiolysis) has been developed as a conservative procedure to reduce or eliminate adhesions or fibrosis [178–180]. A semi-rigid catheter with a flexible tip is placed into the epidural space to mechanically loosen or remove adhesions from the nerve roots. Hypertonic saline can be injected through the catheter at the area of fibrosis to mechanically disrupt adhesions and potentially reduce perineural edema. Hyaluronidase also can be injected to assist with breakdown of scar tissue and allow for better infiltration of a local anesthetic and corticosteroid mixture dispensed through the catheter at the site of nerve root involvement.

The indications for lysis of epidural adhesions include failed back surgery syndrome, chronic intractable back pain, and chronic radicular leg pain from a disc herniation. Local infection and sepsis are absolute contraindications to this procedure because of the potential for hematogenous spread via Batson's plexus. Coagulopathy is another absolute contraindication because of potential compression of the spinal cord or thecal sac from a hematoma.

Technique

The patient is placed in a prone position and the sacral hiatus is identified by palpation and fluoroscopy. A 16-gauge, 3.5-inch styletted needle suitable for catheter placement is inserted and advanced into the sacral hiatus. An anteroposterior fluoroscopic view is obtained to ensure that the needle tip is midline and positioned slightly toward the side of pain just below the S3 foramen. The location of the needle in the epidural space is verified with the injection contrast under biplanar fluoroscopy producing an epidurogram that also identifies the areas of adhesions (Fig. 30A).

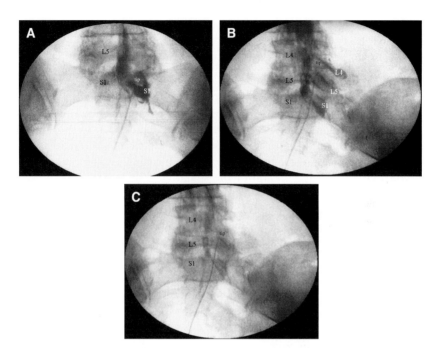

Fig. 30. Epidural lysis of adhesions. (*A*) Contrast injection revealing right-sided adhesions above the S1 nerve root. (*B*) Contrast injection after epidural lysis demonstrates elimination of adhesions. (*C*) Injection of local anesthesia and corticosteroid with subsequent washout of contrast. tip, catheter tip; L4 (black), L4 vertebra; L5 (black), L5 vertebra; S1 (black), S1 vertebra; L4 (white), L4 nerve root; L5 (white), L5 nerve root; S1 (white), S1 nerve root. (*From* Falco FJE, Kim D, Zhu J, et al. Interventional pain management procedures. In: Braddom RL, editor. Physical medicine and rehabilitation e-dition. 3rd edition. Philadelphia: WB Saunders; 2006; with permission.)

A styletted epidural catheter is used to perform the lysis of adhesions. To help steer the catheter in the epidural space, a small bend is made at the distal end of the stylet before it is reinserted into the catheter. The introducer needle stylet is withdrawn and the epidural catheter is carefully inserted through the needle to the level of the S3 sacral foramina. The catheter is steered gently by alternatively rotating the bent stylet from its proximal end and advancing or retracting the catheter to lyse the epidural adhesions under a live fluoroscopy. After mechanical lysis of the adhesions with the catheter, an additional 5 to 10 mL of contrast medium are injected slowly through the catheter to confirm the degree of adhesiolysis (Fig. 30B). Hypertonic saline or hyaluronidase can be injected at this time through the epidural catheter to assist with the removal of scar tissue. A mixture of local anesthesia and corticosteroid is injected after the lysis of adhesions through the catheter at the location of nerve root involvement to provide further therapeutic relief (Fig. 30C). The catheter is removed carefully after finishing the procedure so as not to shear any part of the catheter as it is withdrawn through the needle.

Complications

Possible side effects and complications of this procedure include increasing pain in the injection site or worsening of symptoms, transient increase in back and leg pain, catheter fracture, and ecchymosis or hematoma formation over the sacral hiatus. More severe complications of epidural lysis of adhesions include local infections, sepsis, bleeding and hematoma formation that cause compression of the spinal cord and paralysis, transient nerve compression with temporary paresis, unintended subdural or subarachnoid injection of hypertonic saline, persistent sensory deficit in the lumbar and sacral dermatomes, persistent bowel or bladder dysfunction, and sexual dysfunction. Lysis of adhesions in the cervical or thoracic spine must be performed with caution because of the significant risk for spinal cord trauma.

Efficacy

Epidural lysis of adhesions can reduce pain in 25% or more of patients who have lumbar radiculopathy plus low back pain refractory to conventional therapies for up to 1 year [178,179]. Racz and Holubec [180] reported that 65% of patients had therapeutic pain relief for 1 to 3 months but only 13% of patients had same pain relief for 3 to 6 months. Manchikanti and Bakhit [181] showed that there were no significant differences in pain relief among 1-, 2-, and 3-day procedures. In a prospective, randomized, controlled study, Manchikanti and Pampati [182] demonstrated long-term efficacy of pain relief from this procedure, with 97% of patients experiencing significant pain relief at 3 and 6 months and 47% of patients experiencing relief at 12 months. These patients also showed a significant improvement in mental health and functional status and a reduction in the use of narcotics. There seems to be no significant difference in treatment efficacy between normal saline and hypertonic saline or between hyaluronidase and hypertonic saline [74,178,179]. On the other hand, the use of hypertonic saline might reduce the number of patients who require additional treatments [178].

Summary

Lumbar spine injections play a role in the evaluation and treatment of low back pain and lumbar radiculopathy. These injection procedures have been demonstrated to be effective in determining the pain generator for low back pain. There is still debate as to the long-term pain relief from epidural and intra-articular facet joint injections, and no controlled studies have examined the long-term effects of SI joint injections. Additional investigation is certainly warranted to evaluate further the long-term benefits and determine which patients would benefit the most from these injections. Current evidence validates that these injections provide temporary relief of low back and radicular leg pain up to several months, if not longer. This duration of pain relief creates an opportunity to maximize rehabilitation efforts while symptoms are minimal.

Diagnostic lumbar spine injections can identify patients who are candidates for several intricate interventional procedures that can provide them with long-term low back and leg pain relief. There definitely is a need for more controlled studies to evaluate the long-term effectiveness from these lumbar spine procedures. Future studies also are needed to assess in a controlled manner the impact that these injections and procedures have on rehabilitation and their role in functional restoration of lumbar spine disorders.

References

[1] Biering-Sorenson F. Physial measurements as risk indicators for low-back trouble over a one-year period. Spine 1984;9:106–19.

[2] Frymoyer JW, Pope MH, Constanza MC, et al. Risk factors in low back pain: an epidemiological survey. J Bone Joint Surg Am 1983;65A:213–8.

[3] Svensson HO, Anderson GBJ. Low back pain in 40- to 47-year-old men: I. Frequency of occurrence and impact on medical services. Scand J Rehabil Med 1982;14: 47–53.

[4] Antonakes JA. Claims costs of back pain. Best's Review 1981;82:36–40, 129.

[5] Holbrook TL, Grazier K, Kelsey JL, et al. The frequency of occurrence, impact and cost of selected musculoskeletal conditions in the United States. Park Ridge (IL): American Academy of Orthopaedic Surgeons; 1984. p. 154–6.

[6] National Safety Council. Accident prevention manual for industrial operations. 7th edition. Chicago: National Safety Council; 1974. p. 162–9.

[7] Rowe ML. Preliminary statistical study of low back pain. J Occup Med 1963;5:336.

[8] Rowe ML. Low back pain in industry: a position paper. J Occup Med 1969;11:161.

[9] Valkenburg HA, Haanen HCM. The epidemiology of low back pain. In: White AA III, Gordon SL, editors. Symposium on idiopathic low back pain. St. Louis (MO): Mosby; 1982. p. 9–22.

[10] Chaffin DB, Park KYS. Longitudinal study of low back pain as associated with occupational weight lifting factors. J Am Ind Hyg Assoc J 1973;34:513.

[11] Damkot DK, Pope MH, Lord J, et al. The relationship between work history, work environment and low-back pain in men. Spine 1984;9:395–9.

[12] Frymoyer JW, Pope JW, Constanza MC, et al. Epidemiological studies of low-back pain. Spine 1980;5:419–23.

[13] Kelsey JL, Hardy RJ. Driving of motor vehicles as a risk factor for acute herniated lumbar intervertebral discs. Am J Epidemiol 1975;102:63–73.

[14] Klein BP, Jensen RC, Sanderson LM. Assessment of worker's compensation claims for back strains/sprains. J Occup Med 1984;26:443–8.

[15] Nachemson A. Work for all. Clin Orthop 1983;179:77–82.

[16] Dreyfuss P, Dreyer S, Griffin J, et al. Positive sacroiliac screening tests in asymptomatic adults. Spine 1994;19:1138–43.

[17] Schwarzer AC, Aprill CN, Derby R, et al. Clinical features of patients with pain stemming from the zygapophyseal joints: is the lumbar facet syndrome a clinical entity? Spine 1994;19: 1132–7.

[18] Schwarzer AC, Aprill CN, Derby R, et al. The relative contributions of the disc and zygapophyseal joint in chronic low back pain. Spine 1994;19:801–6.

[19] Boden SD, Davis DO, Dina TS, et al. Abnormal magnetic-resonance scans of the lumbar spine in asymptomatic subjects. J Bone Joint Surg Am 1990;72A:403–8.

[20] Horton WC, Daftari TK. Which disc as visualized by magnetic resonance imaging is actually a source of pain? A correlation between magnetic resonance imaging and discography. Spine 1992;17:S164–71.

[21] Jensen MC, Brant-Zawadzki MN, Obuschowski N, et al. Magnetic resonance imaging of the lumbar spine in people without back pain. N Engl J Med 1994;331:69–73.

[22] Simmons EH, Segil CM. An evaluation of discography in the localization of symptomatic levels in discogenic disease of the spine. Clin Orthop 1975;108:57–69.

[23] Zucherman J, Derby R, Hsu K, et al. Normal magnetic resonance imaging with abnormal discography. Spine 1988;13:1355–9.

[24] Robechhi A, Capra R. L'idrocortisone (composto F): prime esperienze cliniche in campo reumatologico. Minerva Med 1952;98:1259–63.

[25] Lièvre J-A, Bloch-Michel H, Nan G, et al. L'hydrocortisone en injection locale. Rev Rhum Mal Osteoartic 1953;20:310–1.

[26] Goebert HW Jr, Jallo SJ, Gardner WJ, et al. Painful radiculopathy treated with epidural injections of procain and hydrocortisone acetate: results in 113 patients. Anesth Analg 1961;40:130–4.

[27] Hitselberger WE, Witten RM. Abnormal myelograms in asymptomatic patients. J Neurosurg 1968;28:204–6.

[28] Schmorl G. Über knorpelknoten an der hinterflache der wirbelbandscheiben. Fortsch Rontgenstr 1929;40:629–34.

[29] Slipman CW, Sterenfeld EB, Chou LH, et al. The value of radionuclide imaging in the diagnosis of sacroiliac joint syndrome. Spine 1996;21:2251–4.

[30] Wiesel SW, Tsourmas N, Feffer HL, et al. A study of computed-assisted tomography. I. The incidence of positive CAT scans in an asymptomatic group of patients. Spine 1984;9:549–51.

[31] Dougherty JH Jr, Fraser RA. Complications following intraspinal injections of steroids: report of two cases. J Neurosurg 1978;48:1023–5.

[32] Goucke CR, Graziotti P. Extradural abscess following local anaesthetic and steroid injection for chronic low back pain. Br J Anaesth 1990;65:427–9.

[33] Gutknecht DR. Chemical meningitis following epidural injections of corticosteroids. J Am Acad Dermatol 1993;29:890–4.

[34] Knight CL, Burnell JC. Systemic side-effects of extradural steroids. Anaesthesia 1980;35:593–4.

[35] Kushner FH, Olson JC. Retinal hemorrhage as a consequence of epidural steroid injection. Arch Ophthalmol 1995;113:309–13.

[36] Lerner SM, Gutterman P, Jenkins F. Epidural hematoma and paraplegia after numerous lumbar punctures. Anaesthesia 1973;39:550–1.

[37] Nelson DA. Dangers from intraspinal steroid injections [letter]. Arch Neurol 1990;47:255.

[38] Roy-Camille R, Mazel C, Husson JL, et al. Symptomatic spinal epidural lipomatosis induced by long-term steroid treatment: review of the literature and report of two additional cases. Spine 1991;16:1365–71.

[39] Strong WE. Epidural abscess associated with epidural catheterization: a rare event? Report of two cases with markedly delayed presentation. Anesthesiology 1991;74:943–6.

[40] Beliveau P. A comparison between epidural anaesthesia with and without corticosteroids in the treatment of sciatica. Rheumatol Phys Med 1971;11:40–3.

[41] Brown FW. Management of diskogenic pain using epidural and intrathecal steroids. Clin Orthop 1977;129:72–8.

[42] Houten JK, Errico TJ. Paraplegia after lumbosacral nerve root block: report of three cases. Spine J 2002;2:70–5.
[43] Glaser SE, Falco F. Paraplegia following a thoracolumbar transforaminal epidural steroid injection: a case report. Pain Physician 2005;8:309–14.
[44] Windsor RE, Falco FJE. Paraplegia following selective nerve root blocks. International Spinal Injection Society Newsletter 2001;4(1):53–4.
[45] Heavner JE, Racz GB, Jenigiri B, et al. Sharp versus blunt needle: a comparative study of penetration of internal structures and bleeding in dogs. Pain Practice 2003;3:226.
[46] Benzon HT, Brunner EA, Vaisrub N. Bleeding time and nerve blocks after aspirin. Reg Anesth 1984;9:86–9.
[47] Ciocon JO, Galindo-Ciocon D, Amaranath L, et al. Caudal epidural blocks for elderly patients with lumbar canal stenosis. J Am Geriatr Soc 1994;42:593–6.
[48] Bogduk N, Brazenor G, Christophidis N, et al. Epidural use of steroids in the management of back pain. Canberra (Australia): National Health and Medical Research Council; 1994.
[49] Bogduk N, Christophidis N, Cherry D, et al. Epidural steroids in the management of back pain and sciatica of spinal origin: report of the working party on epidural use of steroids in the management of back pain. Canberra (Australia): National Health and Medical Research Council; 1993.
[50] Manchikanti L, Staats PS, Vijay S, et al. Evidence-based practice guidelines for interventional techniques in the management of chronic spinal pain. Pain Physician 2003; 6:63–81.
[51] Goldthwaite GE. The lumbosacral articulation: an explanation of many cases of lumbago, sciatica and paraplegia. Boston Med Surg J 1911;164:365–72.
[52] Putti V. New conceptions in the pathogenesis of sciatic pain. Lancet 1927;2:53–60.
[53] Ghormley RK. Low back pain with special reference to the articular facets, with presentation of an operative procedure. JAMA 1933;101:1773–7.
[54] Manchikanti L, Pampati V, Fellows B, et al. Prevalence of lumbar facet joint pain in chronic low back pain. Pain Physician 1999;2:59–64.
[55] Manchikanti L, Singh V, Pampati V, et al. Evaluation of the relative contributions of various structures in chronic low back pain. Pain Physician 2001;4:308–16.
[56] Mooney V, Robertson J. The facet syndrome. Clin Orthop 1976;115:149–56.
[57] Mooney V, Cairns D, Robertson J. A system for evaluation and treatment of chronic back disability. West J Med 1976;124:370–6.
[58] Ransford AO, Cairns D, Mooney V. The pain drawing as an aid to the psychologic evaluation of patients with low-back pain. Spine 1976;1:127–34.
[59] Bogduk N. Back pain: zygapophyseal blocks and epidural steroids. In: Cousins MJ, Bridenbaugh PO, editors. Neural blockade in clinical anaesthesia and management of pain. 2nd edition. Philadelphia: Lippincott; 1989. p. 263–7.
[60] Derby R, Bogduk N, Schwarzer A. Precision percutaneous blocking procedures for localizing spinal pain. Part 1: The posterior lumbar compartment. Pain Digest 1993;3:89–100.
[61] Revel ME, Listrat VM, Chevalier XJ, et al. Facet joint block for low back pain: identifying predictors of a good response. Arch Phys Med Rehabil 1992;73:824–8.
[62] Schwarzer AC, Aprill CN, Derby R, et al. The false positive rate of single lumbar zygapophyseal joint blocks. Pain 1994;58:195–200.
[63] Dreyfuss P, Schwarzer AC, Lau P, et al. Specificity of lumbar medial branch and L5 dorsal ramus blocks: a computed tomography study. Spine 1997;22:895–902.
[64] Dreyfuss P, Halbrook B, Pauza K, et al. Efficacy and validity of radiofrequency neurotomy for chronic lumbar zygapophyseal joint pain. Spine 2000;25:1270–7.
[65] North RB, Han M, Zahurak M, et al. Radiofrequency lumbar facet denervation: analysis of prognostic factors. Pain 1994;57:77–83.
[66] Rashbaum RF. Radiofrequency facet denervation: a treatment alternative in refractory low back pain with or without leg pain. Orthop Clin North Am 1983;14:569–75.
[67] Silvers HR. Lumbar percutaneous facet rhizotomy. Spine 1990;15:36–40.

[68] Dory MA. Arthrography of the lumbar facet joints. Radiology 1981;140:23–7.

[69] Glover JR. Arthrography of the joints of the lumbar vertebral arches. Orthop Clin North Am 1977;8:37–42.

[70] Lewinnek GE, Warfield CA. Facet joint degeneration as a cause of low back pain. Clin Orthop 1986;213:216–22.

[71] Goldstone JG, Pennant JH. Spinal anaesthesia following facet joint injection: a report of two cases. Anaesthesia 1987;42:754–6.

[72] Thomson SJ, Lomax DM, Collett BJ. Chemical meningism after lumbar facet joint block with local anesthetic and steroids. Anaesthesia 1991;46:563–4.

[73] Erlacher PR. Nucleography. J Bone Joint Surg Br 1952;34B:204–10.

[74] Manchikanti L. Facet joint pain and the role of neural blockade in its management. Curr Rev Pain 1999;3:348–58.

[75] Manchikanti L, Pampati V, Fellows B, et al. The diagnostic validity and therapeutic value of medial branch blocks with or without adjuvants. Curr Rev Pain 2000;4:337–44.

[76] Manchikanti L, Pampati V, Fellows B, et al. The inability of the clinical picture to characterize pain from facet joints. Pain Physician 2000;3:158–66.

[77] Schwarzer AC, Derby R, Aprill CN, et al. The value of the provocation response in lumbar zygapophyseal joint injections. Clin J Pain 1994;10:309–13.

[78] Dreyfuss PH, Dreyer SJ, Herring SA. Contemporary concepts in spine care: lumbar zygapophyseal (facet) joint injections. Spine 1995;20:2040–7.

[79] Carette S, Marcoux S, Truchon R, et al. A controlled trial of corticosteroid injections into facet joints for chronic low back pain. N Engl J Med 1991;325:1002–7.

[80] Blanchard J, Ramamurthy S, Walsh N, et al. Intravenous regional sympatholysis: a double blind comparison of guanethidine, reserpine and normal saline. J Pain Symptom Manage 1990;5:357–61.

[81] Frost FA, Jessen R, Siggard-Anderson J. A controlled double-blind comparison of mepivicaine injection versus saline injection for myofascial pain. Lancet 1980;1:499–500.

[82] Lilius G, Laasonen EM, Myllynen P, et al. Lumbar facet joint syndrome: a randomized clinical trial. J Bone Joint Surg Br 1989;71B:681–4.

[83] Brooke R. The sacroiliac joint. J Anat 1924;58:299–305.

[84] Goldthwaite GE, Osgood RB. A consideration of the pelvic articulations from an anatomical, pathological, and clinical standpoint. Boston Med Surg J 1905;152:593–601.

[85] Mixter WJ, Barr JS. Rupture of the intervertebral disc with involvement of the spinal canal. N Engl J Med 1934;211:210–5.

[86] Bakalim G. Results of radical evacuation and arthrodesis in sacroiliac tuberculosis. Acta Orthop Scand 1966;37:375–86.

[87] Brower AC. Disorders of the sacroiliac joint. Surgical Rounds in Orthopedics 1989;13: 47–54.

[88] Cheng PA. The anatomical and clinical aspects of epidural anesthesia. Curr Res Anesth Analg 1963;42:398–406.

[89] Kuslich SD, Ulstrom CL, Michael CJ. The tissue origin of low back pain and sciatica. Orthop Clin North Am 1991;22:181–7.

[90] Roland MR, Moms RM. A study of the natural history of low back pain. Spine 1983;8: 145–50.

[91] Cohen AS, McNeill JM, Calkins E, et al. The "normal" sacroiliac joint: analysis of 88 sacroiliac roentgenograms. Am J Roentgenol Radium Ther Nucl Med 1967;100:559–63.

[92] Jajic I, Jajic Z. The prevalence of osteoarthritis of the sacroiliac joints in an urban population. Clin Rheumatol 1987;6:39–41.

[93] Resnick E, Niwayama G, Georgen TG. Degenerative disease of the sacroiliac joint. Invest Radiol 1975;10:608–21.

[94] Schwarzer AC, Aprill CN, Bogduk N. The sacroiliac joint in chronic low back pain. Spine 1995;20:31–7.

[95] Haldeman KO, Soto-Hall R. The diagnosis and treatment of sacroiliac conditions by the injection of procaine (novocaine). J Bone Joint Surg 1938;20:675–85.

[96] Hendrix RW, Kane WJ. Simplified aspiration or injection technique for the sacroiliac joint. J Bone Joint Surg Am 1982;64A:1249–52.

[97] Miskew DB, Block RA, Witt PF. Aspiration of infected sacroiliac joint. J Bone Joint Surg Am 1979;61A:1071–2.

[98] Fortin JD, Dwyer AP, West S, et al. Sacroiliac joint: pain referral maps upon applying a new injection/arthrography technique. Part I: Asymptomatic volunteers. Spine 1994; 19:1475–82.

[99] Fortin JD, Aprill CN, Ponthieux B, et al. Sacroiliac joint: pain referral maps upon applying a new injection/arthrography technique. Part II: Clinical evaluation. Spine 1994;19:1483–9.

[100] Pang WW, Mok MS, Lin ML, et al. Application of spinal pain mapping in the diagnosis of low back pain-analysis of 104 cases. Acta Anaesthesiol Sin 1998;36:71–4.

[101] Fortin JD. The sacroiliac joint: a new perspective. J Back Musculoskeletal Rehabil 1993;3: 31–43.

[102] Fortin JD, Falco FJE. The Fortin finger test: an indicator of sacroiliac pain. Am J Orthop 1997;27:477–80.

[103] Maigne JY, Aivaliklis A, Pfefer F. Results of sacroiliac joint double block and value of sacroiliac pain provocation tests in 54 patients with low back pain. Spine 1996;21: 1889–92.

[104] Rosenburg JM, Quint TJ, de Rosayro AM. Computerized tomographic localization of clinically-guided sacroiliac joint injections. Clin J Pain 2000;16:18–21.

[105] Fortin JD, Washington WJ, Falco FJE. Three pathways between the sacroiliac joint and neural structures. AJNR Am J Neuroradiol 1990;20:1429–34.

[106] Steindler A, Luck J. Differential diagnosis of pain low in the back: allocation of the source of pain by procaine hydrochloride method. JAMA 1938;110:106–13.

[107] Hirsch C. Attempt to diagnose the level of disc lesion clinically by disc puncture. Acta Orthop Scand 1948;18:131–40.

[108] Lindblom K. Diagnostic puncture of the intervertebral discs in sciatica. Acta Orthop Scand 1948;17:231–9.

[109] Wise RE, Weiford EC. X-ray visualization of the intervertebral disk. Cleve Clin Q 1951;18: 127–30.

[110] Cloward RB, Busaid LL. Discography: technique, indications and evaluation of normal and abnormal intervertebral discs. AJR Am J Roentgenol 1952;68:552–64.

[111] Antti-Poika I, Soini J, Tallroth K, et al. Clinical relevance of discography combined with CT scanning: a study of 100 patients. J Bone Joint Surg Br 1990;72B:480–5.

[112] Brodsky AE, Binder WF. Lumbar discography: its value in diagnosis and treatment of lumbar disc lesions. Spine 1979;4:110–20.

[113] Colhoun E, McCall IW, Williams L, et al. Provocation discography as a guide to planning operations on the spine. J Bone Joint Surg Br 1988;70B:267–71.

[114] Collins HR. An evaluation of cervical and lumbar discography. Clin Orthop 1975;107:133–8.

[115] Collis JS, Gardner WJ. Lumbar discography: analysis of 600 degenerated disks and diagnosis of degenerative disk disease. JAMA 1961;178:167–70.

[116] Konings J, Veldhuizen AG. Topographic anatomical aspects of lumbar disc puncture. Spine 1988;13:958–61.

[117] Kornberg M. Extreme lateral lumbar disc herniation. Spine 1987;12:586–9.

[118] Crock HV. A reappraisal of intervertebral disc lesions. Med J Aust 1970;1:983–9.

[119] Adams MA, Hutton WC. The relevance of torsion to the mechanical derangement of the lumbar spine. Spine 1981;6:241–8.

[120] Farfan HF, Cossette JW, Robertson GH, et al. The effects of torsion on the lumbar intervertebral joints: the role of torsion in the production of disc degeneration. J Bone Joint Surg Am 1970;52A:468–97.

[121] Farfan HF, Huberdeau RM, Dubow HI. Lumbar intervertebral disc degeneration: the influence of geometrical features on the pattern of disc degeneration. A post mortem study. J Bone Joint Surg Am 1972;54A:492–510.

[122] Gibson MJ, Buckley J, Mawhinney R. Magnetic resonance imaging and discography in the diagnosis of disc degeneration: a comparative study of 50 discs. J Bone Joint Surg Br 1986; 68B:369–73.

[123] Osti OL, Fraser RD, Vernon-Roberts B. Discitis after discography: the role of prophylactic antibiotics. J Bone Joint Surg Br 1990;72B:271–4.

[124] Schneiderman G, Flannigan B, Kingston S, et al. MRI in the diagnosis of disc degeneration: correlation with discography. Spine 1987;12:276–81.

[125] Panagiotacopulas ND, Pope MH, Krag MH, et al. Water content in human intervertebral discs, part I. Measurements by magnetic resonance imaging. Spine 1987;12:912–7.

[126] Aprill C, Bogduk N. High-intensity zone: a diagnostic sign of painful lumbar disc on magnetic resonance imaging. Br J Radiol 1992;65:361–9.

[127] Ricketson R, Simmons JW, Hauser BO. The prolapsed intervertebral disc: the high-intensity zone with discography correlation. Spine 1996;21:2758–62.

[128] Guyer RD, Ohnmeiss DD. Contemporary concepts in spine care: lumbar discography. Position statement from the North American Spine Society and Therapeutic Committee. Spine 1995;18:2048–59.

[129] Falco FJ, Moran JG. Lumbar discography using gadolinium in patients with iodine contrast allergy followed by postdiscography computed tomography scan. Spine 2003;28:E1–4.

[130] Keck C. Discography: technique and interpretation. Arch Surg 1960;80:580–5.

[131] Lindblom K. Technique and results in myelography and disc puncture. Acta Radiol Scand 1950;34:321–30.

[132] Aprill CN. Diagnostic disc injection. In: Frymoyer JW, editor. The adult spine: principles and practice. New York: Raven Press; 1991. p. 403–42.

[133] McCulloch JA, Waddell G. Lateral lumbar discography. Br J Radiol 1978;51:498–502.

[134] Fraser RD, Osti OL, Vernon-Roberts B. Discitis after discography. J Bone Joint Surg Br 1987;69B:26–35.

[135] Fraser RD, Osti OL, Vernon-Roberts B. Iatrogenic discitis: the role of intravenous antibiotics in the prevention and treatment. Spine 1989;14:1025–32.

[136] Adams MA, Dolan P, Hutton WC. The stages of disc degeneration as revealed by discograms. J Bone Joint Surg Br 1986;68B:36–41.

[137] Bernard TN. Lumbar discography followed by computed tomography: refining the diagnosis of low-back pain. Spine 1990;15:690–707.

[138] Derby R, Howard M, Grant J, et al. The ability of pressure controlled discography to predict surgical and non-surgical outcome. Spine 1999;24:364–71.

[139] Schellhas KP, Pollei SR, Gundry CR, et al. Lumbar disc high-intensity zone: correlation of magnetic resonance imaging and discography. Spine 1996;21:79–86.

[140] Sachs BL, Vanharanta H, Spivey MA, et al. Dallas discogram description: a new classification of CT/discography in low-back disorders. Spine 1987;12:287–94.

[141] Vanharanta H, Sachs BL, Spivey MA, et al. The relationship of pain provocation to lumbar disc deterioration as seen by CT/discography. Spine 1987;12:295–8.

[142] Gardner WJ, Wise RE, Hughes CR, et al. X-ray visualization of the intervertebral disk: with a consideration of the morbidity of disk puncture. AMA Arch Surg 1952;64:355–64.

[143] Gresham JL, Miller R. Evaluation of the lumbar spine by diskography and its use in selection of proper treatment of the herniated disk syndrome. Clin Orthop 1969;67:29–41.

[144] Guyer RD, Collier R, Stith WJ, et al. Discitis after discography. Spine 1988;13:1352–4.

[145] Modic MT, Feiglin D, Pirano D, et al. Vertebral osteomyelitis: assessment using MR. Radiology 1985;157:157–66.

[146] Szypryt E, Hardy J, Hinton C, et al. A comparison between magnetic resonance imaging and scintigraphic bone imaging in the diagnosis of disc space infection in an animal model. Spine 1988;13:1042–8.

[147] Johnson RG. Does discography injure normal discs? An analysis of repeat discograms. Spine 1989;14:424–6.

[148] Carragee E, Tanner C, Khurana S, et al. The rates of false-positive lumbar discography in select patients without low back symptoms. Spine 2000;25:1373–81.

[149] Holt EP. The question of lumbar discography. J Bone Joint Surg Am 1968;50A:720–6.

[150] Manchikanti L, Singh V, Pampati V, et al. Provocative discography in low back pain patients with or without somatization disorder: a randomized prospective evaluation. Pain Physician 2001;4:227–39.

[151] Simmons JW, Aprill CN, Dwyer AP, et al. A reassessment of Holt's data on the question of lumbar discography. Clin Orthop 1988;237:120–4.

[152] Walsh TR, Weinstein JN, Spratt KF, et al. Lumbar discography in normal subjects. J Bone Joint Surg Am 1990;72:1081–8.

[153] Lee CK, Vessa P, Lee JK. Chronic disabling low back pain syndrome caused by internal disc derangements: the results of disc excision and posterior lumbar interbody fusion. Spine 1995;20:356–61.

[154] Fries JW, Abodeely DA, Vijungco JG, et al. Computed tomography of herniated and extruded nucleus pulposus. J Comput Assist Tomogr 1982;6:874–87.

[155] Kurobane Y, Takahashi T, Tajima T, et al. Extraforaminal disc herniation. Spine 1986;11: 260–8.

[156] Maezawa S, Muro T. Pain provocation at lumbar discography as analyzed by computed tomography/discography. Spine 1992;17:1309–15.

[157] Moneta GB, Videman T, Kaivanto K, et al. Reported pain during lumbar discography as a function of anular ruptures and disc degeneration. Spine 1994;19:1968–74.

[158] Vanharanta H, Guyer RD, Ohnmeiss DD, et al. Disc deterioration in low-back syndromes. a prospective, multi-center CT/discography study. Spine 1988;13:1349–51.

[159] Grubb SA, Lipscomb HJ, Guilford WB. The relative value of lumbar roentgenograms, metrizamide myelography, and discography in the assessment of patients with chronic low-back syndrome. Spine 1987;12:282–6.

[160] Milette PC, Raymond J, Fontaine S. Comparison of high-resolution computed tomography with discography in the evaluation of lumbar disc herniations. Spine 1990;15:525–33.

[161] Ferrante FM, King LF, Roche EA, et al. Radiofrequency sacroiliac joint denervation for sacroiliac syndrome. Reg Anesth Pain Med 2001;26:137–42.

[162] Munglani R. The longer term effect of pulsed radiofrequency for neuropathic pain. Pain 1999;80:437–9.

[163] Sluijter M, Cosman E, Rittman W III, et al. The effects of pulsed radiofrequency fields applied to the dorsal root ganglion: a preliminary report. Pain Clin 1998;11:109–17.

[164] Chen YC, Lee SH, Saenz Y, et al. Histologic findings of disc, endplate and neural elements post coblation of nucleus pulposus: an experimental nucleoplasty study. Spine J 2003;3: 466–70.

[165] Singh V, Piryani C, Liao K, et al. Percutaneous disc decompression, using coblation (nucleoplasty), in the treatment of discogenic pain. Pain Physician 2002;5:250–9.

[166] Sharps LS, Issac Z. Percutaneous disc decompression using nucleoplasty. Pain Physician 2002;5:121–6.

[167] Derby R. Outcome comparison between IDET, combined IDET nucleoplasty and biochemical injection treatment. Presented at the 10th Annual Scientific Meeting of the International Spinal Injection Society. Austin(TX), September 6–8, 2002.

[168] Chen YC, Lee SH, Chen D. Intradiscal pressure study of percutaneous disc decompression with nucleoplasty in human cadavers. Spine 2003;28:661–5.

[169] Chen YC, Derby R, Lee S. Percutaneous disc decompression in the management of chronic low back pain. Orthop Clin North Am 2004;35:17–23.

[170] Pauza K, Howell S, Dreyfuss P, et al. A randomized, double-blind, placebo-controlled trial evaluating the efficacy of intradiscal electrothermal annuloplasty (IDET) for the treatment

of chronic discogenic low back pain: 6-month outcomes. In Proceedings of the International Spinal Injection Society. Austin, September 7, 2002.

[171] Pauza K, Howell S, Dreyfuss P, et al. A randomized, placebo-controlled trial of intradiscal electrothermal therapy for the treatment of discogenic low back pain. Spine J 2004;4:27–35.

[172] Derby R. Intradiscal electrothermal annuloplasty. Presented at the 13th Annual Meeting of the North American Spine Society. San Francisco, October 28–31, 1998.

[173] Saal JS, Saal JA. Management of chronic discogenic low back pain with a thermal intradiscal catheter: a preliminary report. Spine 2000;25(3):382–8.

[174] Derby R, Chen Y, O'Neill C, et al. Intradiscal electrothermal annuloplasty: a novel approach for treating chronic discogenic back pain. Neuromodulation 2000;3:82–8.

[175] Lagattuta FB, Brady R, Hudoba P, et al. Incidence of intervertebral fusion in patients treated with intradiscal electrothermotherapy. Presented at the Annual Meeting of the American Association of Orthopedic Medicine. Amelia Island, Florida, May 4–6, 2000.

[176] Saal JA, Saal JS. Intradiscal electrothermal treatment for chronic discogenic low back pain: a prospective outcome study with minimum 1-year follow-up. Spine 2000;25:2622–7.

[177] Kapural L, Mekhail N, Korunda Z, et al. Intradiscal thermal annuloplasty for the treatment of lumbar discogenic pain in patients with multilevel degenerative disc disease. Anesth Analg 2004;99:472–6.

[178] Heavner JE. Percutaneous epidural neuroplasty: prospective evaluation of 0.9% NaCl versus 10% NaCl with or without hyaluronidase. Reg Anesth Pain Med 1999;24:202–7.

[179] Racz GB, Heavner JE, Raj PP. Epidural neuroplasty. Semin Anesth 1997;16(4):302–12.

[180] Racz GB, Holubec JT. Lysis of adhesions in the epidural space. In: Racz GB, editor. Techniques of neurolysis. Boston: Kluwer Academic; 1989. p. 57–72.

[181] Manchikanti L, Bakhit CE. Percutaneous lysis of epidural adhesions. Pain Physician 2000; 3:46–64.

[182] Manchikanti L, Pampati V, Fellows B, et al. Role of one day epidural adhesiolysis in management of chronic low back pain. Pain Physician 2001;4:153–66.

**ELSEVIER
SAUNDERS**

Clin Occup Environ Med
5 (3) 703–717

CLINICS IN
OCCUPATIONAL AND
ENVIRONMENTAL
MEDICINE

Surgical Issues in the Injured Worker with Lower Back Pain

Mitchell F. Reiter, MD*, Michael Vives, MD

*Department of Orthopaedic Surgery, The New Jersey Medical School/UMDNJ Newark,
90 Bergen St., DOC Suite 1200, Newark, NJ 07101, USA*

Low back injuries represent the single largest workplace problem in the industrialized world [1]. Proper treatment of patients remains frustratingly difficult, with a significant number of individuals continuing to have persistent impairment despite medical care. This situation has been labeled as one of the most dramatic failures of health care in modern times [2]. The available literature regarding workers with lower back injuries tends to be divided into two major categories. The first group consists primarily of occupational medicine publications that focus on nonspecific diagnoses with a tendency toward minimal intervention and the use of return to work as their primary outcomes endpoint. The second group of publications is made up of articles written by subspecialists that emphasize treatment of specific diagnoses and use general medical outcomes. These two bodies of literature frequently provide differing recommendations regarding treatment, which can lead to difficulty for clinicians who encounter these patients.

When considering surgical issues as opposed to more conservative care in injured workers, it becomes critical to attempt to establish an exact diagnosis. Certain conditions, such as herniated disks or spinal fractures, have fairly well-defined surgical indications and documented results. A few conditions that represent surgical emergencies, such as cauda equina syndrome, must be identified promptly. Clinicians must be able to identify certain red flags in a patient's history or physical examination that should prompt further evaluation and treatment. It is well known that in many patients an exact diagnosis cannot be made, and these patients are usually labeled more vaguely as having nonspecific low back pain or mechanical low back pain. This difficult category of injured workers rarely benefits from surgical

---

* Corresponding author. 20 Lockhern Drive, Livingston, NJ 07039.
E-mail address: ReiterMF@UMDNJ.edu (M.F. Reiter).

1526-0046/06/$ - see front matter © 2006 Elsevier Inc. All rights reserved.
doi:10.1016/j.coem.2006.03.004   *occmed.theclinics.com*

intervention, and they must be identified so that unnecessary surgery with poor outcomes is avoided.

Once surgical emergencies and serious red flags have been excluded, workers with lower back injury should be treated with standard conservative care, which usually includes education, activity modification, analgesic medications, physical therapy, and early return to work [3,4]. Additional treatment options, including transcutaneous electrical nerve stimulation, injection therapies (eg, epidural steroids, facet blocks, sacroiliac injections), chiropractic care, and several forms of back school or work hardening programs, also have been tried with varying success. Although this article discusses the surgical issues that arise in workers with lower back injury, the assumption is that these patients have failed to improve with nonoperative care. Numerous studies have demonstrated worse outcomes with surgical intervention in patients on workers' compensation compared with other patients. Surgery should be undertaken only with careful consideration in injured workers [5–7]. Psychological factors also have been shown to play an important role in patients who receive workers' compensation. The treating physician must consider the possible roles of job dissatisfaction, stress, and secondary gain when formulating a plan of care that might include surgical intervention for an injured worker [8,9].

Red flags and surgical emergencies

The surgical evaluation of workers with lower back injury begins with a standard history and physical examination. Specific historical factors that may influence surgical treatment include the exact mechanism of injury (high- versus low-energy injuries), the employee's type of work, and whether the patient has a history of previous lower back injuries. Patients must be asked if they are experiencing any symptoms of neurologic dysfunction, including presence of numbness, weakness, paresthesias, or any difficulties with bladder or bowel function. The location of a patient's pain is also an important factor in planning treatment. Axial pain has a different differential diagnosis and prognosis than radiculopathy. Physical examination must include a thorough neurologic evaluation of the lower extremities, including motor, sensory, reflex testing, and provocative maneuvers, such as the straight leg raise test and evaluation for Waddell's signs of nonorganic pain. Although some controversy exists on the topic, studies looking at the presence of nonorganic signs of pain have found significantly worse outcome and delay in return to work in patients who exhibit these behaviors [10–12].

After the initial history and physical examination, most workers with lower back injuries can begin a conservative treatment program. There are only a few situations in which additional testing or treatment may be immediately necessary, but the rapid identification of these situations is critical. Any worker with back pain and a high-energy mechanism of injury should undergo lumbar radiographs to evaluate for possible vertebral fracture or subluxation. Although most spinal fractures can be treated nonoperatively with bracing, specialty consultation is recommended when these injuries are identified. Most spinal fractures require advanced imaging with a CT scan or MRI to plan proper treatment. In older workers, the threshold for obtaining a radiograph should be lower because the presence of osteoporosis can allow for spinal fracture with less severe mechanisms of injury.

Any worker with symptoms of bowel or bladder dysfunction requires a much more detailed evaluation. Cauda equina syndrome is clinically defined by bladder or bowel difficulties, saddle anesthesia, with possible lower extremity sensory or motor deficits. This syndrome is most frequently caused by a large lumbar disc herniation that causes significant pressure on the centrally placed sacral nerve root fibers. Difficulties with urination can include retention, frequency, or overflow incontinence [13]. Rectal examination should be performed in all patients with suspected cauda equina syndrome, because the physical finding can include loss of perianal sensation and diminished rectal tone. An urgent MRI scan of the lumbar spine should be obtained in patients followed by immediate surgical consultation and neurologic decompression if necessary. The prognosis for recovery from cauda equina syndrome is dramatically improved with early surgical decompression within 24 to 48 hours of onset [14].

Another situation that requires urgent evaluation and treatment involves patients with a progressive neurologic deficit. When a patient is identified with a clearly progressing neurologic deficit, he or she should be sent to the nearest capable emergency room for treatment. An urgent MRI should be obtained and surgical consultation requested. Some possible causes of progressive neurologic deficits include a massive lumbar disc herniation, spinal fracture, epidural abscess, spinal tumor, or an epidural hematoma. Once the proper diagnosis has been made, patients with these conditions should undergo urgent neurologic decompression.

Although acute fractures, cauda equina syndrome, and progressive neurologic deficits can represent surgical emergencies, another group of patients that requires additional evaluation and potentially surgical referral before initiating conservative care are individuals who have incapacitating low back pain. Patients with severe pain that cannot be well controlled with medication should undergo timely imaging evaluation to rule out serious pathology before pursuing care along standard treatment algorithms. When evaluating patients with intractable pain, red flags that can suggest more ominous pathology should be considered, including a history of cancer, immunosuppression from disease or medication, advanced age, and constitutional symptoms that include fever, chills, weight loss, or malaise. The presence of constant pain that is not relieved by rest, night pain, or pain described as deep or boring in nature also can suggest the presence of more serious pathology, such as a tumor or infection. Ultimately clinicians must use their judgment as to which patients must undergo more advanced imaging studies before initiating treatment (Box 1).

Disc herniation

Lumbar disc herniation is defined by an annular tear or bulge with displacement of the nucleus pulposus. When a disc is described as bulging, it implies that the annulus remains intact. An extruded disc is one in which the nucleus material extends beyond the annulus into the spinal canal. A disc fragment that is no longer in continuity with the disc space is described as sequestered. Patients with a symptomatic lumbar disc herniation typically present with sciatica pain that radiates from the lower back or buttock down into the lower extremity in a dermatomal pattern. This pain may be associated with lower extremity numbness or weakness. The symptoms are typically worsened with sitting, coughing, or sneezing and are improved with standing or laying flat [15]. Physical findings may include motor or sensory deficits and the presence of a tension sign, such as a positive straight leg raise or femoral stretch test.

Barring the presence of one of the red flags, such as cauda equina syndrome, intractable pain, or a progressive neurologic deficit, an injured worker with sciatica-type pain can be managed with standard conservative treatment. Treatment guidelines for the primary and secondary phases of nonoperative care of lumbar disc herniations are well described and have been published by several medical societies, including the North American Spine Society [13]. If a patient with radicular pain fails to respond to initial treatment, consideration should be given to obtaining a lumbar MRI scan

---

Box 1. Historical factors that should prompt further evaluation and situations in which surgical consultation should be strongly considered

Historical red flags
Age over 65
History of cancer
Constitutional symptoms
Immunosuppression
Pain unrelieved by rest
Night pain

Potential surgical emergencies
Cauda equina syndrome
Progressive neurologic deficit
Acute spinal fracture
Incapacitating pain

---

some time between 4 and 12 weeks after the onset of symptoms. MRI scanning allows for excellent visualization of the neurologic elements and is the imaging modality of choice in a patient with a suspected lumbar disc herniation (Fig. 1). CT scanning provides excellent bony detail but is less sensitive for intracanal spinal pathology. CT scan performed in conjunction with myelography provides excellent detail but is invasive and should be reserved for patients in whom an MRI is not possible (eg, patients with pacemaker, intracranial clips, or severe claustrophobia).

The presence of MRI abnormalities in asymptomatic patients is a well-described phenomenon that can lead to confusion for the clinician and patient. In Dr. Boden's classic study of MRI abnormalities in 67 subjects without symptoms of back pain or sciatica, 20% of subjects younger than age 60 had a disc herniation and 36% of subjects over age 60 had a documented disc herniation [16]. When considering surgical treatment in patients with lumbar disc herniation, it is important to remember that the natural history of a symptomatic herniated disc is good. Dr. Weber's landmark study in 1983 on patients with lumbar disc herniations and severe sciatica in whom surgery was being considered found that symptoms were improved at 1 year in 60% of patients treated nonoperatively and in 92% of patients who underwent operative treatment. By 4 years there was no statistically significant difference between the groups, and at 10 years there was no difference [17].

In injured workers with a symptomatic lumbar disc herniation, surgery should be considered only after they have failed to improve with 6 to 12 weeks of conservative care. Indications for surgery in patients who do not experience cauda equina syndrome or a progressive neurologic deficit include severe pain that fails to improve with conservative treatment, significant neurologic deficit, or frequently recurring episodes of sciatica pain.

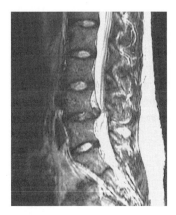

Fig. 1. T2-weighted sagittal MRI sequence demonstrates a large L4-5 disc herniation with significant narrowing of the spinal canal.

Surgery is only an option when a patient's symptoms and physical examination correlate with neurologic compression noted on imaging studies (Box 2). Surgery in the presence of minimal or no neurologic compression has been shown to result in poor outcomes.

The gold standard surgical technique for the treatment of lumbar disc herniations is an open lumbar discectomy, which can be accomplished using loupe magnification or the operating microscope, with the typical incision being approximately 3 cm in length. Variations on the open technique, in which endoscopes are used to allow for direct visualization of the herniated disc, also have demonstrated efficacy. Percutaneous techniques, in which the disc herniation is not addressed directly, including automated percutaneous lumbar discectomy and the use of chymopapain, have been shown to have lower success rates compared with standard discectomy [18]. Most lumbar discectomy surgeries can be performed on an outpatient basis.

Published reports on the success rate of surgical treatment of lumbar disc herniations show a variable success rate. Case series and retrospective reviews tend to show success rates in the 90% to 95% range, whereas prospective studies demonstrate success rates between 73% and 77% [19]. Poorer outcomes have been found in workers' compensation claimants when compared with control patients [20]. The ethical dilemma faced by physicians as to whether a patient's compensation status with the associated lower surgical success rate should preclude him or her from otherwise indicated surgery has no easy answer.

After surgical intervention, minimal activity restrictions are necessary. Most patients can begin a rehabilitation program within a few days of surgery. Return to work criteria are frequently debated, but it has been shown that the risk of reinjury is not increased with early return to work [21,22]. In general, injured workers can attempt return to work in a light duty capacity between 2 and 6 weeks postoperatively, and most patients can return to full duty between 6 and 12 weeks postoperatively. It has been found that most recovery after discectomy surgery occurs in the first 2 months postoperatively and that outcomes at 2 months strongly correlate with a patient's

---

Box 2. Indications for surgery in patients with lumbar disc herniation in which their symptoms, physical findings, and imaging studies correlate

Cauda equina syndrome (urgent)
Progressive neurologic deficit (urgent)
Severe radicular pain despite conservative treatment
Clinically significant neurologic deficit despite conservative treatment
Frequently recurring episodes of radiculopathy despite treatment

result at 1 year postoperatively [23]. With these data in mind, one can infer that most patients will have reached maximum medical improvement within 2 or 3 months of discectomy surgery. At that point, patients who are unable to return to work despite postoperative rehabilitation may benefit from referral to a palliative chronic pain management program. Education of patients regarding return to work timeframes and judicious use of functional capacity evaluations can help expedite care postoperatively and reduce physician-patient conflict.

Lumbar discogenic pain

The treatment of patients with predominantly axial lower back pain is an area fraught with controversy. Sixty percent to 80% of adults experience back pain at some point in their life. Injured workers with lower back pain should be treated with standard conservative measures, with a strong emphasis on continuing activities as normally as possible. Although most patients with acute low back pain improve with conservative treatment, approximately 10% of patients become chronic pain sufferers [13]. Some of these patients with persistent lower back pain after an injury suffer from an internal derangement of the disc. This condition is also known as internal disc disruption, discogenic pain syndrome, or—when the morphologic changes in the disc become further advanced—degenerative disc disease.

Internal disc derangement is defined as one or more pathologic conditions within the disc that cause low back pain with no or minimal deformation of the anatomic contours of the disc. Despite the rising popularity of identifying patients as having discogenic pain, diagnosis and treatment remain controversial [13]. It should be emphasized that no consensus exists on the specific diagnostic criteria that should be used for discogenic pain. The syndrome must be diagnosed by combining a patient's history, physical finding, imaging studies, and the results of discography testing with the exclusion of other known causes of low back pain.

Patients who have discogenic pain tend to be between 20 and 50 years old with chronic lower back pain. They also may have referred pain in the buttocks and thighs in the same sclerotome as the injured disc but typically do not have radiculopathy. Physical examination demonstrates back pain, tenderness, and limited range of motion, but the neurologic examination is usually normal. The classic imaging finding for disc disruption is decreased signal intensity within the disc on T2-weighted MRI sequences. MRI findings of a diffuse disc bulge or a hig- intensity zone in the posterior annulus also can suggest discogenic pain (Fig. 2) [24].

In patients who have had persistent severe back pain for longer than 6 months that has failed to improve with standard treatment and in whom the diagnosis of discogenic back pain is being considered, additional testing may be necessary. In a patient with one or two disrupted discs on MRI, discography testing may provide additional data to support or refute the

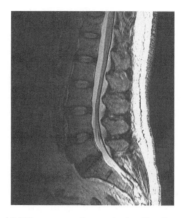

Fig. 2. Sagittal T2-weighted MRI sequence demonstrates disc degeneration at the L5-S1 level, which is evidenced by the decreased signal intensity at L5-S1 as compared with the other lumbar discs.

diagnosis of discogenic back pain. Discography is an invasive and painful test that should be performed only in patients in whom surgical treatment is being considered. Discography testing in patients who are not surgical candidates serves no purpose and subjects patients to unnecessary risk. Discography involves injection of contrast into the abnormal disc to evaluate for annular disruption and, more importantly, to see if injection produces a concordant pain response. An important part of the test is the injection of an adjacent normal disc as a control that should be painless and have a normal nucleogram.

The merits and limitations of discography have been debated in the literature at great length. Although studies have demonstrated its predictive value in diagnosing patients with painful disc disruption, false-positive results make interpretation difficult. Some of the best literature on this topic has been published by Carragee and colleagues [25], who have shown that discography results are the least reliable in patients with chronic pain and abnormal psychometric profiles (the exact population that tends to have discogenic pain syndromes). Because there are no specific criteria for making the diagnosis of internal disc derangement, underdiagnosis and overdiagnosis remain a problem. Some physicians believe that discogenic pain does not exist as a clinical syndrome and that all patients with back pain eventually improve with conservative care. This has been found not to be the case, because a significant number of patients with disc disruption continue to have disabling pain despite treatment. Other physicians are overdiagnosing disc disruption and are performing far too many spinal fusion surgeries.

The current standard surgical treatment option for internal disc disruption involves lumbar interbody fusion surgery, in which the painful disc is excised and the involved segment stabilized. Other less invasive procedures, such as intradiscal electrothermal coagulation or nucleoplasty, are less well proven and remain controversial [26]. More recently, disc replacement has emerged as another treatment option for these patients. Any type of surgery for axial back pain should be considered only in patients who have failed to improve despite 6 months of standard conservative treatment and in whom the imaging and physical findings correlate with provocative discography testing. Surgery has been found to be only modestly successful in patients who have internal disc disruption, and the results in patients who receive workers' compensation tend to be worse than in controls [5,6]. Surgery should be thought of as a last resort for these patients and should be considered only after careful discussion with patients.

The standard surgical treatment for discogenic back pain is lumbar interbody fusion, which can be accomplished via a posterior approach with a posterior lumbar interbody fusion (Fig. 3), an anterior approach with an anterior lumbar interbody fusion (Fig. 4), or a combined anterior and posterior fusion (360° or circumferential fusion). The merits and drawbacks of the various techniques are constantly debated, and that discussion is beyond the scope of this article. Most of these procedures are accomplished using spinal instrumentation, and newer techniques using bone morphogenetic proteins have been shown to increase fusion rates [27]. Although controversy exists regarding the effectiveness of spinal fusion in the treatment of chronic low back pain, a landmark randomized, controlled, multicenter trial that compared lumbar fusion to nonoperative treatment found that in well-selected patients, fusion surgery could diminish pain and decrease disability more effectively that nonoperative treatment [28].

A newer treatment option that recently has been in the media spotlight is that of disc arthroplasty or total disc replacement. The potential advantages of disc replacement include preservation of motion, which may protect the adjacent spinal segments from early deterioration, avoidance of the need

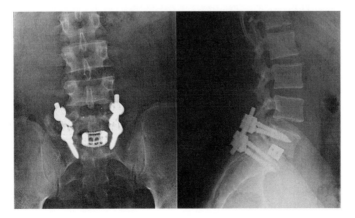

Fig. 3. Anteroposterior and lateral postoperative radiographs of a patient who underwent an L5-S1 posterior lumbar interbody fusion using the transforaminal lumbar interbody fusion technique.

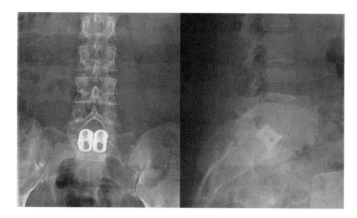

Fig. 4. Anteroposterior and lateral postoperative radiographs of a patient who underwent an L5-S1 anterior lumbar interbody fusion using cages and bone morphogenetic protein.

for fusion with its associated morbidity of harvesting bone graft and risk of nonunion, and the potential for a quicker recovery with early return of motion (Fig. 5). A large prospective, randomized, multicenter US Food and Drug Administration investigational device exemption study of lumbar disc replacement that compared the Charite artificial disc to anterior lumbar interbody fusion recently was published. Using quantitative clinical outcome measures, the study demonstrated that disc replacement was at least equivalent to anterior lumbar fusion surgery. At 24 months postoperatively, disc replacement patients had a 73.7% rate of satisfaction with their results [29].

Tempering the enthusiasm for operative treatment of discogenic back pain that is found in the surgical literature is the knowledge that many

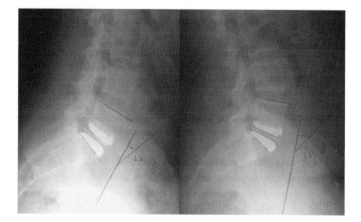

Fig. 5. Flexion and extension radiographs of a patient with a Charite disc replacement at the L5-S1 level. Note that the patient has 11° of intervertebral motion at the level of the total disc arthroplasty.

studies have demonstrated poor outcomes with surgical fusion in the subset of workers' compensation patients [6,30]. Other studies have questioned the efficacy of spinal fusion for back pain altogether. In a Cochrane review of randomized, controlled trials for the treatment of lumbar degenerative disc disease or spondylosis (which the authors regarded as one entity), the authors concluded that there was no scientific evidence about the effectiveness of lumbar fusion for degenerative lumbar disease compared with placebo, the natural history, or conservative treatment [31]. Caught in the middle of this dilemma are clinicians, who face patients with severe low back pain that has failed to improve with standard care and who are unable to return to work. The decision for or against surgery in these patients must take clinical, psychosocial, and economic factors into account. Clinicians also must be realistic in the sense that although fusion surgery may improve a patient's quality of life, return to a physically demanding occupation may be an unrealistic goal [32].

With most newer spinal fusion and disc replacement techniques, stable fixation of the spine is achieved immediately. Postoperative outpatient rehabilitation usually can be started some time between 2 and 6 weeks after surgery. Return to work in a modified duty capacity typical occurs between 3 and 4 months postoperatively. A reasonable expectation for a patient achieving maximum medical improvement after lumbar fusion surgery is at the 6-month timeframe. As with lumbar discectomy surgery, reasonable patient expectations, pre-emptively discussing timeframes for return to work with patients, and use of functional capacity evaluations can help with a smooth transition of patients back to productivity.

Spinal stenosis and spondylolisthesis

The diagnosis of spinal stenosis or spondylolisthesis sometimes is made in workers with a lower back injury. Spinal stenosis is the clinical syndrome of narrowing of the spinal canal that results in symptoms of back, buttocks, or leg pain with characteristic provocative and palliative features (Fig. 6) [13]. Spondylolisthesis is the anterior displacement of one vertebra on the vertebra below it, which can be the result of degenerative disease or a developmental defect in the pars interarticularis portion of the vertebra. Although stenosis and spondylolisthesis are not typically traumatically induced, their presence can be aggravated by an injury leading to the onset of clinical symptoms.

The management of injured workers diagnosed with spinal stenosis or spondylolisthesis follows the same nonoperative treatment algorithm used for other lower back injuries. The natural history of spinal stenosis is not well defined, but clearly in the face of an acute exacerbation, many patients return to their baseline asymptomatic status. In a study by Johnsson and colleagues [33] of 32 patients who were advised to have operative treatment but who were managed with observation only, 47% had clinical

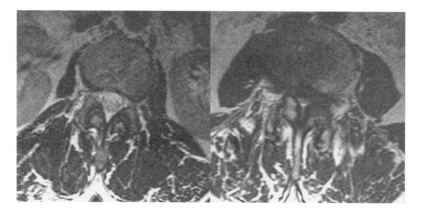

Fig. 6. T2-weighted axial MRI sequences demonstrate a normal canal size and severe spinal stenosis with significant compression of the neurologic elements.

improvement, 38% had no change in symptoms, and 16% experienced worsening of their symptoms over a mean duration of follow-up of 4 years.

Because the risk of symptom progression is low and it develops slowly, surgical intervention for injured workers with spinal stenosis or spondylolisthesis should be considered only when a patient's symptoms are severe and nonoperative treatment has been maximized. Most patients who require surgical treatment of spinal stenosis can be treated solely with a decompressive lumbar laminectomy. There are certain situations in which a concomitant lumbar fusion must be considered, including the presence of spondylolisthesis, significant scoliosis, or instability in the areas that require decompression. Fusion also should be considered in patients with severe back pain and degenerative disease in the area undergoing laminectomy.

The short-term outcomes of lumbar laminectomy surgery are relatively good. In one series, a good or excellent outcome was reported for 272 (62%) of 438 patients [34]. Satisfactory outcomes also can be achieved in patients who have degenerative spondylolisthesis and stenosis and are undergoing laminectomy and fusion [35]. The results of surgery in the workers' compensation patient population are not as satisfying. In a study by Herno and colleagues [36] that looked specifically at return to work after surgical treatment of lumbar spinal stenosis, only 37% of women and 41% of men returned to work. Studies also have shown that results of lumbar laminectomy surgery do deteriorate with time, with one study finding that 20% of patients with an initially good result had an unsatisfactory outcome at a mean of 8.2 years postoperatively [37].

Summary

Despite all of the controversies that exist regarding the surgical treatment of injured workers, certain firm surgical indications do exist. Clinicians must work to develop a systematic approach to these patients, including obtaining a careful history, performing a thorough physical examination, and judiciously using imaging studies. Urgent situations must be identified promptly and treatment provided. Once these grave situations have been ruled out, most patients can be treated safely with standard conservative measures. In patients who fail to improve, an attempt should be made to localize the source of their pain. Patients with specific diagnoses who have failed to improve despite exhaustive nonoperative management and who meet exacting surgical criteria can benefit dramatically from operative intervention.

When treating these patients one must keep in mind that workers' compensation claims are much more complex than simply identifying the physical injury and providing effective medical or physical treatment alone. Occupational low back pain is multidimensional in nature and requires the recognition of other social, legal, cultural, organizational, and economic factors that contribute to the genesis of illness and disability [38]. These factors add to the considerable ambiguity that exists as to the optimal diagnostic criteria, management, and outcomes measures that should be used for workers who have lower back injuries. Prospective investigations that address the contribution of physician, patient, legal, and financial factors are needed to help elucidate further the optimal treatment of these complex patients. Until these studies are performed, clinicians must use the available evidence to provide sound and ethical treatment while minimizing complications and morbidity in their patients who have lower back injuries.

References

[1] Frymoyer JW. Back pain and sciatica. N Engl J Med 1988;318(5):291–300.
[2] Waddell G, Burton AK. Occupational health guidelines for the management of low back pain at work: evidence review. Occup Med (Lond) 2001;51(2):124–35.
[3] Frank JW, Kerr MS, Brooker AS, et al. Disability resulting from occupational low back pain. Part I: What do we know about primary prevention? A review of the scientific evidence on prevention before disability begins. Spine 1996;21(24):2908–17.
[4] Frank JW, Brooker AS, DeMaio SE, et al. Disability resulting from occupational low back pain. Part II: What do we know about secondary prevention? A review of the scientific evidence on prevention after disability begins. Spine 1996;21(24):2918–29.
[5] Franklin GM, Haug J, Heyer NJ, et al. Outcome of lumbar fusion in Washington State workers' compensation. Spine 1994;19(17):1897–903 [discussion: 1904].
[6] Greenough CG, Taylor LJ, Fraser RD. Anterior lumbar fusion: a comparison of noncompensation patients with compensation patients. Clin Orthop Relat Res 1994;300:30–7.
[7] Hansson TH, Hansson EK. The effects of common medical interventions on pain, back function, and work resumption in patients with chronic low back pain: a prospective 2-year cohort study in six countries. Spine 2000;25(23):3055–64.
[8] Papageorgiou AC, Macfarlane GJ, Thomas E, et al. Psychosocial factors in the workplace: do they predict new episodes of low back pain? Evidence from the South Manchester Back Pain Study. Spine 1997;22(10):1137–42.
[9] Svensson HO, Andersson GB. The relationship of low-back pain, work history, work environment, and stress: a retrospective cross-sectional study of 38- to 64-year-old women. Spine 1989;14(5):517–22.

[10] Gaines WG Jr, Hegmann KT. Effectiveness of Waddell's nonorganic signs in predicting a delayed return to regular work in patients experiencing acute occupational low back pain. Spine 1999;24(4):396–400 [discussion: 401].

[11] Kummel BM. Nonorganic signs of significance in low back pain. Spine 1996;21(9):1077–81.

[12] Waddell G, McCulloch JA, Kummel E, et al. Nonorganic physical signs in low-back pain. Spine 1980;5(2):117–25.

[13] Fardon DF. North American Spine Society. Orthopaedic knowledge update: spine 2. 2nd edition. Rosemont (IL): American Academy of Orthopaedic Surgeons; 2002.

[14] Kohles SS, Kohles DA, Karp AP, et al. Time-dependent surgical outcomes following cauda equina syndrome diagnosis: comments on a meta-analysis. Spine 2004;29(11):1281–7.

[15] Frymoyer JW, Ducker TB. The adult spine: principles and practice. New York: Raven Press; 1997.

[16] Boden SD, Davis DO, Dina TS, et al. Abnormal magnetic-resonance scans of the lumbar spine in asymptomatic subjects: a prospective investigation. J Bone Joint Surg Am 1990; 72(3):403–8.

[17] Weber H. Lumbar disc herniation: a controlled, prospective study with ten years of observation. Spine 1983;8(2):131–40.

[18] McCulloch JA. Focus issue on lumbar disc herniation: macro- and microdiscectomy. Spine 1996;21(24 Suppl):45S–56S.

[19] Postacchini F. Management of herniation of the lumbar disc. J Bone Joint Surg Br 1999; 81(4):567–76.

[20] Klekamp J, McCarty E, Spengler DM. Results of elective lumbar discectomy for patients involved in the workers' compensation system. J Spinal Disord 1998;11(4):277–82.

[21] Carragee EJ, Han MY, Yang B, et al. Activity restrictions after posterior lumbar discectomy: a prospective study of outcomes in 152 cases with no postoperative restrictions. Spine 1999; 24(22):2346–51.

[22] Carragee EJ, Helms E, O'Sullivan GS. Are postoperative activity restrictions necessary after posterior lumbar discectomy? A prospective study of outcomes in 50 consecutive cases. Spine 1996;21(16):1893–7.

[23] Hakkinen A, Ylinen J, Kautiainen H, et al. Does the outcome 2 months after lumbar disc surgery predict the outcome 12 months later? Disabil Rehabil 2003;25(17):968–72.

[24] Luoma K, Vehmas T, Riihimaki H, et al. Disc height and signal intensity of the nucleus pulposus on magnetic resonance imaging as indicators of lumbar disc degeneration. Spine 2001; 26(6):680–6.

[25] Carragee EJ, Tanner CM, Khurana S, et al. The rates of false-positive lumbar discography in select patients without low back symptoms. Spine 2000;25(11):1373–80 [discussion: 1381].

[26] Webster BS, Verma S, Pransky GS. Outcomes of workers' compensation claimants with low back pain undergoing intradiscal electrothermal therapy. Spine 2004;29(4):435–41.

[27] Burkus JK, Sandhu HS, Gornet MF, et al. Use of rhBMP-2 in combination with structural cortical allografts: clinical and radiographic outcomes in anterior lumbar spinal surgery. J Bone Joint Surg Am 2005;87(6):1205–12.

[28] Fritzell P, Hagg O, Wessberg P, et al. 2001 Volvo Award Winner in Clinical Studies: lumbar fusion versus nonsurgical treatment for chronic low back pain. A multicenter randomized controlled trial from the Swedish Lumbar Spine Study Group. Spine 2001;26(23):2521–32 [discussion: 2532].

[29] Blumenthal S, McAfee PC, Guyer RD, et al. A prospective, randomized, multicenter Food and Drug Administration investigational device exemptions study of lumbar total disc replacement with the CHARITE artificial disc versus lumbar fusion. Part I: evaluation of clinical outcomes. Spine 2005;30(14):1565–75 [discussion: E1387–1591].

[30] Hodges SD, Humphreys SC, Eck JC, et al. Predicting factors of successful recovery from lumbar spine surgery among workers' compensation patients. J Am Osteopath Assoc 2001;101(2):78–83.

[31] Gibson JN, Waddell G, Grant IC. Surgery for degenerative lumbar spondylosis. Cochrane Database Syst Rev 2000;3:CD001352.

[32] Kwon BK, Vaccaro AR, Grauer JN, et al. Indications, techniques, and outcomes of posterior surgery for chronic low back pain. Orthop Clin North Am 2003;34(2):297–308.

[33] Johnsson KE, Rosen I, Uden A. The natural course of lumbar spinal stenosis. Clin Orthop Relat Res 1992;279:82–6.

[34] Airaksinen O, Herno A, Turunen V, et al. Surgical outcome of 438 patients treated surgically for lumbar spinal stenosis. Spine 1997;22(19):2278–82.

[35] Herkowitz HN, Kurz LT. Degenerative lumbar spondylolisthesis with spinal stenosis: a prospective study comparing decompression with decompression and intertransverse process arthrodesis. J Bone Joint Surg Am 1991;73(6):802–8.

[36] Herno A, Airaksinen O, Saari T, et al. Pre- and Postoperative factors associated with return to work following surgery for lumbar spinal stenosis. Am J Ind Med 1996;30:473–8.

[37] Postacchini F, Cinotti G, Gumina S, et al. Long-term results of surgery in lumbar stenosis: 8-year review of 64 patients. Acta Orthop Scand Suppl 1993;251:78–80.

[38] Lemstra M, Olszynski WP. The effectiveness of standard care, early intervention, and occupational management in workers' compensation claims: part 2. Spine 2004;29(14):1573–9.

**ELSEVIER
SAUNDERS**

Clin Occup Environ Med
5 (3) 719–740

CLINICS IN
OCCUPATIONAL AND
ENVIRONMENTAL
MEDICINE

Impairment and Disability Rating in Low Back Pain

Richard T. Katz, MD

Department of Clinical Neurology (Physical Medicine and Rehabilitation), Washington University School of Medicine, 4660 Maryland Avenue, Suite 250, St. Louis, MO 63108, USA

"The first thing we do, let's kill all the lawyers." William Shakespeare

Many publications emphasize the theoretical relationship between impairment, disability, and the workplace. This article is intended to provide the reader with some framework in this regard, but its main intent is to create a practical how-to guide in the evaluation of impairment and disability that result from low back pain (LBP). The article is designed to help the reader deal with five questions:

1. What are impairment, disability, and handicap?
2. What background information do I need before entering the field of independent medical evaluations (IME) and disability ratings?
3. How do I help my partially disabled patient return to work?
4. How do I rate permanent partial and total disability?
5. What makes the IME different from any other evaluation?

What are impairment, disability, and handicap?

The definitions of impairment, disability, and handicap are key to the disability evaluation construct. The World Health Organization has offered widely accepted definitions of these three concepts that are worthy of review. Impairment is an abnormality of structure, appearance, or function at the end-organ level [1]. In our context of LBP, it is a herniated disc, a rotated hemipelvis, osteomyelitis of the spine, metastatic prostatic cancer, soft tissue pain, or myofascial pain.

Disability is the inability to perform an activity because of an abnormality of the person as a whole [1]. When a patient can no longer lift "twenty

E-mail address: pianodoctor@pol.net

1526-0046/06/$ - see front matter © 2006 Elsevier Inc. All rights reserved.
doi:10.1016/j.coem.2006.03.001

ton per day" (eg, throw 400 sacks that weigh 100 pounds each per day), he or she is disabled for performing that particular job. When a nurse can no longer bend over and stoop on a frequent basis, which most job analyses require for a ward nurse, he or she no longer can work full duty and must be placed temporarily or permanently on light duty.

A handicap is an environmentally defined abnormality that reflects societal bias experienced by the individual trying to fulfill a role [1]. If a registered nurse were not expected to lift heavy weights regularly, stand, or stoop, he or she would not be disabled for the job. It is our handicap or expectation placed on an individual that he or she is expected to do so.

In 2001, the World Health Organization abandoned the construct of impairment, handicap, and disability and promoted a new model. The new model describes body functions and structures. Impairments are the loss or deviations in these functions and structures. Also described are activities and limitations in performing those roles and participation and restrictions thereto. In this author's opinion, the new model is possibly more politically correct but offers little in the way of new insight.

Although the World Health Organization models offer a conceptual model, in the real world these terms are used differently. Insurance companies use the term "disabled" to imply that a person no longer can perform the substantial and material duties of an occupation. To be disabled in the context of the Social Security Administration means that a person must be disabled for "all substantial gainful activity" to receive benefits from this agency. A ballerina who drops an iron on her right great toe while ironing her tutu and crushes the digit most likely has concluded her career as a dancer and is disabled from this occupation in the eyes of her long-term disability carrier. The Social Security Administration would not see her as disabled and would point out several occupations to which the dancer could still apply herself.

Finally, there are important modifiers to the concept of disability. When a patient who has LBP has an acute musculoskeletal back injury, we may place the patient on temporary disability, but permanent disability is unlikely. When treatment for LBP has continued without improvement for more than 12 months, many professional would consider that a patient's temporary disability has become a permanent disability. A disability rating is then required by many workers' compensation jurisdictions, which determine if a patient's disability is total (100% of the whole person) or some fraction thereof (partial disability).

The terms "impairment" and "disability" are used somewhat interchangeably and incorrectly. For example, physicians may be asked in certain jurisdictions (eg, Illinois) to use the American Medical Association "Guides to the Evaluation of Permanent Impairment" to provide a disability rating, although the title and introduction to the book clearly state it was intended to rate impairment and not disability [2]. This fact remains unchanged in the expected 2007 release of the sixth edition of the guide. The reason is simple: different jurisdictions rate and provide compensation for physical impairments differently. There is no way the guide could satisfy the rules of disability ratings in these different settings.

What background information is useful when entering the disability evaluation arena?

The history of legislation relating to the concept of disability dates back several hundred years to the English Poor Laws of 1601 and 1834 [3]. These laws were designed with the need to protect individuals with special needs (ie, children, elderly, infirm, impaired) within English society during the decline of feudalism. Within the prior feudal system, charity from community members took care of persons with special needs.

Germany was a second model for state-sponsored programs for people who were unable to care for themselves. As industry developed in the mid 1800s, Chancellor Otto von Bismarck believed that social insurance would instill patriotism and loyalty in the newly forged German State, and it was enacted through policies such as the German Invalidity and Pension Law of 1889. This introduced the concept of disability as a function of lost earning capacity. In the United States, two major programs have served as the bedrock of disability social insurance: workers' compensation and Social Security disability, which are discussed more fully later.

Prevalence and costs of low back pain disability

The prevalence of disability varies widely in different western countries. For example, the United States, Canada, and Great Britain have a prevalence of approximately 2% to 3%, West Germany and the Netherlands have 4%, and Sweden has climbed to an astonishing 8% of the population. In Britain, the disability rates for chronic LBP are increasing exponentially [4].

Physicians who are interested in occupational health are keenly aware of the relationship between impairment and disability. On one hand, we wish to support patients who have severe impairments (eg, head injury, spinal cord injury, severe fractures). Our government should provide a social safety net for these patients. On the other hand, many patients who have LBP seek disability support from this same social safety net, often without any clear pathologic condition. If 8% of the working age population is on disability (many of them because of LBP), it places a huge burden on the remaining persons in the work force. We realize that LBP is one of the most common causes of disability in westernized societies, which highlights the terrible importance in dealing with these issues. The prevalence of work disability in the United States by state was summarized in a recent report (Table 1).

Table 1

Disabled persons aged 18 to 64 as a percentage of resident population

State	Resident population	Population on disability	% of resident population
United States	176,953,784	5,971,315	3.4
Alabama	2,747,771	151,019	5.5
Alaska	407,453	8,519	2.1
Arizona	3,132,603	102,083	3.3
Arkansas	1,623,669	92,073	5.7
California	21,144,215	518,301	2.5
Colorado	2,838,260	69,281	2.4
Connecticut	2,138,791	66,093	3.1
Delaware	494,467	17,732	3.6
District of Columbia	389,112	9,939	2.6
Florida	9,711,553	364,808	3.8
Georgia	5,317,873	189,458	3.6
Hawaii	756,108	17,299	2.3
Idaho	795,680	24,756	3.1
Illinois	7,854,830	218,364	2.8
Indiana	3,865,854	133,360	3.4
Iowa	1,763,303	58,164	3.3
Kansas	1,682,561	50,361	3.0
Kentucky	2,558,726	152,624	6.0
Louisiana	2,711,760	114,851	4.2
Maine	827,889	41,702	5.0
Maryland	3,360,657	85,750	2.6
Massachusetts	4,098,275	146,665	3.6
Michigan	6,302,087	229,910	3.6
Minnesota	3,175,948	83,460	2.6
Mississippi	1,731,872	104,508	6.0
Missouri	3,447,893	149,097	4.3
Montana	559,496	19,973	3.6
Nebraska	1,041,866	31,058	3.0
Nevada	1,309,842	37,164	2.8
New Hampshire	814,471	27,167	3.3
New Jersey	5,435,114	151,947	2.8
New Mexico	1,109,372	38,214	3.4
New York	11,960,990	411,582	3.4
North Carolina	5,128,840	230,612	4.5
North Dakota	400,951	11,314	2.8
Ohio	7,140,951	242,215	3.4
Oklahoma	2,122,509	79,520	3.7
Oregon	2,169,403	67,931	3.1
Pennsylvania	7,568,159	271,650	3.6
Rhode Island	660,302	27,644	4.2
South Carolina	2,541,428	123,656	4.9
South Dakota	462,843	14,502	3.1
Tennessee	3,618,725	172,301	4.8
Texas	13,086,904	320,035	2.4
Utah	1,348,158	26,449	2.0
Vermont	401,335	15,064	3.8
Virginia	4,578,340	154,452	3.4
Washington	3,789,913	107,888	2.8

Table 1 (*continued*)

State	Resident population	Population on disability	% of resident population
West Virginia	1,128,452	76,814	6.8
Wisconsin	3,388,628	102,719	3.0
Wyoming	312,582	9,267	3.0

From US Census Bureau. Disabled beneficiaries and dependents master beneficiary record file. Washington, DC: US Census Bureau; 2001.

The costs to society of this "wealth of disability," much related to LBP, are simply staggering [5]. Costs include medical expenditures, lost wages, lost production, consumer cost increases, employee retraining, and litigation. The costs of workers' compensation claims by case are listed by state in Table 2.

The total cost for LBP disability is also staggering but may be difficult to estimate because of various factors. Webster cited a figure of between $26 and $56 billion in 1988 and more than $70 billion in 1992 [6,7]. A small percentage of claims (approximately 5%) accounts for a large percentage of total disability days (approximately 85%). Progress has been made in reducing the most expensive length of disability claims [8]. Medical costs previously made up approximately one third of workers' compensation costs but currently make up > 55% of total losses [9].

Workers' compensation

The Workmen's Compensation Program was a social program enacted state by state in the United States from 1910 through 1949, with the intent of addressing accidental injuries in the workplace. The critical language of workers' compensation statutes was that employees must suffer "accidental...personal injury...out of and in the scope of employment." This language highlights one of the most difficult aspects of workers' compensation law and LBP. LBP is an essentially ubiquitous condition, yet statutes indicate that LBP must arise clearly through the course of employment.

Another key concept in the workers' compensation statutes is that of no-fault or tort immunity. In exchange for an employer caring for an injured worker, the worker offers the employer tort immunity from legal suit in response to being injured. Workers' compensation usually offers a worker between 50% and 70% of preinjury wages as an incentive to return to work. Box 1 summarizes coverage and benefits under workers' compensation.

Compensation varies greatly among states. Some states provide scheduled awards based on a physician-determined disability rating or the permanent partial loss of function of the body part or person as a whole. Other states compensate on a nonscheduled fashion as a function of the loss of

Table 2
Average cost of workers' compensation case, 2002

Rank	State	Amount ($)
1	Louisiana	11,817
2	New York	11,793
3	California	11,788
4	Alaska	10,384
5	Texas	9,689
6	Florida	9,447
7	Delaware	8,897
8	Hawaii	8,658
9	Alabama	8,593
10	Montana	8,382
11	Rhode Island	8,158
12	Vermont	8,039
13	Connecticut	8,010
14	Maryland	7,797
15	Illinois	7,762
16	South Carolina	7,293
17	Nevada	6,843
18	Missouri	6,838
19	New Hampshire	6,808
20	New Jersey	6,648
21	Tennessee	6,617
22	Georgia	6,545
23	North Carolina	6,527
24	Oklahoma	6,522
25	Pennsylvania	6,516
26	Oregon	6,406
27	Virginia	6,262
28	Colorado	6,161
29	Mississippi	6,080
30	Massachusetts	5,967
30	Kentucky	5,844
32	Nebraska	5,698
33	New Mexico	5,643
34	Minnesota	5,488
35	Iowa	5,058
36	Michigan	4,987
37	Kansas	4,911
38	Arizona	4,639
39	Wisconsin	4,253
40	Maine	3,998
41	Idaho	3,975
42	South Dakota	3,741
43	Utah	3,683
44	Arkansas	3,521
45	Indiana	3,093
	North Dakota	NA
	Ohio	NA
	West Virginia	NA
	Washington	NA
	Wyoming	NA

Data from the National Council on Compensation Insurance. Average cost of a workers' compensation case, 2001–2002. Albany (NY): The Public Policy Institute of NYS, Inc. Available at: http://www.ppinys.org/reports/jtf2004/workerscomp.htm. Accessed July 13, 2006.

Box 1. Coverage under workers' compensation

Medical expenses: all acute, most chronic, some other (eg, YMCA to swim), medical supplies, psychological, some travel.
Employer insurer must accept an injured worker "as is" (ie, must cover exacerbation of pre-existing emotional problems).
  Short-term disability beyond specified interval (3–6 days)
  Permanent disability assessed when (1) individual returns to work or (2) maximum healing has occurred
  Rehabilitation services (some states only)
  Some states allow employer/carrier to choose the doctor, others allow employee complete choice
  Insurance carriers always have right to obtain IME

---

the ability to be gainfully employed in a part of the workplace as a function of the disability.

The physician has five key responsibilities when determining disability under workers' compensation statutes:

(1) Is there a causal relationship between the injury and the impairment?
(2) Has the patient completed the healing period?
(3) Is there a permanent impairment (covered later)?
(4) What are the work capacity and restrictions (covered later)?
(5) Can the worker return to the same job, a similar job with modifications, a similar job with a different employer, a different employer or receive on-the-job training with same employer or receive job retraining?

When a worker wishes to file for permanent impairment under workers' compensation statutes, the worker is responsible for filing a "first report of injury" to the insurance carrier and state agency. It is reviewed by a hearing officer employed by the state industrial commission. Objective data are obtained from medical consultation, and a physician is asked to quantify the medical impairment or disability according to the rules of the state.

Social Security

Social Security is the second major system for providing a social safety net for persons with disability. This federal program was first enacted in 1935 as the Social Security Act, an old-age pension program. The Social Security Disability insurance program (known as Title II) was created in 1954 and funded disability through wage deductions, which any salaried person knows well from pay stubs. The Supplemental Security Income program of 1973 (known as Title XVI) was intended to provide a safety net for persons who had not worked long enough to be eligible for SSDI. Unlike SSDI, this program is funded through taxes and not payroll deductions. In order for a worker to become eligible for Social Security disability benefits, he or she must have a disability defined as "the inability to engage in any substantial gainful activity by reason of any medically determinable physical or mental impairment(s) which can be expected to result in death or which has lasted or can be expected to last for a continuous period of not less than 12 months."

When an injured worker files for Social Security benefits, he or she applies to the local Social Security district office. The Disability Determination Agency initially disallows 70% of all claims. Upon appeal to an administrative law judge, 20% of denials are reviewed and 50% are reversed. A worker then has the right to appeal to the Social Security Appeals Council Review and may litigate within the federal court system.

Other disability programs

Although most physicians are aware of the workers' compensation statutes and Social Security disability programs, they may not be aware of special programs in existence for other specific populations. Three million federal employees are protected under the Federal Employees' Compensation Act of 1916, and approximately 500,000 harbor workers (but not seamen) are protected under the Longshoreman and Harbor Workers' Compensation Act of 1927. Benefits for veterans and their families can be obtained through the Veterans Administration, and benefits vary based on whether the disability was service or non–service connected. Railroad workers and seaman are protected under the Federal Employers' Liability Act but have no formal workers' compensation law. They must sue their employers to obtain disability benefits.

In Canada, the provinces are responsible for Workmen's Compensation Boards, and employers must purchase coverage from these boards, which compensate for 75% to 90% of net earnings. The method of determining impairment rating varies by province but may be based on Bell's Tables or the AMA guides.

How do I determine if my patient who has low back pain can return to work?

Physicians are often asked to determine when and to what job patients who have LBP may return. Physicians can do so based solely on their clinical judgment, or they may rely on a functional capacity evaluation (FCE). An FCE is a quantified physical ability test in which various parameters are measured over time: how long and how much a given patient can perform in a given day in regards to strength, flexibility, endurance, lifting, carrying, pushing, pulling, bending, crawling, sitting, standing, walking, and ascending steps or ladders. These parameters are quantified in terms of weight and frequency. Terms used to modify frequency include occasional ($\leq 33\%$ of the day), frequent (34%–66% of the day), and constant or frequent ($\geq 67\%$ or more of the day). Although there is an intuitive attractiveness to FCE, there is debate over whether these tests are reproducible and the degree to which they are limited by patient motivation. An excellent review of this subject is provided by Matheson [10]. In this author's opinion, an FCE in a highly cooperative patient may be of value. In a patient with poor motivation, it is expensive and often invalid.

The key question with FCE is "does physical testing predict successful return to work?" Although there are proponents and detractors of physical capacity testing, the value of pre-employment testing in predicting injury is lacking. Although we intuitively believe that increased physical abilities on pre-employment testing would be associated with lesser future injury, this has not been the case in several well-designed clinical studies [11,12]. We frequently designate that a patient may or may not return to work based on strength requirements (Table 3).

Generally, physicians who offer return to work restrictions cannot be found negligent if a worker is reinjured unless (1) a physician made false statements in the report or (2) physician recommendations were made recklessly [13].

Americans with Disabilities Act

The Americans with Disabilities Act (ADA), Public Law 101-335, was signed into law on July 26, 1992 under the first Bush administration. The ADA defines disability as a "physical or mental impairment that substantially limits one or more of the major life activities of the individual, or a record of such an impairment, or being regarded as having such an impairment." The ADA has five major sections, called titles, and Title I deals with employment (Box 2).

Table 3
Strength requirements classification

Degree of strength	Amount of lifting/carrying	Posture, other activities
Sedentary work	Occasional: ≤ 10 lb	Primarily sitting; walking and standing at most occasionally
Light work	≤ 20, ≤ 10 lb frequently	Significant walking/standing or primarily sitting, but requiring pushing and pulling of arm and/or leg controls
Medium work	≤ 50 lb, ≤ 50 lb frequently	Unspecified
Heavy work	≤ 100 lb, ≤ 50 lb frequently	Unspecified
Very heavy work	> 100 lb, ≥ 50 lb frequently	Unspecified

Adapted from United States Department of Labor. Dictionary of Occupational Titles. Washington, DC: US Department of Labor; 1977.

Box 2. Americans with Disabilities Act

(1) No major employer or labor organization may discriminate against a qualified individual with a disability as relates to terms, conditions, or privileges of employment.

(2) A qualified individual with a disability is a disabled person who, with or without reasonable accommodation, can perform the essential functions of the job being sought.[a] The employer decides essential job functions and is advised to develop a written, detailed job description.

(3) "Reasonable accommodation" may include making an existing facility more accessible for persons with disabilities or job restructuring by modifying work schedules, equipment, or environment.[b] Only accommodations that would impose "undue hardship" on the organization are exempted.

(4) Discrimination against disabled persons is outlawed in every aspect of the employment process, including pre-employment examination inquiries related to the disability, medical examinations to screen out workers, and the limiting or classifying of job applicants to adversely affect job opportunity. Ability to perform job-specific functions (as opposed to generic inquiries about physical, sense organ, or cognitive limitations) may, however, be considered in a decision to hire. An employer also may require a post-hiring examination and may make the employer offer contingent on the results of that examination if (a) all entering employees are subjected to the same examination, (b) information obtained is collected confidentially, and (c) criteria for performance acceptability are related to essential job functions.

(5) A major defense against a charge of discrimination under the ADA is that an employer's selection criteria that seem to screen out an individual with a disability are job related, consistent with business necessity, and not compensated for by reasonable accommodation.

(6) An individual who is currently engaged in the illegal use of drugs is not considered a "qualified individual with a disability."

(7) Compliance with the terms of Title I are expected by July 26, 1992 for employers with 25 or more employees and by July 26, 1994 for employers with 15 to 24 employees.

---

[a] "Essential" is determined on a case-by-case basis.

[b] "Reasonable" accommodation for physical/mental limitations is only required if an individual is otherwise qualified. Eighty percent for reasonable accommodations cost contractors <$500; many were free. Employer may deny reasonable accommodation because of (1) financial hardship and (2) business necessity.

From Americans with Disabilities Act. Public Law 101-336. Federal Register 1990;327–78.

The ADA is intended to protect persons who can perform the essential functions of a job with reasonable accommodation. Employers may not inquire about potential employees' impairment or medical history when they apply for a job. Upon offering a potential employee a job, a medical examination may be performed. The position may be withdrawn if the medical officer, based on receiving more information about the worker's abilities, impairments, or past medical history, believes that the particular position offered would be a direct threat to the health of the worker or other employees. For example, consider a patient with a herniated nucleus pulposa treated conservatively within the last 3 months who applies for a job that requires lifting 70 pounds 50 times per day. Most physicians would feel comfortable with the decision that the worker would not be able physically to perform the job without a direct threat to his or her own health. If the worker sued the employer, it is hoped that the court would uphold the company decision. Similarly, if a worker had an uncontrolled seizure disorder and the job required him or her to operate a cherry picker that held other workers, most experts would agree that the risk of seizure while operating the machine would be a direct threat to the workers in the compartment.

What about a worker who needs to lift moderate weights? Can an employer make a reasonable accommodation? Could some type of machine or coworker help to perform certain activities that would let the employee complete the essential functions of the job? These are the crucial issues relating to LBP and the ADA, and to date no final decision has been reached. Physicians are sometimes in the position of determining whether a worker can enter employment or return to employment based on an inadequate job analysis (also called a job description), which may inadequately document the physical abilities required for the job. Johns and colleagues [12] described a simple model that they defended successfully in regard to LBP and direct threat. A worker is considered high risk (likely direct threat) if he or she has three or more LBP episodes in the last 5 years involving lost time or treatment. A worker is moderate risk (possible direct threat) if there are one to two documented LBP episodes in the last 5 years. A low-risk employee (remote direct threat) has had no episodes in the last 5 years.

How do I rate permanent disability?

If a patient is injured in a workers' compensation setting, the first thing to do is find out the laws in the state. These laws can be obtained by searching the state's Website, contacting a human resources department, or speaking to an attorney who handles workers' compensation. There are certain periods of time in which a worker must notify an employer of the injury (waiting period) and a certain period after which compensation begins (waiting period). States vary in whether physician care is employer or employee directed. In Illinois, workers may select a practitioner of their choice (including, but not limited to, physician, surgeon, osteopath, chiropractor), whereas in Missouri the insurance underwriter selects the physician (or other practitioner) to whom the patient must go for care if costs are to be assumed by the workers' compensation insurer. Certain states, such as Florida, Minnesota, and California, have their own schedules for rating disability, and a physician should consult those statutes before proceeding. Veterans are rated according to their own schedule, which can be found in the *Federal Register* [14].

American Medical Association guides

In many jurisdictions, physicians are asked to provide a disability rating, and the best available document (and one that often is mandated by that state's workers' compensation statute) is the "AMA Guides to the Evaluation of Permanent Impairment." The fifth edition of the guide was published in 2001, and the sixth edition is underway. The guide is not a scientific document based on demographic or epidemiologic data but is rather a "Delphi" panel of informed experts who have formed a relative consensus. An effort was made to include a greater variety of experts for the fifth edition, including expert physicians of different ethnic and cultural backgrounds, and to receive input from the judges and attorneys who are active within the field of disability and its legislation. The sixth edition will make an attempt to integrate functional assessment into the impairment rating, whereas previous editions have focused more on diagnosis-based ratings.

The AMA guide began to take form in the 1950s and evolved into a widely recognized impairment rating document used in 40 of 53 jurisdictions, according to a 1991 AMA survey. The proportion is approximately the same currently. Although experts who are familiar with the guide often complain of its inadequacies, it can be argued that there is no superior document available. The guide rates impairments (not disabilities, schedule for compensation, or employability) for each organ system in the body, but this discussion focuses only on impairments of the lumbosacral spine.

A suitable period of time must elapse before an impairment is considered to be permanent—generally 12 months according to the current guide. Raters must determine within their jurisdiction how long patients must remain at the "therapeutic plateau" before they are considered to be at maximal medical improvement, also called permanent and stationary.

The concept of regional versus whole-person impairment is incorporated into the guide. Impairments of the hand or foot (regional impairments) must be converted to whole-person impairments using certain tables. Spine impairments are simple (in this respect); all are based on impairments of the whole person.

Spine rating models in the fifth edition

Before the fourth edition of the guide, the primary method of determining spine impairment was based on range of motion (ROM) with an additional set of modifying diagnoses, which proved to be highly unsatisfactory. Most physicians who have performed disability rating realize that spinal ROM is a highly variable phenomena even in a normal population, and its relationship to impairment is almost (although not entirely) nonexistent. The contributors to the musculoskeletal chapter of the fourth edition elected to use the ROM model as an alternate to a diagnosis-related estimate (DRE) model, also called the injury model, and indicated that the ROM model is to be used only when the injury model is not applicable. This approach continued in the fifth edition of the guide but is expected to change in the sixth edition (in which ROM testing for the spine is deemphasized).

One of the principal arguments in creating the ROM model was whether one could measure spinal ROM accurately during clinical examination. Proponents of Loebl measurements (also known as inclinometry) believed that it could be achieved reliably and convinced the AMA panel that it should be a major emphasis in the quantification of low back disability [15]. Clinical experience proved markedly different, however. Observations after the third edition of the AMA guide demonstrated that the majority of physicians did not know what inclinometry was, and few (if any) physicians used it on any regular basis. Many factors complicated the accurate assessment of ROM: patient fear of injury, lack of desire to cooperate, and, most importantly, reproducibility [16,17].

The DRE model is used when a distinct injury occurred and is currently the preferred method of spinal rating. It has the advantages of simplicity and ease of application, and high interrater reliability is likely (but unproven). The fifth edition uses clinical findings and spinal radiology to place patients in a DRE category (Table 4). Clinical findings include muscle spasm, muscle guarding, asymmetry of spinal motion, nonverifiable radicular root pain, loss of reflexes, weakness and loss of sensation, atrophy, radiculopathy, electrodiagnostic verification of radiculopathy, alteration of motion segment integrity, cauda equina syndrome, and urodynamic tests. The attempt to clarify the controversial issue of muscle spasms is not entirely successful. Nonverifiable root pain is defined as nerve root pain that has an unexplained origin and is without objective corroboration.

A major change has been made in the rating of radiculopathy within the DRE model in the fifth edition. Patients who are treated successfully in a conservative manner for documented radiculopathy are rated as a category II, not category III. Category III is for patients who remain symptomatic after conservative or surgical treatment or who underwent surgical treatment and improved. The AMA guide rewards patients who underwent surgical intervention, although they may experience more prompt and complete resolution of their pain than was otherwise possible with conservative treatment.

DRE categories have a range rather than a fixed value. For example, a patient with surgically treated radiculopathy (category III) ranges from 10% to 13% impairment, in contrast to the fourth edition ratings of a patient,

Table 4
Impairment categories for the lumbosacral spine

DRE category	Physical examination and test findings	Spinal radiology	Whole person impairment
Category I	No significant physical findings	No significant radiologic findings	0
Category II	Muscle spasm/guarding, asymmetric loss of ROM, nonverifiable radiculopathy, no alteration of MSI, resolved radiculopathy with conservative management	Compression fracture 25%, posterior element fracture without dislocation, spinous or transverse process fracture	5–8
Category III	Signs of radiculopathy, electrodiagnostic confirmation of radiculopathy, resolved radiculopathy with surgical management	20%–50% compression fracture, healed posterior element fracture that disrupts the spinal canal	10–13
Category IV	Muscle guarding and pain, no neurologic findings necessary	LOMSI noted on flexion-extension films, 50% compression fracture, fracture dislocations without neurologic compromise	20–23
Category V	Meets criteria for categories III and IV	Fracture 50% compression of one vertebral body with unilateral neurologic compromise	25–28

Abbreviations: LOMSI, loss of motion segment integrity; ROM, range of motion.
From American Medical Association. Guides to the evaluation of permanent impairment. 5th edition. Chicago (IL): American Medical Association; 2001.

which were fixed at a single value of 10%. The DRE model remains hierarchical, that is, a fusion is always rated higher than a surgically treated radiculopathy, which is always rated higher than a strain. A patient with persistent and painful sacroiliac torsion is rated lower than an operated radiculopathy with total resolution of symptoms. This categorical hierarchy without overlap of rating values between categories is artificial and counterintuitive.

Physical findings in LBP are explained better in the fifth edition. For example, the requirements for positive straight leg raise are discussed (eg, pain that starts at 60° of hip flexion does not suggest radicular pain) [18], and the hamstring reflex has been included as an indicator of the L5-S1 reflex arc. The discussion of radiology in the fifth edition is broader and more factually based. The wide range of degenerative changes that increase in frequency by decade are emphasized, hopefully laying to rest the ill-informed opinions that degenerative changes are closely linked to low back complaints. One chapter makes a solid effort to highlight the findings of disc bulge, spondylolysis, herniation, aging changes, and spondylolisthesis in the normal population without LBP.

Spinal cord injury is no longer rated in the spine chapter but rather in the chapter on the neurological system. This change is a distinct improvement, because in previous editions one could score ratings differently using alternative tables. New ratings for the pelvis, previously addressed in the lower extremity chapter, are included in that same chapter. Pelvic ratings vary from 0% to 15% depending on the extent of fracture, dislocation, and healing.

The fifth edition tried to improve on the construct from the fourth edition of loss of motion segment integrity. In the fifth edition, segmental motion can be either increased (generally caused by acute trauma) or decreased (caused by congenital or spontaneous fusion, developmental changes, fracture, healing, healed infection, or surgical arthrodesis). Unfortunately, the relative importance of increased segmental motion in settings other than the acute trauma patient is not addressed. Such patients are often considered candidates for fusion, despite the absence of normal data as to expected degrees of segmental motion in various decades of life. The translational and angular definitions of loss of motion segment integrity also have been changed arbitrarily. Translational changes on flexion-extension films currently must be only 4.5 mm to indicate instability. Angular motion changes more than $15°$ are considered abnormal at L1-2, L2-3, and L3-4, $>20°$ at L4-5, and $>25°$ at L5-S1, in contrast to lesser numbers referenced in the fourth edition.

The ROM model is still used in the fifth edition in certain scenarios:

- If it is statutorily mandated
- If there was no injury or injury was "uncertain"
- If there is multilevel involvement at the same spinal region (multiple fractures, herniations, multiple level stenosis/radiculopathy)
- If there is alteration of motion segment integrity at multiple levels
- If there is recurrent radiculopathy caused by new or recurrent disk herniation or injury at the same level
- If there are multiple episodes of "other pathology" that alter motion segment integrity or radiculopathy

Patient measurements must meet certain reproducibility criteria to accept the inclinometry readings. If inconsistency persists, the measurements are considered invalid and then no impairment rating can be offered. Measurements in the lumbosacral region include flexion, extension, and lateral flexion. These specific impairments are then combined with specific spine disorders, such as fractures, disk lesions, spondylolysis, spondylolisthesis, spinal stenosis, instability, and whether surgery was performed. According to this model, the more surgeries a patient had, the greater was the impairment rating. Techniques using one or two goniometers were described in the fourth edition, but only the two-goniometer method was approved in the fifth edition.

As with previous editions of the AMA guide, the fifth edition suffers from lack of evidence-based data to support or refute the validity of the spinal impairment ranges assigned by DRE or ROM methodology, which continues to be a major shortcoming (and will remain so in the sixth edition).

Long-term disability insurance and Social Security

It is estimated that 40 million Americans are protected by long-term disability, largely through their workplace. There are no uniform criteria when a person becomes disabled for LBP according to their long-term disability insurer. Typically an insurer asks a treating physician for information about lifting, bending, and stooping, and the physician may feel somewhat awkward about answering these questions unless an FCE has been performed.

An important feature of long-term disability policies is whether there is own-occupation versus any-occupation coverage. Own-occupation coverage provides insured persons with disability benefits (typically in the range of 60% of normal salary reimbursement to provide incentive to return to work) if they are not able to provide the essential elements of their particular job. A neurosurgeon would receive reimbursement if no longer able to perform surgery, even if other physician responsibilities could be completed. Any-occupation coverage means, within limits, employees would be reimbursed only if they could no longer perform meaningful work in any related occupation. Again, the criteria vary according to the insurer. Less expensive group long-term disability plans tend to have own-occupation coverage for approximately 2 years, and then the worker must be disabled from any occupation to receive further benefits. More expensive individual long-term disability plans tend to have more restrictive own-occupation provisions.

Criteria for determining disability for spine disorders according to Social Security are actually strict and are presented in Box 3 [19]. Whether a patient is issued disability benefits versus how strictly he or she conforms to these criteria is another issue entirely.

Upon examination of these Social Security guidelines, any expert observer realizes the administration has outlined spinal disability for neurologic LBP. How do we understand the many persons who are "out on Social Security" without these diagnoses? As noted earlier in the discussion concerning Social Security, the ability to obtain social support depends not only on the specific spinal pathology but also on the fortitude with which one seeks the award.

Independent medical evaluation, disability evaluation, and court testimony

The most important statement that can be made in discussing the role of the disability evaluating physician is for the physician to ask himself or herself, "How do I remain objective in assessing this patient?" The disability evaluating physician is placed in an ethical dilemma [20]. If a patient is in

---

Box 3. Social Security guidelines for disorders of the spine 2005

Disorders of the spine (eg, herniated nucleus pulposus, spinal arachnoiditis, spinal stenosis, osteoarthritis, degenerative disc disease, facet arthritis, vertebral fracture) that result in compromise of a nerve root (including the cauda equina) or the spinal cord. With:

A. Evidence of nerve root compression characterized by neuroanatomic distribution of pain, limitation of motion of the spine, motor loss (atrophy with associated muscle weakness or muscle weakness) accompanied by sensory or reflex loss and, if there is involvement of the lower back, positive straight leg raise test (sitting and supine).

OR

B. Spinal arachnoiditis, confirmed by an operative note or pathology report of tissue biopsy, or by appropriate medically acceptable imaging, manifested by severe burning or painful dysesthesia, which results in the need for changes in position of posture more than once every 2 hours.

OR

C. Lumbar spinal stenosis that results in pseudoclaudication, established by findings on appropriate medically acceptable imaging, manifested by chronic nonradicular pain and weakness, and resulting in ability to ambulate effectively.

---

our own practice, can we offer a disability rating in an objective fashion? Are we biased toward erring on the side of our patient? If we see a patient at the behest of a workmen's compensation carrier or insurer who regularly refers business to our practice, can we provide an unbiased assessment? Is our patient the customer or the insurer? If we give a report that is unfavorable to the referring insurer or attorney, will he or she ever refer another patient?

Independent medical evaluation

When we see a patient for an IME, certain features of the interaction are distinct from our traditional patient evaluation. First, and most importantly, you are not assuming care of the patient. You must make this statement orally to the patient and document the oral warning in your report. Make it clear that the evaluation is for IME purposes and there is no ongoing physician-patient relationship. Have the patient sign a disclosure indicating that he or she understands that the evaluation is only for the purpose of an IME and you will not assume care.

IMEs are often obtained for the purpose of workers' compensation or for the solicitation of expert testimony in a tort liability case. A tort is a breech of duty that gives rise to an action for damages. There are four components of tort liability:

(1) a legal duty existed (party A had a responsibility to your injured patient)
(2) there was a breech of that duty
(3) there was a proximate or direct cause (ie, the accident on the part of Party A caused the impairment)
(4) harm or damage occurred (in this case to your patient)

The concept of causality or proximate (direct) cause is key and often places the examiner in an ethical dilemma. When there is loss of limb because of an accident, a physician feels comfortable in stating that A (eg, nail gun piercing popliteal artery) caused B (eg, below-knee amputation). Because LBP is such a ubiquitous phenomenon, however, how often can one state that a particular job-related injury clearly caused the LBP, especially in light of more than 20 years of imaging studies that delineate the high number of radiologic spinal abnormalities in asymptomatic adults?

The standard exists, and the IME physician is asked to comment on causality. The physician generally is asked, "Within a reasonable degree of medical certainty, Doctor, can you state that A caused B?" The real question the attorney is asking you is, "Is it more likely than not (more than 50% probability) that A caused B?" If you can say yes, you are satisfying the legal requirement that it is "probably true," which is the level of certainty that the attorney is requesting. It is not the standard of "beyond a reasonable doubt" that holds in criminal cases. If you answer that A possibly caused B, the real meaning of your statement is that it is less than likely (<50% probability) that A caused B and would suggest evidence against causality.

Your expert role in an IME has eight steps:

(1) Give a diagnosis and severity of the condition
(2) Determine causality
(3) Determine if necessary tests have been performed
(4) Suggest any additional tests that you believe are required to complete the evaluation
(5) Determine whether maximal medical improvement has been reached
(6) Determine an impairment rating
(7) Determine apportionment
(8) Determine what restrictions are needed

Some of these steps require additional commentary. Maximal medical improvement refers to the point when you believe a patient's condition is either resolved or has reached a plateau. It is the time when impairment ratings should be performed because the condition is considered permanent. There should be no expectation of change over the next year to rate a patient using the guide. Certain jurisdictions may have their own rules. Patients who undergo complex surgeries may not reach maximal medical improvement for several years.

Although impairment rating presents an ethical dilemma, the concept of apportionment is additionally precarious. IME physicians may be asked, "Doctor, you felt the patient's back condition is worthy of a 20% whole person impairment. But the patient had back injuries in 1986, 1992, 1994, and 1996! How much of that 20% do you apportion to each injury?" It is safe to say that there is no scientific way to do this.

Physicians may be asked to provide restrictions for a patient regarding lifting, carrying, and stooping. Although the limitations of FCE were addressed briefly, restricting patients in the workplace without at least attempting such an evaluation is precarious. If a patient participates in such an evaluation and you feel that the results do not reflect his or her best effort, one can still offer more liberal restrictions and comment on the level (or lack) of motivation of the patient participating in the FCE.

An additional wrinkle in certain workers' compensation jurisdictions is legislation creating a second injury fund, which is a special fund meant to encourage employment of individuals with pre-existing disabilities. Suppose you performed an IME on a patient who had LBP with three separate injuries in 1986, 1992, and 1997. The patient was employed in Missouri (where second injury fund legislation applies), and his third injury was during the course of employment with a new employer. You rate and apportion the three injuries as 5%, 5%, and 10% permanent partial disability rated at the level of the whole person. When compensation is made to the injured worker, the second injury fund recompenses (up to a ceiling) for monies related to the first two injuries. The importance of second injury fund legislation has been eroded by the ADA.

Medicolegal interface

Finally, IME physicians may be asked, in their role as expert evaluators, to participate in depositions and trial appearances [21–23]. Depositions come in two varieties—discovery and evidentiary. Discovery depositions offer the plaintiff and defendant attorneys a chance to hear what the other's experts have to say and hopefully to lay out what the weight of truth is for each side. The rules of evidence do not apply in discovery deposition, and the physician's testimony can be introduced into the courtroom only if it conflicts with testimony the physician offers at the time of trial. In distinction, evidentiary depositions represent legal testimony according to the formal rules of evidence and may be videotaped in lieu of the physician appearing at trial. The physician's testimony may be read verbatim at the trial (or the videotape played) as part of the trial record.

Physicians may be intimidated at the thought of answering questions from an attorney, but as long as they understand the ground rules, they need not be. The first rule of survival is to remember that all of your time is billable, so keep close track of it. The second rule of survival is to learn more about giving effective testimony. The following list may be of help:

- Prepare your qualifications carefully. Put together an attractive curriculum vitae that lists your many qualifications, extensive experience, numerous talks, and papers and presentations. Stress your diversity of experience in academia and private practice. Attorneys often desire a physician with the wealth of knowledge from the academic world who also knows the real world of private practice.
- During discovery testimony, make sure you have prepared thoroughly and reviewed the details of the case. Your report should document all pertinent history and physical findings so that when the case comes to deposition months or years later, your summary completely and effectively summarizes the case. In contrast, busy attorneys may be asked to pinch hit for one another and may be less than up-to-date on many of the issues about which they are asking questions.
- Have an independent recollection of each patient aside from your written report. An inexpensive way to do so is to photocopy a picture identification of all patients when they first see you.
- Know the role of each person in the room. At times there are many attorneys and assistants, and you should understand which person represents what interest. This knowledge may help you understand the angle from which a certain question is posed.
- Keep your testimony consistent. Make sure you answer the question the same way each time, because if you do not, the attorney attempts to make you look less than credible by comparing your courtroom response with your deposition transcript.
- Honesty is required, and brevity is desired. Your answers during depositions should be short and on point if possible. Yes or no is a fine response. Save your scholarly dissertations for the jury. Do not educate opposing counsel about how much you know and how many articles you have read. Let them do their own homework.
- Wait for the entire question to be asked. Physicians love to answer questions before the sentence is finished. You want to be certain you are asking the correct question, and you want to see if the attorney who has retained you wishes to make an objection.
- Articles are great to quote on rounds but not in testimony. First, you do not want to cite all the literature on a particular subject because that is handing over information to the other side. Second, do not admit that any source is definitive. The medical literature is always in flux and must be tempered by your own extensive knowledge and experience. Finally, if you quote articles in court that you did not mention in deposition, the attorney may complain that that information was not previously discovered in deposition, thus depriving him or her of the opportunity to read those papers.
- Know who is looking at you. In deposition, no one is (other than the attorneys and court reporter). Your goal should be to give short, concise answers that precisely express your opinion. Use sophisticated English,

and speak in the best grammar possible so that you make a strong impression on someone who reads your transcript. In court, however, looks count. Dress neatly and conservatively. Look professional and confident. Be sincere, and make eye contact. Speak to the jury; they respect physicians. Teach but do not preach. Use appropriate audiovisual materials.

Upon completing the questions by the attorney who referred the patient to you or retained by the insurer who sought your opinion, depositions may seem easy. The true art, however, is surviving cross-examination by the attorney on the other side. The adversarial attorney has a goal to make you look bad. A few comments are helpful to survive cross-examination.

- You are the batter; swing only if it is in the strike zone. You are entitled to understand any question to you. Within limits, answer questions only if they make sense. Be polite but firm if they do not. Explain limitations in current knowledge but do not apologize for them.
- "A man's got to know his limitation." This quote from Dirty Harry is from a bygone era but applies to both genders of physicians. Know when to limit your testimony. You are not a psychologist but you can use the results of psychological testing. You are not a vocational rehabilitation specialist but you can state that the patient you examined with two spinal fusions will never again lift 100 pounds. You cannot list all the possible jobs in the workplace from which the patient is currently excluded. A vocational rehabilitation specialist could.
- Beware of sucker questions. Often the attorney tries to trap you with unreasonable questions. Avoid unreasonable hypothetical questions. Answer yes or no only when the logical construct allows you to. There is no favorable yes or no response to "Did you stop beating your wife?" State your whole opinion to the question posed, and try not to let the attorney limit you. Beware of leading questions with which the attorney is trying to take you down the primrose path. Stick to your guns when you are right; you know the medical literature better than the attorney (or you should). In medicine we say nothing is always or never, so beware when the attorney uses these modifiers. Beware when the lawyer starts quoting literature and becoming the expert witness. Make sure that when the attorney repeats what you said, it is really what you said!
- Do not let the attorney undermine your credibility and allegiance. You do not know the answer to every possible question; do not think you need to. You may not be able to answer an impossibly broad question. When the attorney tries to undermine your opinion based on the inadequacy of your 2-hour evaluation, state that a 2-hour evaluation was adequate for you as a physician to reach your opinion. Finally, the lawyer often tries to make you seem to be a hired gun. The strategy is to make your opinion appear biased. State carefully that you work for plaintiff and defense (if true). You are paid for your time, not your testimony. Your skills are for sale, and you provide them to any ethical person

or party. You do not do medicolegal work for most of your practice (hopefully this is true), but it represents a fixed percentage of your time commitment during your work week.

References

[1] World Health Organization. International classification of impairments, disabilities, and handicaps. Geneva: World Health Organization; 1980.
[2] American Medical Association. Guides to the evaluation of permanent impairment. 5th edition. Chicago (IL): American Medical Association; 2001.
[3] Hadler NM. Disabling backache: an international perspective. Spine 1995;20:640–9.
[4] Waddell G. LBP: a 20th century health care enigma. Spine 1996;21:2820–5.
[5] van Tulder MW, Koes BW, Bouter LM. Cost of illness study of back pain in the Netherlands. Pain 1995;62:233–40.
[6] Webster BS, Snook SH. The cost of compensable low back pain. J Occup Med 1990;32:13–5.
[7] Webster BS, Snook SH. Cost of 1989 workers' compensation LBP claims. Spine 1994;19: 1111–6.
[8] Hashemi L, Webster BS, Clancy EA. Trends in disability duration and cost of workers' compensation low back pain claims 1988–1996. J Occup Environ Med 1998;40:1110–9.
[9] National Council on Compensation Insurance. Average cost of a workers' compensation case, 2001–2002. Albany (NY): The Public Policy Institute of NYS, Inc. Available at: http://www.ppinys.org/reports/jtf2004/workerscomp.htm. Accessed July 13, 2006.
[10] Matheson LN. Functional capacity evaluation. In: Demeter SL, Andersson GBJ, Smith GM, editors. Disability evaluation. 2nd edition. St. Louis (MO): Mosby; 2003. p. 748–68.
[11] Kaplan GM, Wurtele SK, Gillis D. Maximal effort during functional capacity evaluations: an examination of psychological factors. Arch Phys Med Rehabil 1996;77:161–4.
[12] Mooney V, Kenney K, Leggett S, et al. Relationship of lumbar strength in shipyard workers to workplace injury claims. Spine 1996;21:2001–5.
[13] Johns RE, Elegante JM, Teynor PD, et al. Fitness for duty. In: Demeter SL, Andersson GBJ, Smith GM, editors. Disability evaluation. 2nd edition. St. Louis (MO): Mosby; 1996. p. 709–38.
[14] Pensions, bonuses and veterans' relief. Part 4. Schedule for rating disabilities. Federal Register 1994;38:339–445.
[15] Mayer T, Tencer A, Kristoferson S, et al. Use of noninvasive techniques for quantification of spinal range of motion in normal subjects and chronic low back dysfunction patients. Spine 1984;9:588–95.
[16] Merritt JL, McLean TJ, Erickson RD, et al. Measurement of trunk flexibility in normal subjects: reproducibility of three clinical methods. Mayo Clin Proc 1986;61:192–7.
[17] Rondinelli R, Murphy J, Esler A, et al. Estimation of normal lumbar flexion with surface inclinometry: comparison of three methods. Am J Phys Med Rehabil 1992;71:219–24.
[18] Deyo RA, Rainville J, Kent DL. What can the history and physical examination tell us about low back pain? JAMA 1992;268:760–5.
[19] Social Security Administration Office of Disability Programs. Disability evaluation under Social Security. Washington, DC: Social Security Administration; 2005. Publication Number 64–039, ICN 468600.
[20] Carey TS, Hadler NM. Role of the primary physician in disability determination for Social Security Insurance and Workers' Compensation. Ann Intern Med 1986;104:706–10.
[21] Bonfiglio RP, Bonfiglio RL. Medical testimony in workers' compensation matters. Phys Med Rehabil Clin N Am 1992;3(3):665–76.
[22] Johnston W. Importance of communication between physician and attorney. Phys Med Rehabil Clin N Am 1992;3(3):677–94.
[23] Hirsch G, Beach G, Cooke C, et al. Relationship between performance on lumbar dynamometry and Waddell Score in a population with LBP. Spine 1991;16:1039–43.

ELSEVIER
SAUNDERS

Clin Occup Environ Med
5 (3) 741–746

CLINICS IN
OCCUPATIONAL AND
ENVIRONMENTAL
MEDICINE

Index

Note: Page numbers of article titles are in **boldface** type.

A

Acetaminophen, for acute low back pain, 643–644

ADA. See *Americans with Disabilities Act (ADA).*

Adenomatous Polyp Prevention on Vioxx (APPROVe) study, 646

Adhesion(s), epidural lysis of, in low back pain management, 691–694. See also *Epidural lysis of adhesions, in low back pain management.*

Aerobic training, in prevention of acute low back pain, 620–622

Age, as risk factor for occupational low back pain, 510–511

"AMA Guides to the Evaluation of Permanent Impairment," 730

Americans with Disabilities Act (ADA), 727–729

Anthropometry, as risk factor for occupational low back pain, 511

Antidepressant(s), tricyclic, for acute low back pain, 651

Anti-inflammatory drugs, nonsteroidal (NSAIDs)
COX-2 selective, for acute low back pain, 646–647
for acute low back pain, 644–646

APPROVe study. See *Adenomatous Polyp Prevention on Vioxx (APPROVe) study.*

B

Back pain
in workplace, prevalence of, 502–504
low, occupational, prevention strategies for, **529–544.**
See also *Low back pain, occupational, prevention strategies for.*

workers' compensation claims related to, 529

Back schools, in prevention of occupational low back pain, 530–531

Baclofen, for acute low back pain, 648

Bed rest, for acute low back pain, 616–617

Bending, risk factors for, 517

Bone scintigraphy, in low back pain diagnosis, 575–577

C

Cardiovascular conditioning, in prevention of acute low back pain, 620–622

Carisoprodol, for acute low back pain, 648

Celecoxib, for acute low back pain, 646–647

Celecoxib Long-term Arthritis Safety Study (CLASS), 646

CLASS. See *Celecoxib Long-term Arthritis Safety Study (CLASS).*

Colchicine, for acute low back pain, 651

Compensation, workers', disability due to low back pain and, 723–725

Computed tomography (CT), in low back pain diagnosis, 577–578

Corticosteroid(s), for acute low back pain, 650

CT. See *Computed tomography (CT).*

Cyclobenzarpine, for acute low back pain, 648

D

Degenerative disc disease, diagnosis of, imaging studies in, 585

Diagnosis-related estimate (DRE) model, 731

Diazepam, for acute low back pain, 648

doi:10.1016/S1526-0046(06)00062-8

Disability(ies)
    defined, 719–721
    permanent, rating of, 729–734

Disability insurance, long-term, Social
    Security and, 734

Disability rating, in low back pain, **719–740.**
    See also *Low back pain, disability
    rating in.*

Disc herniation, in injured worker, surgical
    issues related to, 706–709

Discogenic pain, lumbar, in injured
    workers, surgical issues related to,
    709–713

Discography, lumbar
    in low back pain diagnosis, 578–581
    in low back pain management,
        671–680. See also *Lumbar
        discography, in low back pain
        management.*

Dorsal root ganglia, pain related to,
    management of, radiofrequency
    neurolysis techniques in, 684–685

DRE model. See *Diagnosis-related estimate
    (DRE) model.*

E

Education, in prevention of occupational
    low back pain, 530–532

Electrodiagnosis, in low back pain
    evaluation, **591–613.** See also *Low
    back pain, evaluation of,
    electrodiagnosis in.*

Electromyography (EMG), surface, in low
    back pain evaluation, 607–608

Electrothermal therapy, intradiscal, in low
    back pain management, 689–691. See
    also *Intradiscal electrodermal therapy,
    in low back pain management.*

EMG. See *Electromyography (EMG).*

Epidural injections, lumbar, in low back
    pain management, 656–662. See also
    *Lumbar epidural injections, in low back
    pain management.*

Epidural lysis of adhesions, in low back
    pain management, 691–694
    complications of, 693–694
    efficacy of, 694
    indications for, 691–692
    technique, 692–693

Ergonomics, in prevention of occupational
    low back pain, 533–535

Ethanercept, for acute low back pain, 651

Exercise
    in prevention of acute low back pain,
        615–632
        aerobic training, 620–622
        background of, 615–616
        cardiovascular conditioning,
            620–622
        described, 619–620
        flexibility training, 625–626
        future directions in, 626–628
        strength training, 622–625
        vs. usual care options, 618–620
    in prevention of occupational low back
        pain, 532–533
    spinal stabilization, for injured
        workers, **633–642.** See also
        *Injured workers, spinal
        stabilization exercises for.*

F

Federal Employees' Compensation Act of
    1916, 726

Flexibility training, in prevention of acute
    low back pain, 625–626

G

Ganglion(a), dorsal root, pain related to,
    management of, radiofrequency
    neurolysis techniques in, 684–685

Gender, as risk factor for occupational low
    back pain, 510–511

Genetic(s), as risk factor for occupational
    low back pain, 509–510

Gygapophyseal joint injections, in low back
    pain management, 662–668
    complications of, 667
    efficacy of, 667–668
    indications for, 662–663
    technique, 663–667

H

Handicap, defined, 720

Heavy physical work, risk factors for,
    515–516

Herniation, disc, in injured workers,
    surgical issues related to, 706–709

I

IDD. See *Internal disc disruption (IDD).*

Imaging studies, in low back pain diagnosis,
    571–589. See also *Low back pain,
    diagnosis of, imaging studies in.*

Impairment, defined, 720–721

Impairment rating, in low back pain, **719–740.** See also *Low back pain, disability rating in.*

Independent medical evaluation, in disability rating in low back pain, 734–737

Injured workers
    low back pain in, surgical issues related to, **703–717.** See also *Low back pain, in injured workers, surgical issues related to.*
    spinal stabilization exercises for, **633–642**
        stage one, 638
        stage three, 639–641
        stage two, 638

Insurance, disability, long-term, Social Security and, 734

Internal disc disruption (IDD), 672

Intradiscal electrothermal therapy, in low back pain management, 689–691
    complications of, 691
    efficacy of, 691
    indications for, 689
    technique, 689–691

L

Late responses, in low back pain evaluation, 598–599

Lifting, as risk factor for occupational low back pain, 516–517

Lifting techniques, in prevention of occupational low back pain, 530

Longshoreman and Harbor Workers' Compensation Act of 1927, 726

Long-term disability insurance, Social Security and, 734

Low back pain
    acute
        background of, 615–616
        bed rest for, 616–617
        clinical guidelines for, 616
        management of, **643–653**
            acetaminophen in, 643–644
            colchicine in, 651
            corticosteroids in, 650
            ethanercept in, 651
            muscle relaxants in, 647–648
            NSAIDs in, 644–646

            COX-2 selective, 646–647
            opioids in, 649–650
            sarpogrelate hydroxychloride in, 651
            tricyclic antidepressants in, 651
            willow bark extract in, 651–652
        prevention of, exercise in, **615–632.** See also *Exercise, in prevention of acute low back pain.*
    diagnosis of, imaging studies in, **571–589**
        bone scintigraphy, 575–577
        common radiographic views, 572–574
        CT, 577–578
        in degenerative disc disease, 585
        lumbar discography, 578–581
        lumbar spine radiography, 574–575
        MRI, 581–585
        myelography, 578
        preplacement radiography, 585–586
        standard radiographs, 572
        ultrasound, 586
    disability rating in, **719–740**
        ability to return to work, determining factors in, 726–729
        background information in, 721–726
        costs related to, 721–723
        independent medical evaluation in, 734–737
        medicolegal interface in, 737–740
        permanent disability, 729–734
        prevalence of, 721–723
        Social Security and, 725–726
        workers' compensation due to, 723–725
    evaluation of, electrodiagnosis in, **591–613**
        indications for, 608–610
        late responses, 598–599
        NEE in, 599–605
        nerve conduction studies, 593–597
        quantitative sensory testing, 607
        spinal nerve root stimulation, 605
        SSEPs, 605–607
        surface EMG, 607–608
    in injured workers
        disc herniation, 706–709
        lumbar discogenic pain, 709–713

Low back pain (*continued*)
  prevalence of, 703–704
  red flags, 704–706
  spinal stenosis, 713–714
  spondylolisthesis, 713–714
  surgical emergencies, 704–706
  surgical issues related to, **703–717**
  management of
    epidural lysis of adhesions in,
      691–694
    injections and intervention
      procedures in, **655–702.** See
      also specific procedures,
      e.g., *Lumbar epidural
      injections.*
    intradiscal electrothermal
      therapy in, 689–691
    lumbar discography in, 671–680
    lumbar epidural injections in,
      656–662
    nucleoplasty in, 685–688
    radiofrequency neurolysis
      techniques in, 680–685
    sacroiliac joint injections in,
      668–671
    zygapophyseal joint injections in,
      662–668
  natural history of, 507–508
  occupational, **545–569**
    causes of, 506–507, 545
    epidemiology of, **501–528**
    patient history in, 545–552
      chief complaint in, 546
      current illness history in,
        546–548
      family history in, 550
      past medical and surgical
        history in, 548–550
      review of systems in, 552
      social history in, 550–552
    physical examination in, 552–566
      flexibility in, 556–557
      inspection in, 552–553
      neurologic assessment in,
        557–559
      nonorganic signs in, 563–566
      palpation in, 556
      provocative maneuvers in,
        559–562
      range of motion in, 553–556
    prevention strategies for, **529–544**
      back schools, 530–531
      education and training,
        530–532
      ergonomics, 533–535
      exercise, 532–533
      goals of, 529–530
      levels of, 529
      lifting techniques, 530

      lumbar orthotics, 537–538
      management training,
        531–532
      risk factor modification, 535
      worker selection, 535–537
    risk factors for, 508–518
      age, 510–511
      anthropometry, 511
      bending, 517
      gender, 510–511
      genetics, 509–510
      lifting, 516–517
      lumbar spine mobility, 514
      muscle strength, 514–515
      personal, 508–512
      physical fitness, 513–514
      posture, 515
      psychosocial factors,
        511–512
      smoking, 515
      static work postures, 516
      structural abnormalities,
        512–515
      twisting, 517
      whole–body vibration,
        517–518
      work–related factors,
        515–518
  prevalence of, 655

Lumbar discogenic pain, in injured worker,
  surgical issues related to, 709–713

Lumbar discography
  in low back pain diagnosis, 578–581
  in low back pain management,
    671–680
    complications of, 676–678
    efficacy of, 678–680
    indications for, 671–673
    technique, 673–676

Lumbar epidural injections, in low back
  pain management, 656–662
  complications of, 661–662
  efficacy of, 662
  indications for, 656
  technique, 656–661

Lumbar facet joint, pain of, management
  of, radiofrequency neurolysis
  techniques in, 680–683

Lumbar orthotics, in prevention of
  occupational low back pain,
  537–538

Lumbar spine mobility, as risk factor for
  occupational low back pain, 514

Lumbar spine radiography, in low back
  pain diagnosis, 574–575

M

Magnetic resonance imaging (MRI), in low back pain diagnosis, 581–585

Management training, in prevention of occupational low back pain, 531–532

Medical evaluation, independent, in disability rating in low back pain, 734–737

Medicolegal interface, in disability rating in low back pain, 737–740

Metaxalone, for acute low back pain, 648

Methocarbamol, for acute low back pain, 648

Mobility, lumbar spine, as risk factor for occupational low back pain, 514

MRI. See Magnetic resonance imaging (MRI).

Muscle relaxants, for acute low back pain, 647–648

Muscle strength, as risk factor for occupational low back pain, 514–515

Myelography, in low back pain diagnosis, 578

N

NEE. See Needle electromyographic examination (NEE).

Needle electromyographic examination (NEE), in low back pain evaluation, 599–605

Nerve conduction studies, in low back pain evaluation, 593–597
1994 Agency for Health Care Policy, 648

North American Spine Society, 673

NSAIDs. See Anti-inflammatory drugs, nonsteroidal (NSAIDs).

Nucleoplasty, in low back pain management, 685–688
complications of, 688
efficacy of, 688
indications for, 685
technique, 686–687

O

Occupational low back pain, 545–569. See also Low back pain, occupational.
prevention strategies for, 529–544. See also Low back pain, occupational, prevention strategies for.

Opioid(s), for acute low back pain, 649–650

Orthotics, lumbar, in prevention of occupational low back pain, 537–538

P

Pain
back, low, occupational, prevention strategies for, 529–544. See also Low back pain, occupational, prevention strategies for.
discogenic, lumbar, in injured worker, surgical issues related to, 709–713

Physical fitness, as risk factor for occupational low back pain, 513–514

Physical work, heavy, as risk factor for occupational low back pain, 515–516

Posture
as risk factor for occupational low back pain, 515
static work, as risk factor for occupational low back pain, 516

Preplacement radiography, in low back pain diagnosis, 585–586

Psychosocial factors, as risk factor for occupational low back pain, 511–512

Q

Quantitative sensory testing, in low back pain evaluation, 607

R

Radiofrequency neurolysis techniques, in low back pain management, 680–685
of dorsal root ganglia, 684–685
of lumbar facet joint, 680–683
of sacroiliac joint, 683–684

Radiography, in low back pain diagnosis
common views, 572–574
lumbar spine, 574–575
preplacement, 585–586
standard, 572

Range of motion (ROM) model, 730–732

Risk factor modification, in prevention of occupational low back pain, 535

Rofecoxib, for acute low back pain, 646–647

S

Sacroiliac joint, pain of, management of, radiofrequency neurolysis techniques in, 683–684

Sacroiliac joint injections, in low back pain management, 668–671

Sacroiliac (*continued*)
complications of, 671
efficacy of, 671
indications for, 668–670
technique, 670

Sarpogrelate hydroxychloride, for acute low back pain, 651

School(s), back, in prevention of occupational low back pain, 530–531

Scintigraphy, bone, in low back pain diagnosis, 575–577

Smoking, risk factors for, 515

Social Security
disability due to low back pain and, 725–726
long-term disability insurance and, 734

Social Security Act, 725

Social Security Disability insurance program, 725

Somatosensory evoked potentials (SSEPs), in low back pain evaluation, 605–607

Spinal nerve root stimulation, in low back pain evaluation, 605

Spinal stabilization exercises, for injured workers, **633–642.** See also *Injured workers, spinal stabilization exercises for.*

Spinal stenosis, in injured worker, surgical issues related to, 713–714

Spine, stabilizers of
dynamic, 635–637
passive, 634–635

Spondylolisthesis, in injured worker, surgical issues related to, 713–714

SSDI, 725–726

SSEPs. See *Somatosensory evoked potentials (SSEPs).*

Stabilizer(s), of spine
dynamic, 635–637
passive, 634–635

Static work postures, as risk factor for occupational low back pain, 516

Stenosis(es), spinal, in injured worker, surgical issues related to, 713–714

Strength, muscle, as risk factor for occupational low back pain, 514–515

Strength training, in prevention of acute low back pain, 622–625

Structural abnormalities, as risk factor for occupational low back pain, 512–515

Supplemental Security Insurance program of 1973, 725

Surface EMG, in low back pain evaluation, 607–608

T

Tizanidine, for acute low back pain, 648

Training
in prevention of occupational low back pain, 530–532
management, in prevention of occupational low back pain, 531–532

Tricyclic antidepressants, for acute low back pain, 651

Twisting, as risk factor for occupational low back pain, 517

U

Ultrasound, in low back pain diagnosis, 586

V

Vibration, whole-body, as risk factor for occupational low back pain, 517–518

VIGOR trial. See *Vioxx Gastrointestinal Outcomes Research (VIGOR) trial.*

Vioxx Gastrointestinal Outcomes Research (VIGOR) trial, 646

W

Whole-body vibration, as risk factor for occupational low back pain, 517–518

Willow bark extract, for acute low back pain, 651–652

Work, physical, heavy, as risk factor for occupational low back pain, 515–516

Worker(s)
injured. See *Injured workers.*
selection of, in prevention of occupational low back pain, 535–537

Workers' compensation, disability due to low back pain and, 723–725

Workmen's Compensation Boards, 726

Workplace
back pain in, prevalence of, 502–504
low back pain in, **545–569.** See also *Low back pain, occupational.*